Clinical Psychiatry

Editor

LEO SHER

MEDICAL CLINICS
OF NORTH AMERICA

www.medical.theclinics.com

Consulting Editor
JACK ENDE

January 2023 • Volume 107 • Number 1

ELSEVIER

1600 John F. Kennedy Boulevard • Suite 1800 • Philadelphia, Pennsylvania, 19103-2899

http://www.theclinics.com

MEDICAL CLINICS OF NORTH AMERICA Volume 107, Number 1
January 2023 ISSN 0025-7125, ISBN-13: 978-0-323-96065-6

Editor: Taylor Hayes
Developmental Editor: Arlene Campos

Medical Clinics of North America (ISSN 0025-7125) is published bimonthly by Elsevier Inc., 360 Park Avenue South, New York, NY 10010-1710. Months of publication are January, March, May, July, September, and November. Business and editorial offices: 1600 John F. Kennedy Boulevard, Suite 1800, Philadelphia, PA 19103-2899. Periodicals postage paid at New York, NY, and additional mailing offices. Subscription prices are USD $332.00 per year (US individuals), $786.00 per year (US institutions), $100.00 per year (US Students), $416.00 per year (Canadian individuals), $1023.00 per year (Canadian institutions), $200.00 per year for (foreign students), $100.00 per year for (Canadian students), $461.00 per year (foreign individuals), and $1023.00 per year (foreign institutions). To receive student/resident rate, orders must be accompanied by name of affiliated institution, date of term, and the signature of program/residency coordinator on institution letterhead. Orders will be billed at individual rate until proof of status is received. Foreign air speed delivery is included in all Clinics' subscription prices. All prices are subject to change without notice. **POSTMASTER:** Send address changes to *Medical Clinics of North America*, Elsevier Health Sciences Division, Subscription Customer Service, 3251 Riverport Lane, Maryland Heights, MO 63043. **Customer Service: Telephone: 1-800-654-2452** (U.S. and Canada); **1-314-447-8871** (outside U.S. and Canada). **Fax: 314-447-8029. E-mail: journalscustomerserviceusa@ elsevier.com** (for print support); **journalsonlinesupport-usa@elsevier.com** (for online support).

Reprints. For copies of 100 or more of articles in this publication, please contact the Commercial Reprints Department, Elsevier Inc., 360 Park Avenue South, New York, NY 10010-1710. Tel.: 212-633-3874; Fax: 212-633-3820; E-mail: reprints@elsevier.com.

Medical Clinics of North America is also published in Spanish by McGraw-Hill Interamericana Editores S. A., P.O. Box 5-237, 06500 Mexico, D.F., Mexico.

Medical Clinics of North America is covered in *MEDLINE/PubMed (Index Medicus), Current Contents, ASCA, Excerpta Medica, Science Citation Index,* and *ISI/BIOMED.*

PROGRAM OBJECTIVE
The goal of the *Medical Clinics of North America* is to keep practicing physicians up to date with current clinical practice by providing timely articles reviewing the state of the art in patient care.

TARGET AUDIENCE
All practicing physicians and other healthcare professionals.

LEARNING OBJECTIVES
Upon completion of this activity, participants will be able to:
1. Review the factors that are linked to psychiatric disorders and suicide.
2. Explain the appropriate use of strategies, assessment, and screening tools for use by health care clinicians of all specialties in diagnosing and treating psychiatric disorders and reducing the risk of suicide.
3. Discuss the importance of using a multidisciplinary, systematic approach to diagnosing and treating psychiatric disorders, as well as lowering the risk of suicide.

ACCREDITATION
The Elsevier Office of Continuing Medical Education (EOCME) is accredited by the Accreditation Council for Continuing Medical Education (ACCME) to provide continuing medical education for physicians.

The EOCME designates this journal-based CME activity for a maximum of 11 *AMA PRA Category 1 Credit*(s)™. Physicians should claim only the credit commensurate with the extent of their participation in the activity.

All other healthcare professionals requesting continuing education credit for this enduring material will be issued a certificate of participation.

DISCLOSURE OF CONFLICTS OF INTEREST
The EOCME assesses conflict of interest with its instructors, faculty, planners, and other individuals who are in a position to control the content of CME activities. All relevant conflicts of interest that are identified are thoroughly vetted by EOCME for fair balance, scientific objectivity, and patient care recommendations. EOCME is committed to providing its learners with CME activities that promote improvements or quality in healthcare and not a specific proprietary business or a commercial interest.

The planning committee, staff, authors and editors listed below have identified no financial relationships or relationships to products or devices they or their spouse/life partner have with commercial interest related to the content of this CME activity:
Andrea Aguglia, MD, PhD; Andrea Amerio, MD, PhD; Mario Amore, MD; Rivka Benyaminov, BA; María Dolores Braquehais, MD, PhD; Jessica A. Burket, PhD; Alexander Bystritsky, MD, PhD; Carl I. Cohen, MD; Alessandra Costanza, MD; Nolan Dang, BS; Stephen I. Deutsch, MD, PhD; Margaret Distler, MD, PhD; Andrea Escelsior, MD, PhD; Justin Faden, DO; Jess G. Fiedorowicz, MD, PhD; Matthew Ganeles; Aliza Grossberg, MD, MPH; Jonathan Haroon, BS; Kurt Kroenke, MD; Helen Lavretsky, MD, MS; Luca Magnani, MD; Addie N. Merians, PhD; Dilys Ngu, MD; Katerina Nikolitch, MD, CM, MSc; Erika Nurmi, MD, PhD; Maria A. Oquendo, MD, PhD; Merlin Packiam; Robert H. Pietrzak, PhD, MPH; Valeria Placenti, MD; Collin Price, MD; Manumar Rahman, MD; Michael Reinhardt, MD; Timothy Rice, MD; Gayatri Saraf, MD; Gianluca Serafini, MD, PhD; Leo Sher, MD; Tobias Spiller, MD; Norman M. Spivak, BS; Andrew Swenson; Doreen Thomas-Payne, MSN, BSN, RN, PMHNP-BC; Alice Trabucco, MD; Scott A. Turnbull, DO; Sebastián Vargas-Cáceres, MD

The planning committee, staff, authors, and editors listed below have identified financial relationships or relationships to products or devices they or their spouse/life partner have with commercial interest related to the content of this CME activity:
Leslie Citrome, MD, MPH: Consultant: AbbVie, Allergan, Acadia Pharmaceuticals Inc., Adamas Pharmaceuticals, Alkermes, Angelini, Astellas, Avanir, Axsome, BioXcel Therapeutics Inc., Boehringer Ingelheim International GmbH, Cadent Therapeutics, Eisai, Enteris BioPharma, HLS Therapeutics, Impel, Intra-Cellular Therapies, Janssen Pharmaceuticals, Karuna Therapeutics, Lundbeck, Lyndra Therapeutics, Merck, Neurocrine Biosciences, Novartis AG, Noven, Otsuka, Relmada Therapeutics, Reviva Pharmaceuitcals Inc., Sage Therapeutics, Inc., Sunovion Pharmaceuticals Inc., Supernus Pharmaceuticals Inc., Teva Pharmaceuticals; Speaker: AbbVie, Allergan, Acadia, Alkermes, Angelini, Eisai, Intra-Cellular Therapies, Janssen Pharmaceuticals, Lundbeck, Neurocrine Biosciences, Noven, Otsuka, Sage Therapeutics, Sunovion Pharmaceuticals, Takeda, Teva Pharmaceuticals; Stock Ownership: Bristol-Myers Squibb, Lilly, Johnson & Johnson, Merck, Pfizer Inc., Reviva Pharmaceuticals

Ilan Harpaz-Rotem, PhD: Independent Contractor: Boehringer Ingelheim International GmbH

John H. Krystal, MD: Consultant: Aptinyx, Inc., Atai Life Sciences, AstraZeneca Pharmaceuticals, Biogen, Idec, MA, Biomedisyn Corporation, Bionomics, Limited (Australia), Boehringer Ingelheim International GmbH, Cadent Therapeutics, Inc., Clexio Bioscience, Ltd., COMPASS Pathways, Limited, United Kingdom, Concert Pharmaceuticals, Inc., Epiodyne, Inc., EpiVario, Inc., Greenwich Biosciences, Inc., Heptares Therapeutics, Limited (UK), Janssen Research & Development, Jazz Pharmaceuticals, Inc., Otsuka, Perception Neuroscience Holdings, Inc., Spring Care, Inc., Sunovion Pharmaceuticals, Inc., Takeda Industries, Taisho Pharmaceutical Co., Ltd; Advisor: Biohaven Pharmaceuticals, BioXcel Therapeutics, Inc., Cadent Therapeutics, Inc., Cerevel Therapeutics, LLC, EpiVario, Inc., Eisai, Inc., Lohocla Research Corporation, Novartis Pharmaceuticals Corporation, PsychoGenics, Inc., RBNC Therapeutics, Inc., Tempero Bio, Inc., Terran Biosciences, Inc.; Stock Ownership: Biohaven Pharmaceuticals, EpiVario, Inc., RBNC Therapeutics, Inc., Sage Pharmaceuticals, Spring Care, Inc., Terran Biosciences, Inc. Tempero Bio, Inc.; Research Support: AstaZeneca Pharmaceuticals, Novartis Pharmaceutical Corporation

Marco Solmi, MD, PhD: Consultant: Angelini, Lundbeck, Otsuka

UNAPPROVED/OFF-LABEL USE DISCLOSURE
The EOCME requires CME faculty to disclose to the participants;
1. When products or procedures being discussed are off-label, unlabelled, experimental, and/or investigational (not US Food and Drug Administration [FDA] approved); and
2. Any limitations on the information presented, such as data that are preliminary or that represent ongoing research, interim analyses, and/or unsupported opinions. Faculty may discuss information about pharmaceutical agents that is outside of FDA-approved labelling. This information is intended solely for CME and is not intended to promote off-label use of these medications. If you have any questions, contact the medical affairs department of the manufacturer for the most recent prescribing information.

TO ENROLL
To enroll in the *Medical Clinics of North America* Continuing Medical Education program, call customer service at 1-800-654-2452 or sign up online at http; //www.theclinics.com/home/cme. The CME program is available to subscribers for an additional annual fee of USD 324.00.

METHOD OF PARTICIPATION
In order to claim credit, participants must complete the following;
1. Complete enrolment as indicated above.
2. Read the activity.
3. Complete the CME Test and Evaluation. Participants must achieve a score of 70% on the test. All CME Tests and Evaluations must be completed online.

CME INQUIRIES/SPECIAL NEEDS
For all CME inquiries or special needs, please contact elsevierCME@elsevier.com.

MEDICAL CLINICS OF NORTH AMERICA

FORTHCOMING ISSUES

March 2023
Women's Health
Melissa McNeil, *Editor*

May 2023
Hepatology: An Update
Anand V. Kulkarni and K. Rajender Reddy,
Editors

July 2023
An Update in Nephrology
Jeffrey Turner and Ursula Brewster, *Editors*

RECENT ISSUES

November 2022
Pulmonary Diseases
Daniel M. Goodenberger, *Editor*

September 2022
**Nutrition in the Practice of Medicine: A
Practical Approach**
David S. Seres, *Editor*

July 2022
**Communication Skills and Challenges in
Medical Practice**
Heather Hofmann, *Editor*

MEDICAL CLINICS OF NORTH AMERICA

Contributors

CONSULTING EDITOR

JACK ENDE, MD, MACP
The Schaeffer Professor of Medicine, Perelman School of Medicine, University of
Pennsylvania, Philadelphia, Pennsylvania, USA

EDITOR

LEO SHER, MD
Professor, Department of Psychiatry, Icahn School of Medicine at Mount Sinai, New York,
New York, USA

AUTHORS

ANDREA AGUGLIA, MD, PhD
Department of Neuroscience, Rehabilitation, Ophthalmology, Genetics, Maternal and
Child Health (DINOGMI), Section of Psychiatry, University of Genoa, IRCCS Ospedale
Policlinico San Martino, Genoa, Italy

ANDREA AMERIO, MD, PhD
Department of Neuroscience, Rehabilitation, Ophthalmology, Genetics, Maternal and
Child Health (DINOGMI), Section of Psychiatry, University of Genoa, IRCCS Ospedale
Policlinico San Martino, Genoa, Italy

MARIO AMORE, MD
Professor, Department of Neuroscience, Rehabilitation, Ophthalmology, Genetics,
Maternal and Child Health (DINOGMI), Section of Psychiatry, University of Genoa, IRCCS
Ospedale Policlinico San Martino, Genoa, Italy

RIVKA BENYAMINOV, BA
Medical Student, SUNY Downstate Health Sciences University, Brooklyn, New York, USA

MARÍA DOLORES BRAQUEHAIS, MD, PhD
Clinical Chief, Integral Care Program for Health Care Professionals, Galatea Clinic, Galatea
Foundation, Psychiatry, Mental Health and Addiction Research Group, Vall d'Hebron
Research Institute (VHIR), Vall d'Hebron University Hospital, Vall d'Hebron Hospital
Campus, Barcelona, Spain

JESSICA A. BURKET, PhD
Assistant Professor of Biology and Neuroscience, Department of Molecular Biology and
Chemistry, Christopher Newport University, Newport News, Virginia USA

ALEXANDER BYSTRITSKY, MD, PhD
Department of Psychiatry and Biobehavioral Sciences, David Geffen School of Medicine,
UCLA, Los Angeles, California, USA

LESLIE CITROME, MD, MPH
Clinical Professor of Psychiatry and Behavioral Sciences, New York Medical College, Valhalla, New York, USA

CARL I. COHEN, MD
Distinguished Service Professor and Co-Director, SUNY Downstate Health Sciences University, Brooklyn, New York, USA

ALESSANDRA COSTANZA, MD, PD (Privatdozent)
Department of Psychiatry, Faculty of Medicine, University of Geneva (UNIGE), Geneva, Switzerland, Faculty of Biomedical Sciences, University of Italian Switzerland (USI), Lugano, Switzerland

NOLAN DANG, BS
Department of Psychiatry and Biobehavioral Sciences, David Geffen School of Medicine, UCLA, Los Angeles, California, USA

STEPHEN I. DEUTSCH, MD, PhD
Emeritus Professor, Department of Psychiatry and Behavioral Sciences, Eastern Virginia Medical School, Norfolk, Virginia, USA

MARGARET DISTLER, MD, PhD
Department of Psychiatry and Biobehavioral Sciences, David Geffen School of Medicine, UCLA, Los Angeles, California, USA

ANDREA ESCELSIOR, MD, PhD
Department of Neuroscience, Rehabilitation, Ophthalmology, Genetics, Maternal and Child Health (DINOGMI), Section of Psychiatry, University of Genoa, IRCCS Ospedale Policlinico San Martino, Genoa, Italy

JUSTIN FADEN, DO
Associate Professor of Psychiatry, Lewis Katz School of Medicine, Temple University, Philadelphia, Pennsylvania, USA

JESS G. FIEDOROWICZ, MD, PhD
Department of Psychiatry, The Ottawa Hospital, Ottawa Hospital Research Institute, School of Epidemiology and Public Health, The University of Ottawa, Ottawa, Ontario, Canada

MATTHEW GANELES
Department of Molecular, Cell and Developmental Biology, UCLA, Los Angeles, California, USA

ALIZA GROSSBERG, MD, MPH
Department of Psychiatry, Icahn School of Medicine at Mount Sinai, New York, New York, USA

JONATHAN HAROON, BS
Department of Psychiatry and Biobehavioral Sciences, David Geffen School of Medicine, UCLA, Los Angeles, California, USA

ILAN HARPAZ-ROTEM, PhD
Clinical Neurosciences Division, United States Department of Veterans Affairs, National Center for Posttraumatic Stress Disorder, West Haven, Connecticut, USA; Department of Psychiatry, Yale School of Medicine, New Haven, Connecticut, USA

Contributors ix

KURT KROENKE, MD
Indiana University School of Medicine, Regenstrief Institute, Indianapolis, Indiana, USA

JOHN H. KRYSTAL, MD
Clinical Neurosciences Division, United States Department of Veterans Affairs, National Center for Posttraumatic Stress Disorder, West Haven, Connecticut, USA; Department of Psychiatry, Yale School of Medicine, New Haven, Connecticut, USA

HELEN LAVRETSKY, MD, MS
Department of Psychiatry and Biobehavioral Sciences, David Geffen School of Medicine, UCLA, Los Angeles, California, USA

LUCA MAGNANI, MD
Department of Neuroscience, Rehabilitation, Ophthalmology, Genetics, Maternal and Child Health (DINOGMI), Section of Psychiatry, University of Genoa, IRCCS Ospedale Policlinico San Martino, Genoa, Italy

ADDIE N. MERIANS, PhD
Clinical Neurosciences Division, United States Department of Veterans Affairs, National Center for Posttraumatic Stress Disorder, West Haven, Connecticut, USA; Department of Psychiatry, Yale School of Medicine, New Haven, Connecticut, USA

DILYS NGU, MD
Fellow in Geriatric Psychiatry, SUNY Downstate Health Sciences University, Brooklyn, New York, USA

KATERINA NIKOLITCH, MD, CM, MSc
Department of Psychiatry, The University of Ottawa, The Ottawa Hospital, Ottawa Hospital Research Institute, Institute for Mental Health Research, Ottawa, Ontario, Canada

ERIKA NURMI, MD, PhD
Department of Psychiatry and Biobehavioral Sciences, David Geffen School of Medicine, UCLA, Los Angeles, California, USA

MARIA A. OQUENDO, MD, PhD
Department of Psychiatry, Perelman School of Medicine at the University of Pennsylvania, Philadelphia, Pennsylvania, USA

ROBERT H. PIETRZAK, PhD, MPH
Clinical Neurosciences Division, United States Department of Veterans Affairs, National Center for Posttraumatic Stress Disorder, West Haven, Connecticut, USA; Department of Psychiatry, Yale School of Medicine, New Haven, Connecticut, USA

VALERIA PLACENTI, MD
Department of Neuroscience, Rehabilitation, Ophthalmology, Genetics, Maternal and Child Health (DINOGMI), Section of Psychiatry, University of Genoa, IRCCS Ospedale Policlinico San Martino, Genoa, Italy

COLLIN PRICE, MD
Department of Psychiatry and Biobehavioral Sciences, David Geffen School of Medicine, UCLA, Los Angeles, California, USA

MICHAEL REINHARDT, MD
Assistant Professor and Director, SUNY Downstate Health Sciences University, Brooklyn, New York, USA

MANUMAR RAHMAN, MD
Research Assistant, SUNY Downstate Health Sciences University, Brooklyn, New York, USA

TIMOTHY RICE, MD
Department of Psychiatry, Icahn School of Medicine at Mount Sinai, New York, New York, USA

GAYATRI SARAF, MD
Department of Psychiatry, The University of Ottawa, The Ottawa Hospital, Ottawa Hospital Research Institute, Ottawa, Ontario, Canada

GIANLUCA SERAFINI, MD, PhD
Professor, Department of Neuroscience, Rehabilitation, Ophthalmology, Genetics, Maternal and Child Health (DINOGMI), Section of Psychiatry, University of Genoa, IRCCS Ospedale Policlinico San Martino, Genoa, Italy

LEO SHER, MD
Professor, Department of Psychiatry, Icahn School of Medicine at Mount Sinai, New York, New York, USA

MARCO SOLMI, MD, PhD
Department of Psychiatry, The Ottawa Hospital, Ottawa Hospital Research Institute, School of Epidemiology and Public Health, The University of Ottawa, Ottawa, Ontario, Canada

TOBIAS SPILLER, MD
Clinical Neurosciences Division, United States Department of Veterans Affairs, National Center for Posttraumatic Stress Disorder, West Haven, Connecticut, USA; Department of Psychiatry, Yale School of Medicine, New Haven, Connecticut, USA

NORMAN M. SPIVAK, BS
UCLA-Caltech Medical Scientist Training Program, Department of Psychiatry and Biobehavioral Sciences, David Geffen School of Medicine, UCLA, Los Angeles, California, USA

ANDREW SWENSON
Department of Psychiatry and Biobehavioral Sciences, David Geffen School of Medicine, UCLA, Los Angeles, California, USA

ALICE TRABUCCO, MD
Department of Neuroscience, Rehabilitation, Ophthalmology, Genetics, Maternal and Child Health (DINOGMI), Section of Psychiatry, University of Genoa, Genoa, Italy

SCOTT A. TURNBULL, DO
Department of Internal Medicine, Kirk Kerkorian School of Medicine, UNLV, Las Vegas, Nevada, USA

SEBASTIÁN VARGAS-CÁCERES
Adult Mental Health Service, Benito Menni Mental Health Services, L'Hospitalet de Llobregat, Catalonia, Spain

Contents

> Depression and suicidal behavior are 2 complex psychiatric conditions of significant public health concerns due to their debilitating nature. The need to enhance contemporary treatments and preventative approaches for these illnesses not only calls for distillation of current views on their pathogenesis but also provides an impetus for further elucidation of their novel etiological determinants. In this regard, inflammation has recently been recognized as a potentially important contributor to the development of depression and suicidal behavior. This review highlights key evidence that supports the presence of dysregulated neurometabolic and immunologic signaling and abnormal interaction with microbial species as putative etiological hallmarks of inflammation in depression as well as their contribution to the development of suicidal behavior. Furthermore, therapeutic insights addressing candidate mechanisms of pathological inflammation in these disorders are proposed.

> Bipolar disorder is characterized by recurrent mood episodes, affecting 1% to 2% of the population. Although its defining features are manic and hypomanic episodes, its course is dominated by depressive syndromes. Diagnosis can be challenging owing to symptom overlap with other disorders. Management goals include early and complete remission of acute episodes and the prevention of relapse between episodes. We present an overview of bipolar disorder and its subtypes, including algorithms and suggestions for screening, assessment, and management.

> Schizophrenia is a disabling condition impacting approximately 1% of the worldwide population. Symptoms include positive symptoms (eg, hallucinations, delusions), negative symptoms (eg, avolition, anhedonia), and cognitive impairment. There are likely many different environmental and pathophysiologic etiologies involving distinct neurotransmitters and neurocircuits. Pharmacologic treatment at present consists of dopamine

receptor antagonists, which are reasonably effective at treating positive symptoms, but less effective at treating cognitive and negative symptoms. Nondopaminergic medications targeting alternative receptors are under investigation. Supportive psychosocial treatments can work in tandem with antipsychotic medications and optimize patient care.

Initial studies suggested that the fluctuations in the quantity, variety, and composition of the gut microbiota can significantly affect disease processes. This change in the gut microbiota causing negative health benefits was coined dysbiosis. Initial research focused on gastrointestinal illnesses. However, the gut microbiome was found to affect more than just gastrointestinal diseases. Numerous studies have proven that the gut microbiome can influence neuropsychiatric diseases such as Parkinson's disease, Alzheimer's disease, and multiple sclerosis.

Post-traumatic stress disorder (PTSD) is characterized by symptoms of re-experiencing, avoidance, negative alterations in cognition and mood, and marked alterations in arousal and reactivity following exposure to a traumatic event. PTSD can be assessed by structured interviews and screening measures in psychiatric and nonpsychiatric settings. Evidence-based psychotherapies are the first-line treatment of PTSD, with cognitive behavioral therapies, such as prolonged exposure, cognitive processing therapy, and eye movement desensitization and reprocessing having the largest body and highest quality of evidence. Serotonin reuptake inhibitors are the first-line pharmacologic treatments for PTSD and are often used in conjunction with other therapeutic interventions.

The BALB/c mouse displays hypersensitivity to behavioral effects of MK-801 (dizocilpine), a noncompetitive N-methyl-d-aspartic acid (NMDA) receptor "open-channel" blocker, and shows both no preference for an enclosed stimulus mouse over an inanimate object and reduced social interaction with a freely behaving stimulus mouse. NMDA receptor agonist interventions improved measures of social preference and social interaction of the BALB/c mouse model of autism spectrum disorder (ASD). A "proof of principle/proof of concept" translational 10-week clinical trial with 8-week of active medication administration was conducted comparing 20 DSM-IV-TR-diagnosed older adolescent/young adult patients with ASD randomized to once-weekly pulsed administration (50 mg/d) versus daily administration of d-cycloserine (50 mg/d). The results showed that d-cycloserine, a partial glycine agonist, was well tolerated, the 2 dosing strategies did not differ, and improvement was noted on the "lethargy/social withdrawal" and "stereotypic behavior" subscales of the Aberrant Behavior Checklist. NMDA receptor activation contributes to the regulation of mTOR signaling, a pathologic point of convergence in several monogenic syndromic forms of ASD. Furthermore, both NMDA receptor hypofunction and imbalance between NMDA receptor activation mediated by GluN2B and GluN2A-containing NMDA receptors occur as "downstream" consequences of several genetically unrelated abnormalities associated with ASD. NMDA receptor-subtype selective "positive allosteric modulators (PAMs)" are particularly appealing medication candidates for future translational trials.

Most suicides have a diagnosable psychiatric disorder, most frequently, a mood disorder. Psychosocial issues and neurobiological abnormalities such as dysregulation in stress response systems contribute to suicidal behavior. All psychiatric patients need to be screened for the presence of suicidal ideation. Clinicians are expected to gather information about patient's clinical features and to formulate decisions about patient's dangerousness to self and the treatment plan. As psychiatric disorders are a major risk factor for suicide their pharmacologic and psychological treatment is of utmost importance to prevent suicide. Restriction of access to lethal means is important for suicide prevention.

COVID-19 has increased the interest in the wellbeing of health professionals (HPs) as they have experienced stress, loss, and fatigue-related symptoms. Research evidence from previous epidemics points to an increase in the prevalence of affective, anxiety, and addictive disorders among them. HPs are trained to care for others and to recover from severe stressors. However, they tend to neglect self-care and have difficulties in seeking appropriate help when need it. This new scenario becomes an opportunity to promote a new culture of professionalism whereby caring for the caregivers becomes a priority both at a personal and institutional level.

Cognitive-behavioral therapy (CBT) is a form of psychological treatment that is based on the underlying assumption that mental disorders and psychological distress are maintained by cognitive factors, that is, that general beliefs about the world, the self, and the future contribute to the maintenance of emotional distress and behavioral problems. The overall goal of CBT is to replace dysfunctional constructs with more flexible and adaptive cognitions. The most relevant cognitive-behavioral techniques in clinical practice are: i. Cognitive Restructuring (also known as the ABCDE method) is indicated to support patients dealing with negative beliefs or thoughts. The different steps in the cognitive restructuring process are summarized by the letters in the ABCDE acronym that describe the different stages of this coaching model: Activating event or situation associated with the negative thoughts, Beliefs and belief structures held by the individual that explain how they perceive the world which can facilitate negative thoughts, Consequences or feelings related to the activating event, Disputation of beliefs to allow individuals to challenge their belief system, and Effective new approach or effort to deal with the problem by facilitating individuals to replace unhelpful beliefs with more helpful ones. ii. Problem-Solving (also known as SOLVE) to raise awareness for specific triggers, and evaluate and choose more effective options. Each letter of the SOLVE acronym identifies different steps of the problem-solving process: Select a problem, generate Options, rate the Likely outcome of each option, choose the Very best option, and Evaluate how well each option worked. For example, a suicide attempt is reconceptualized as a failure in problem-solving. This treatment approach attempts to provide patients with a better sense of control over future emerging problems. iii. Re-attribution is a technique that enables patients to replace negative self-statements (eg, "it is all my fault") with different statements where responsibility is attributed more appropriately. Furthermore, decatastrophizing may help subjects, especially adolescents decide whether they may be overestimating the catastrophic nature of the precipitating event, and by allowing them to scale the event severity they learn to evaluate situations along a continuum rather than seeing them in black and white. iv. Affect Regulation techniques are often used with suicidal adolescents to teach them how to recognize stimuli that provoke negative emotions and how to mitigate the resulting emotional arousal through self-talk and relaxation.

Depression and Suicidal Behavior in Adolescents

Aliza Grossberg and Timothy Rice

Depression commonly onsets in adolescence, affecting approximately 1 in 4 female adolescents and 1 in 10 males in the United States. Adolescent depression is a significant risk factor for suicide, the cause of over a third of all American adolescent deaths. Adolescent depression is introduced alongside its developmental and gendered considerations with a focus on important risk factors of adolescent depression, including nonsuicidal self-injury, adverse childhood experiences, and substance abuse. Protective factors and contemporary special topics of the COVID-19 pandemic and social media use are reviewed. Therapeutic options and clinical barriers are highlighted before a summary of findings and conclusion.

Frailty: A Multidimensional Biopsychosocial Syndrome

Carl I. Cohen, Rivka Benyaminov, Manumar Rahman, Dilys Ngu, and Michael Reinhardt

The original conceptual landscape of frailty has evolved into a complex, multidimensional biopsychosocial syndrome. This has broadened the field to now include social and behavioral scientists and clinicians from a wide range of specialties. This article aims to provide an updated overview of this conceptual change by examining the emerging definitions of physical, cognitive, social, and psychological frailty; the tools used for diagnosis and assessment of these domains; the epidemiology of the domains; their pathogenesis, risk factors, and course; frameworks for prevention and treatment; and unresolved issues affecting the field.

Foreword
Exciting Times

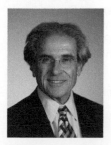

Jack Ende, MD, MACP
Consulting Editor

Primary care physicians and other practitioners hardly need to be convinced of the importance of psychiatry in their practices. Psychiatric disorders are common in primary care. These disorders may underlie or contribute to the problems patients bring to their internists and family physicians. Many patients are reluctant to be referred to a mental health professional, or as our Guest Editor, Leo Sher, points out in his Preface, mental health professionals may not be available. Not surprisingly, therefore, knowledge of psychiatric disorders and treatment of the same have come to be considered core knowledge for internists and family physicians. Psychiatric topics are included in continuing medical education programs for office-based and hospital-based physicians. They are part of the curriculum and requirements for internal medicine and family medicine residency training. At long last, we are finally moving away from the silo model of illness being either somatic or psychiatric. Oftentimes it is both. All this means is that primary care providers need to be able to recognize psychiatric disorders in their practice and, in many cases, manage these disorders, and certainly, they need to know when to refer.

The current issue of *Medical Clinics of North America*, "Management of Psychiatric Disorders and Suicidal Behavior in the Twenty-First Century," is a wonderful resource for primary care providers. Not only does it provide up-to-date information about some of the most important psychiatric disorders we see in our practices but also it provides information about intriguing new discoveries in psychiatry, such as the role of inflammation in depression, the importance of the microbiome in affective disorders, and the promising role that NMDA receptors play in psychiatric disorders and how that may lead to pharmacologic strategies for autism and perhaps also dementia.

Med Clin N Am 107 (2023) xv–xvi
https://doi.org/10.1016/j.mcna.2022.09.002
0025-7125/23/© 2022 Published by Elsevier Inc.

Psychiatry in the twenty-first century is as exciting as any field in medicine. I trust this issue will further your knowledge of psychiatry and its importance in primary care practice.

Jack Ende, MD, MACP
Perelman School of Medicine of the
University of Pennsylvania
5033 West Gates Pavilion
3400 Spruce Street
Philadelphia, PA 19104, USA

E-mail address:
jack.ende@pennmedicine.upenn.edu

Preface

Management of Psychiatric Disorders and Suicidal Behavior in the Twenty-First Century

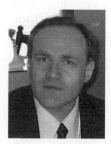

Leo Sher, MD
Editor

Over the past decades, diagnosis and treatment of psychiatric disorders have advanced enormously. Scientific achievements, including advances in biochemistry and neuroimaging, led to the development of new methods of diagnosis and treatment of mental illnesses. Effective medications offer opportunities for individuals with psychiatric disorders to lead full and fruitful lives. Today is definitely the best time in human history for patients and families who face mental disorders. The recognition of the global importance of psychiatric disorders has put mental health firmly on the international public health agenda. However, there are significant problems regarding the care of psychiatric patients.

According to the US National Institute of Mental Health, nearly one-fifth of adults in the United States have a psychiatric disorder. Providing care for the population of patients with psychiatric conditions in the United States is challenging and likely to become even more problematic in the near future. According to a 2017 New American Economy Report, more than 60% of all counties in the United States, including 80% of all rural counties, do not have a single psychiatrist. Therefore, non-mental-health medical professionals need to treat psychiatric conditions. Diagnosis and treatment of psychiatric disorders and suicide prevention interventions are relevant to all clinicians.

The increasing prevalence of comorbid psychiatric and physical disorders is an issue of great concern. I care for hospitalized patients with psychiatric disorders, and each day I encounter patients with the simultaneous presence of psychiatric and physical illnesses. This comorbidity frequently worsens the prognosis of all the diseases. For example, when depression occurs in people with diabetes, their blood sugar control gets much worse. Patients with comorbid depression and diabetes

Med Clin N Am 107 (2023) xvii–xviii
https://doi.org/10.1016/j.mcna.2022.05.001
0025-7125/23/© 2022 Published by Elsevier Inc.

tend to have higher blood glucose readings, worse insulin resistance, and higher rates of diabetes complications, such as blood vessel damage. The collaboration between psychiatrists and nonpsychiatric physicians is vital for effective management of co-morbid psychiatric and physical disorders, and suicide prevention.

Suicidal behavior remains a major medical and public health issue. Primary care physicians and other nonpsychiatrists may play an important role in suicide prevention efforts. Studies of individuals who died by suicide found that most persons had a health care visit in the year prior to the death, and about half of them made a health care visit within 1 month of the death, frequently to a primary care clinic. It is important to educate non-mental-health medical professionals how to identify individuals who may be at risk for suicide. Also, educating nonpsychiatric physicians to better diagnose and treat major depression and other psychiatric disorders may prevent suicides and nonfatal suicide attempts.

This issue of *Medical Clinics of North America* is dedicated to Clinical Psychiatry. The authors have put together a collection of scholarly articles discussing different aspects of contemporary psychiatry. I hope that the articles in this issue of *Medical Clinics of North America* will be helpful for all medical professionals and promote intellectual debates.

Leo Sher, MD
Icahn School of Medicine at Mount Sinai
JJP VAMC
130 West Kingsbridge Road
Bronx, NY 10468, USA

E-mail address:
Leo.Sher@mssm.edu

The Role of Inflammation in the Pathophysiology of Depression and Suicidal Behavior
Implications for Treatment

Gianluca Serafini, MD, PhD[a,b,]*,
Alessandra Costanza, MD, PD (Privatdozent)[c,d],
Andrea Aguglia, MD, PhD[a,b], Andrea Amerio, MD, PhD[a,b],
Alice Trabucco, MD[a], Andrea Escelsior, MD, PhD[a,b],
Leo Sher, MD[e,f,g], Mario Amore, MD[a,b]

KEYWORDS

- Depression • Suicidal behavior • Suicide • Biomarkers • Inflammation
- Neuro-inflammation • Treatment

KEY POINTS

- Inflammation is a prominent feature in depression and suicidal behavior (SB) etiopathogenesis.
- It has different origins.
- Neuroendocrine abnormalities can be involved in depression- and SB-associated inflammation.
- Immune dysregulation can also result in inflammation in these psychiatric conditions.
- Dysbiosis and infection, furthermore, can contribute.

[a] Department of Neuroscience, Rehabilitation, Ophthalmology, Genetics, Maternal and Child Health DINOGMI, Section of Psychiatry, University of Genoa, Genoa, Italy; [b] IRCCS Ospedale Policlinico San Martino, Largo Rosanna Benzi 10, Genoa 16132, Italy; [c] Department of Psychiatry, Faculty of Medicine, University of Geneva (UNIGE), Geneva, Switzerland, Faculty of Biomedical Sciences, Università della Svizzera Italiana (USI), Lugano, Switzerland; [d] Department of Psychiatry, Faculty of Biomedical Sciences, University of Italian Switzerland (USI), Lugano, Switzerland; [e] James J. Peters VA Medical Center, Bronx, NY, USA; [f] Department of Psychiatry, Icahn School of Medicine at Mount Sinai, New York, NY, USA; [g] Department of Psychiatry, New York, NY, USA
* Corresponding author.
E-mail address: gianluca.serafini@unige.it

Med Clin N Am 107 (2023) 1–29
https://doi.org/10.1016/j.mcna.2022.09.001
0025-7125/23/© 2022 Elsevier Inc. All rights reserved.
medical.theclinics.com

INTRODUCTION: PATHOBIOLOGY OF DEPRESSION AND SUICIDAL BEHAVIOR

Neuropsychiatric illnesses represent a significant cause of mortality worldwide,[1] with more than 30% increase in recent years. Among these conditions with high socioeconomic cost and health burden, mental health conditions, such as major depressive disorders (MDD) and suicide behavior (SB) have emerged as diseases of important public health concerns due to their chronic and disabling nature.[2–4] Despite being one of the most common mood disorders that affect more than 350 million people worldwide,[5] the pathophysiology of MDD remain elusive.[6] Similarly, as a leading cause of death in youth, suicide has not yet been completely understood from an etiological perspective. Therefore, further understanding of the risk factors for the development and progression of MDD and SB is pivotal to improving the diagnosis and treatment of affected individuals.

Despite various attempts to define psychiatric hallmarks of MDD,[7] clinical symptoms and pathological features of depression vary among different patient subpopulations and are often complicated by comorbidities of somatic illnesses and demographic factors.[8] From an anatomical perspective, MDD is associated with abnormalities in areas of emotional regulation in the brain, such as the prefrontal cortex and amygdala.[9] Nevertheless, no neurobiological markers are of clinical usefulness for the diagnosis and prediction of MDD.[10] Neurobiological signature of SB is also of significant research and clinical interests, with the proposal of various molecular and genetic determinants.[11–13] However, it is difficult to delineate the which dysfunctional pathway is specific to SB or common among psychiatric disorders. Notably, SB is frequently associated with MDD and other mood disorders.[14–16]

Current treatments for MDD remain unsatisfactory, with a substantial proportion of depressed patients exhibiting unresponsiveness to first-generation antidepressants, including monoamine inhibitors (MAOI), selective serotonin reuptake inhibitors (SSRI), and tricyclic agents (TCA).[17] Contemporary preventative approaches for SB are also limited. Notably, emerging evidence has pointed to an association between the presence of inflammatory pathology as a hallmark of drug-refractory depression[18] as well as a risk factor of SB,[19–24] prompting significant research interests in the exploration of the underlying mechanisms of inflammation in these neuropsychiatric conditions. Overall, the hypothesis that inflammatory markers may be indicators of MDD, SB risk in MMD, or even SB in the absence of major psychiatric conditions has been supported by different experimental paradigms and clinical correlates.[23,25] Nevertheless, the extent and mechanism by which specific inflammatory abnormalities contribute to our current understanding of the complex pathophysiology of MDD and SB remain unknown. This review aims to provide a concise synthesis of the current evidence for the involvement of inflammation in MDD and SB development from neuroendocrinological, immunological, and microbial standpoints, along with possible implications for therapeutic treatments.

CHARACTERISTICS AND ORIGINS OF INFLAMMATION IN DEPRESSION
Characteristics of Inflammation in Depression

The involvement of inflammation in the pathophysiology of depression was supported by various observations. First, patients with inflammatory somatic diseases are more likely to develop depression.[26,27] Second, some proinflammatory immunotherapy, such as IFN-α, induced depressive symptoms.[28,29] As such, extensive efforts have been put forward to comprehensively characterize the presence of inflammatory markers in various types of specimens from depressed subjects.

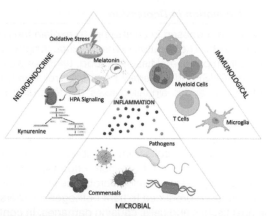

Fig. 1. Putative etiologies of pathological inflammation in depression and suicide.

Among different neurobiological hypotheses, genome-wide association studies have been carried out to identify candidate genes that are linked to depression vulnerability.[30,31] Notably, various genetic networks of inflammation have been identified, with variants in cytokines and inflammatory mediators as the most reproducible findings.[32] For example, polymorphisms in IL-1β, TNF-α, CCL2, and CRP have been linked to higher depression severity.[33–35] Decreased IL-6 methylation status was also noted in depressed patients with higher circulating IL-6.[36] In congruence with these genetic analyses, levels of various innate immunity-associated inflammatory molecules, such as IL-6, TNF-α, and CRP,[37–39] were elevated in MDD patients' sera. In contrast, information regarding cytokines associated with adaptive immunity was limited, with some discrepancies among the reports. For example, cytokines, such as IFN-γ[38] and IL-4,[40] showed decreases in protein and/or mRNA levels in blood samples of patients with MDD in some studies. However, increased IFN-α/IL-4 ratio or elevated levels of Th1 (IFN-α) and Th2 (IL-4) cytokines have also been observed.[41–43] Of note, the role of Th17 cytokine (IL-17A) has gained significant attention in depression research, given its promotion of depressive behaviors in animal models,[44,45] its elevation in MDD patients' sera,[38] and some promising efficacy of IL-17A blockade in psoriasis-associated depression.[46] Some anti-inflammatory cytokines have also been implicated in depression, with the documentation of increases in TGF-β and IL-10,[38,47] suggesting a potential compensatory mechanism for a defective response of the host to elevated inflammation. Alternatively, these cytokines have also been implicated in treatment-resistant depression.[48] Furthermore, some studies showed that inflammation was not a unifying pathology among all types of depression, while another investigation of treatment-naive depressed subjects demonstrated that the majority of these patients exhibited some inflammatory features.[49] Patient cohort characteristics (size, female prevalence), antidepressant exposure and responsiveness[50,51] might account for these discrepancies. Furthermore, nonmelancholic depression was linked with an inflammatory state,[52] which was only observed during acute exacerbation of melancholic depression.[53] While most studies reported inflammatory findings from the circulation of depressed patients, neuroinflammation has also been noted in MDD, with increased expression of IL-6 and TNF-α in the cerebrospinal fluid (CSF) and brain tissues.[54]

Putative Origins of Inflammation in Depression

Various theories have been proposed in an attempt to explain the presence of inflammation in depressed patients. These putative mechanistic insights were derived from analyses of specimens from peripheral tissues (blood, urine) as well as those from the central nervous system (CNS) and generally point toward a unifying hypothesis for simultaneous alterations in various signaling axes as described later in discussion (**Fig. 1**).

Neuroendocrinological origin

Oxidative stress. Oxidative stress results from an imbalance between reactive oxygen species (ROS) synthesis and antioxidant defense response.[55] Both reactive oxygen species and antioxidants are produced during aerobic cellular metabolism in the mitochondria. While the formers are produced to fight pathogen invaders, they can also be directed toward the host tissues and cells, causing damages. In contrast, antioxidants comprise many structurally and functionally diverse molecules to neutralize the activity of ROS in both enzymatic and nonenzymatic manners.

The CNS is particularly susceptible to oxidative stress due to its high oxygen demand with limited antioxidant production and a high content of lipid peroxidation substrates (transition metal and polyunsaturated fatty acids [PUFAs]).[56,57] In this regard, mitochondrial dysfunction and oxidative stress-induced DNA damages in the CNS have also been linked to depressive disorders.[58,59] Levels of various antioxidants, including glutathione peroxidase, vitamin E, erythrocyte superoxide dismutase, and glutathione reductase were reduced in the brain specimens of depressed subjects.[59–63] In the blood samples of MDD subjects, similar changes were also noted, along with increased levels of oxidative stress markers, such as lipid peroxidation products (F2-isoprostanes and malondialdehyde), thiobarbituric acid reactive substances, deoxyguanosine, and uric acid.[60,64–66]

Mechanistically, oxidative stress can cause mitochondrial damage, and the ensuing inflammatory reactions against damaged mitochondrial components exacerbate mitochondrial dysfunction, leading to increased production of ROS, which could also trigger inflammasome activation and inflammation-induced cell death, heightening oxidative stress.[67,68] These hypotheses were supported by both experimental evidence and clinical correlates. In rats, chronic exposure to stressors induced oxidative stress and inflammation while suppressing antioxidant production.[69] Further, lipid peroxidation was also highly increased in a model of stress-induced depression in various tissues[70] including the brain. In humans, childhood maltreatment was associated with adult risk of depression and concurrent increases in inflammation and oxidative stress.[71] Reduction in antioxidant levels in the blood of depressed patients are also linked to elevated levels of circulating inflammatory cytokines.[63] Collectively, these findings suggested that the vicious interplay between oxidative stress and inflammation is an etiological component of MDD.

Hypothalamic–pituitary–adrenal axis. In response to stress, corticotropin-releasing hormone (CRH) and arginine vasopressin (AVP) from the hypothalamus triggers the release of adrenocorticotropic hormone (ACTH) from the anterior pituitary gland, prompting the secretion of cortisol (glucocorticoid) from the adrenal cortex.[72] The hypothalamic–pituitary–adrenal axis (HPA) hyperactivity has been implicated in the development of depression from multiple lines of evidence. First, more than 40–60% of depressed patients experienced hypercortisolemia or other abnormalities of the HPA axis,[73] such as reduction in the ACTH release and elevation in the CRH secretion. Increased cortisol secretion was associated with acute and severe MDD and might contribute to depression-associated psychosis via its potentiation of dopaminergic signaling.[74] Second, increased cortisol was also noted in animal models of stress-induced depression and inhibition of cortisol production could suppress depressive behaviors.[75–78] Third, in postpartum depression (PPD), which affects up to 20% of mothers, overactivity/impaired suppression of HPA axis has been observed in pregnant women as well as in animal models of PPD.[79]

While increased secretion of cortisol might potentiate depression via its possible destructive action on the hippocampus,[79,80] hypercortisolemia-induced glucocorticoid receptor (GR) desensitization[81,82] has also been linked to increased symptoms of depression. Notably, this defective cortisol response might provide a mechanistic connection between HPA dysregulation and the development of inflammatory pathology in MDD.[83] In this regard, while cortisol is known to exert an anti-inflammatory activity,[84] repeated stimulation of GR results in resistance of immune cells to this canonical function of cortisol, heightening the propensity for inflammation. Furthermore, inflammasome activation[48,85] in depressed patients might worsen glucocorticoid desensitization by caspase-1 mediated cleavage of GR.[86]

Kynurenine metabolism. Kynurenine is a product of tryptophan catabolism via the indoleamine 2,3-dioxygenase (IDO) enzymatic pathway. This pathway has been implicated in various putative etiologies of MDD.[87] It has been hypothesized that the activation of kynurenine metabolism results in a reduced availability of tryptophan for the synthesis of serotonin, a neuroprotective factor in depression,[88] leading to increased susceptibility to depressive disorders. Consistent with this idea, a clinical study revealed that acute tryptophan depletion triggered mild depressive symptoms in recovered depressed patients.[89] Furthermore, kynurenine activation was observed in various types of depression, such as IFN-α induced depression,[90] PPD,[91] cardiovascular disease-associated depression,[92] and drug-resistant depression.[93] Notably, in IFN-α induced depression, kynurenine/tryptophan ratio showed decreases in both plasma and CSF and correlated with depression severity.[94] Consistent with these clinical findings, depressive-like behaviors could be induced by L-kynurenine and blocked by an IDO inhibitor.[95–97]

Besides this hypothesis, alteration in the ratio between neurotoxic metabolites of the kynurenine pathway, such as 3-hydroxykynurenine, 3-hydroxyanthranilic acid, and quinolinic acid (QA), and neuroprotective metabolites, such as kynurenic acid (KYN) and picolinic acid, might also contribute to MDD development.[98–100] In fact, increased quinolinic acid was observed in the brain of depressed subjects and reduced cortical thickness in patients with MDD was linked to increased levels of neurotoxic metabolites of the kynurenine pathway.[101,102] Conversely, hippocampal and amygdala volumes were positively correlated with the kynurenic acid/quinolinic acid ratio in serum samples of patients with MDD.[103] Kynurenic acid also exerted an antidepressant effect in animal studies.[104]

Notably, a reciprocal interaction between inflammation and kynurenine metabolism might exist in the development of MDD. On one hand, the activation of the kynurenine pathway is triggered by inflammatory stimuli.[105] On the other hand, various toxic metabolites in this pathway could also result in neurotoxicity-induced neuroinflammation, further propagating pathological activation of kynurenine signaling.

Melatonin signaling. A prominent feature of MDD is the disruption of the rhythmicity of the sleep-wakefulness cycle, in which abnormalities in the neuroendocrine hormone melatonin have been observed. This neuroactive molecule is produced by the pineal gland during darkness, and thus, promotes healthy sleep. Animals lacking melatonin receptors reportedly exhibited depression and anxiety-like behaviors.[106] In humans, a single nucleotide polymorphism in the brain-expressed melatonin receptor has been linked to depression symptoms,[107] prompting the possibility that depressed patients have weaker response to melatonin.[108] In fact, altered production and secretion patterns of melatonin have been reported in various forms of depression.[109]

The protective effect of melatonin against depression might occur via its modulation of neuroplasticity in the hippocampus,[110] a brain area highly implicated in mood pathologies. Alternatively, a connection between melatonin and inflammatory pathology of these neuropsychiatric conditions could be inferred from its immunomodulatory functions. Under inflamed conditions, melatonin could inhibit the activation and migration of various inflammatory immune cells, such as monocytes, macrophages, microglia,[111] and neutrophils.[112] In fact, an inverse correlation between plasma level of melatonin and depression-associated inflammatory markers has been observed.[113,114] Various animal studies and clinical reports also documented an anti-inflammatory effect of melatonin.[115] Therefore, dysregulated production and responses to melatonin might further exacerbate inflammatory pathology in depression. Nevertheless, caution must be taken regarding the interpretation of these findings as a proinflammatory activity of melatonin has been observed under noninflamed states.[115] Additionally, this molecule might not protect against high-grade inflammation.

Immunologic origin

Increasing evidence has suggested that the immune system is a critical regulator of MDD.[116] Various hypotheses regarding the immunologic etiology of depression have been proposed, including the immunosuppression[117] and sickness behavior theories,[118] and most recently, the implication of myeloid cell-mediated hyperinflammation.[119] In this regard, peripheral immune abnormalities have been observed in MDD. Reduced T cell function and numbers in depressed subjects were described in some reports.[120-122] NK cell frequencies and activities were also decreased in patients with MDD.[123,124] These findings supported the immunosuppression hypothesis of depression. However, other studies demonstrated the expansion of CD4+ T helper cells and Th17 cells in depressed subjects,[125-127] particularly those with high risk of SB. These discrepancies suggested that dynamic immune activation phenotype might be associated with various stages of depression. Furthermore, increases in circulating numbers of monocytes and neutrophils were noted in depressed subjects, providing corroborating evidence for the myeloid cell hypothesis of depression. According to this hypothesis, hyperactivation of these innate immune cells accounts for the elevated expression of various prototypical inflammatory mediators in this disease.

Recently, abnormalities in CNS immunity have been explored in MDD with the emerging understanding of the role of microglia in neuroinflammation. Microglia are CNS resident innate immune cells that guard the brains against pathogens and support neurodevelopmental processes. However, their aberrant production of various inflammatory mediators has been noted in patients with MDD. In fact, microglial activation has been linked to increased IL-6, IL-8, and TNF-α levels in brain tissues and CSF of subjects with MDD. Infection-associated depressive symptoms were also associated with microglial reactivity.[128] However, regional reduction of microglial activity was also found in depressed subjects,[129,130] suggesting that complex temporal regulation of the activation of these cells might occur in this disease. Notably, an alternative explanation for the presence of microglial reactivity in early tracing studies of TSPO in major depression has recently been proposed. In this regard, the TSPO signal might represent the infiltration of peripheral monocytes and macrophages into the CNS,[131] rather than reflecting the local activation of microglia. In support of this provocative perspective about the potential loss of the blood–brain barrier integrity in MDD, reduced numbers of astrocytes, a neural cell population involved in the regulation of the blood–brain barrier permeability, have been observed in depressed subjects.[132]

While these diverse changes in the immunophenotype of depressed patients pointed to a unifying theme about the involvement of the immune system in the inflammatory pathology of this disorder, further mechanistic investigations in both experimental models and human specimens are required to delineate the precise involvement of anatomically distinct immune cell populations (peripheral vs. CNS cell subsets as well as resident cells of specific brain regions) in the onset, development, and exacerbation of MDD.

Microbial origin

Microbiome. The microbiome, consisting of all microbes living in the host body, has an intricate connection with the nervous system. Notably, microbial dysbiosis has been linked to morphological impairment in brain areas involved in mood disorders, such as amygdala and hippocampus.[133] Consistent with this finding, microbial dysbiosis has been observed in depression. For example, patients with MDD exhibited alterations in the intestinal microbiome.[134–136] Conversely, alterations in the intestinal microbiome, particularly in subjects with inflammatory bowel syndrome, are associated with symptoms of depression and anxiety.[137] In experimental models of depression, microbes from depressed patients could trigger depression-like behaviors in animals,[138] and animals subjected to chronic stress showed the altered composition of the intestinal microbiome. Notably, these microbial alterations in animals with depression-like behaviors could be reversed by microbial transfers or prebiotic/probiotic supplementation.[139,140] Furthermore, some studies demonstrated that the antidepressant effect of microbial transfer was associated with a reduction in inflammation,[141,142] suggesting that microbial dysregulation might promote the development of depression via the induction of inflammatory signaling. Mechanistically, dysbiosis might result in compromised intestinal barrier integrity, exposing the immune system to inflammatory stimuli from the environment. A distribution shift in microbes might also result in excessive release of immunostimulatory products, such as microbe-associated molecular patterns (MAMPs) and metabolites, causing inflammation. Concurrently, anti-inflammatory products from microbes, such as short-chain fatty acids (SCFAs), might be reduced in depressed patients as a result of dysbiosis,[143] predisposing these individuals to inflammatory pathology. Lastly, relayed immunostimulatory signaling from the periphery to the CNS with the resultant neuroinflammation, might also represent a mechanism by which microbial dysbiosis contributes to neuroinflammatory pathology in MDD.

Infection. Associations between infection and mental disorders were first noted in a case series of influenza patients in 1958.[144] Multiple observations over the past several decades indicate that there is a link between infections and psychiatric conditions[145–149] This association prompted the development of various hypotheses to explain this phenomenon. While some neurotropic microbes could directly affect the CNS, a common feature of microbial infection is the elicitation of inflammation from the immune system, which might predispose infected subjects to depression.[150] Mechanistically, type-1 interferons, including IFN-α, are often elicited by viral and bacterial infections, and this cytokine is known to induce depression symptoms. Alternatively, the production of classical inflammatory cytokines (IL-1, IL-6, TNF-α) by the immune system in response to the pathogens might also contribute to the development of depression. In fact, herpes virus, EBV, CMV, Borna disease virus, and gastroenteritis-related virus are associated with depressive symptoms.[151] Influenza A, B, and C, and H7N9 (bird flu) infections have been linked to depression.[152,153] Furthermore, depression and other mental health-related issues were also documented in patients infected with MERS and SARS.[154] Notably, COVID-19 severity, evidenced by elevated levels of inflammatory cytokines (IL-1, IL-6, TNF-α), is associated with depressive symptoms.[155,156] Interestingly, bidirectional interaction between depression and infection might exist as depressed patients have been reported to be more susceptible to various types of infection.[157,158] Therefore, this pathological interplay between infection with depression might further increase the risk of corecurrence of these illnesses in the affected patients.

CHARACTERISTICS AND ORIGINS OF INFLAMMATION IN SUICIDE BEHAVIOR DEVELOPMENT

One of the first evidence supporting the link between inflammation and SB was the documentation of SB in subjects receiving cytokine treatment for their somatic illnesses.[159] Subsequent studies revealed that an imbalance between pro- (IL-1β, IL-2, IL-6, TNF-α) and anti-inflammatory cytokine (IL-4, IL-10) levels correlated with functional changes in brain regions that control emotion, motivation, and reward, and ultimately, SB-associated behavioral changes.[23,24,160–162] These cytokines could modulate distinct biological functions, including neurotransmitter signaling, neuroplasticity, and neurodegenerative processes.[163–166] Furthermore, major signaling axes with notable dysregulations in MDD were also documented in the development of SB, even in the absence of major psychiatric illnesses. For example, neuroendocrinological abnormalities,[167] including enhanced oxidative stress,[24] dysregulated HPA and kynurenine signaling[168]; SB,[93] reduced melatonin production,[169–171] have been linked to the pathophysiology of SB. Similarly, immunological abnormalities[22] as well as microbial dysbiosis[172] and infection[19] have been postulated as major contributors to pathological inflammation in SB development (see **Fig. 1**). However, discrepancies regarding these findings exist because of methodological differences and, possibly, other factors. Particularly, given the diverse categorization strategies for the patient populations in suicide studies, careful consideration of mechanistic implications from the primary findings is required. The sections later in discussion will provide a brief overview of clinical observations regarding the role of inflammation in SB development in different types of studies.

Studies of Patients with a History Suicide Attempts vs. Healthy Controls

Alterations in brain cytokine levels have been noted in patients with a history of suicide attempts (SA). Compared to healthy controls, elevated IL-6 in the CSF was linked to a history of SA, particularly violent SA.[173] Notably, an increase in CSF IL-6 was correlated with alterations in serotonergic (measured by 5-hydroxyindolacetic acid) and dopaminergic (measured by homovanillic acid) signaling. In contrast, CSF IL-6 showed no differences between patients with SA and health controls in another cohort study that control for male sex and medication-free status,[174] while VEGF and IL-8 were markedly reduced in patients with SA. This association between reduced VEGF and history of SA was also confirmed in serum analysis in a 13-year longitudinal study.[175] Polymorphisms of the neuroprotective chemokine IL-8 were also detected in patients with SA as compared to healthy controls.[176]

In the circulation, increased IL-6 and TNF-α and decreased IL-2 levels were observed in patients with SA as compared to healthy controls.[177] In contrast, soluble IL-2R, a marker of T cell activation, was elevated in patients with SA and showed a trend of correlation with the ratio of norepinephrine–epinephrine in 24-h urine and hydroxy-3-methoxymethylglycol levels in plasma and CSF.[178] Adding to the complexity of IL-2 signaling in SA development, a study of social exclusion by,[179] revealed that alterations in serum IL-2 was not associated with SA, but was implicated in the activation of the right anterior cingulate cortex, insula, and orbitofrontal cortex. Furthermore, the serum level of another inflammatory cytokine, IL-1β, was associated with right orbitofrontal cortex activation during social exclusion, rather than with SA.

Notably, abnormalities in the proinflammatory metabolic pathway of kynurenine were reported in patients with SA. In this regard, increased expression of neurotoxic QA and decreased expression of neuroprotective KYN were observed in the CSF of patients with SA as compared to healthy controls.[180] Increased plasma level of KYN was also documented in patients with SA as compared to healthy controls.[181] Furthermore, increased expression of neopterin, a marker of IFN-γ activation, was associated with higher KYN: tryptophan (TRP) ratio in this study, confirming that inflammatory activation was associated with kynurenine catabolism.

Studies of Patients with a History Suicide Attempts vs. those with Suicidal Ideation

Interestingly, some evidence suggested that pathological inflammation was connected to the history of SA, but not active suicidal ideation (SI). In this regard, IL-8 represented a genetic risk factor for a history of SA, but not active SI, particularly in women.[182] Lower hair cortisol level was a distinct feature of patients with SA, but not those with SI.[183] In this study, patients with SA also showed lower GR expression and increased levels of CRP and TNF-α as compared to those with SI and heathy controls. Furthermore, changes in nitro-oxidative stress, as compared to healthy controls, were more strongly associated with SA than with SI.[184] Collectively, these findings suggested that alterations in inflammatory signaling might be the precipitating factor for progression from SI to SA.

Studies of Patients with a History Suicide Attempts vs. those Non-suicidal Depressed

Few studies have examined changes in inflammatory pathology between nondepressed suicidal patients and depressed patients without SA/SI. Nevertheless, subjects at risk for suicide may be biologically distinguished from depressed individuals without such a risk.[185] For example, inflammatory pathology (serum IL-1β, IL-6, and TNF-α) was more pronounced in patients with SA as compared to nonsuicidal depressed subjects.[177,186,187] Lower serum IL-2 was also observed in patients with SA as compared to nonsuicidal depressed patients.[177]

Studies of Suicidal Behavior Risk in Depressed Patients

Distinct inflammatory pathology has been observed in suicidal depressed patients. In this regard, MDD patients with SI had higher inflammatory scores than both nonsuicidal patients with MDD and healthy controls.[188] TNF-α −308G > A polymorphism was also linked to an enhanced risk of SA[189] in MDD. However, discrepancies exist regarding these findings as reductions in IL-1β,[190] IL-6,[191] and TNF-α[192] were documented in suicidal depressed patients as compared to nonsuicidal depressed patients. TNF-α was also suggested as a biomarker of MDD that is responsive to venlafaxine treatment, rather than suicide.[50] Regarding adaptive immune activation, depressed suicidal patients might have a pro-Th1 response, whereas nonsuicidal depressed patients were linked to a pro-Th2 immune profile.[193] However, a Th2-biased cytokine profile in the sera was observed in MDD patients with SA in another study.[191] Serum IL-2, a marker of T cell activation, levels were also reduced in MDD patients with SA as compared to healthy control and nonsuicidal depressed subjects.[191] Alteration in immune trafficking was also present in depressed suicidal subjects. In this regard, MDD patients with SI also exhibited lower serum levels of CCL2/CCL5 and higher level of CCL11 than healthy controls.[194] While these observations required further validation, they suggest that dynamic changes in cytokine expression occur during the development of SA in patients with MDD.

Studies of Subjects who Died by Suicide vs. Other Causes

Postmortem studies have provided some important information regarding the presence of inflammatory signatures in the brain of suicide victims. Compared to healthy controls, patients with MDD who completed suicides exhibited increased in IL-1β, IL-6, TNF-α, and lymphotoxin A levels and decreased IL-10 and IL-1 receptor antagonists (IL-1RA) levels in the prefrontal cortex (PFC).[18,195] Similarly, IL-6 was elevated in the brain of asphytic suicide victims.[196] Sex-specific pattern of cytokine alterations in the orbitofrontal cortex was also noted in suicide victims, with increased IL-4 in women and increased IL-13 in men.[197] Regarding HPA abnormalities, glucocorticoid receptor-α (GR-α) expression was reduced in the dorsolateral PFC of young adolescent who died by suicide, regardless of psychiatric diagnoses, as compared to health controls.[198] Furthermore, morphological changes in microglia were noted in the brain of suicide victims, with some discrepancies, most likely due to the effect of death on microglial reactivity and the sampling method (i.e., CSF vs. brain tissues/regions).[199] Increased macrophage accumulation was also noted in the dorsal anterior cingulate cortex of individual who died of suicide, with elevated expression of CD45, IBA1, and CCL2.[200] However, reduced CCL2 and other macrophage chemokines (MIP-1β, eotaxin, MCP-4, TARC) were observed in another study.[201]

Markers of oxidative stress and HPA signaling can distinguish between suicidal depressed vs. nonsuicidal depressed patients. In depressed subjects with increasing suicide risk, increased ACTH and cortisol responses have been observed as compared to nonsuicidal depressed subjects.[202] Reduced expression of antioxidants (superoxide dismutase 1/2 [SOD1/2], GPX1) were observed in MDD subjects with SA as compared to nonsuicidal depressed subjects.[203] Increased oxidative stress (nitrogen oxide, lipid hydroperoxides and) and reduced total plasma total antioxidant potential (TRAP) were concurrently observed with increased systemic inflammation in MDD patients with SA as compared to those without SA.[204]

THERAPEUTIC INSIGHTS

Observations of the presence of inflammation in MDD and SB warranted clinical examinations of the effectiveness of anti-inflammatory medications for these psychiatric illnesses.

Many trials have focused on the use of nonsteroidal anti-inflammatory drugs (NSAIDs), which showed promising antidepressant activity. For example, NSAIDs as a monotherapy or adjunct treatment along with conventional antidepressants exhibited clinical effectiveness.[205] While these anti-inflammatory agents have generally good safety profiles, cautions must be taken in the interpretation of these findings due to several reasons. First, many trials included patients with comorbid somatic illnesses of inflammatory nature (psoriasis, arthritis, etc.), which might limit the generalization of the findings.[206] Second, conflicting results regarding the efficacies of NSAIDs also existed, which might be related to medication classification (inclusion of aspirin as an NSAIDs).[207] Regarding suicide, whether the inhibition of inflammation could protect against the development of SB remains to be determined. Of clinical relevance, NSAIDs have been suggested to be efficacious in reducing SB risks, providing the first evidence for the clinical effectiveness of anti-inflammatory drugs in suicide prevention.[208]

Along with these findings, the aforementioned discussion of various potential etiologies of MDD- and SB-associated inflammation provided a strong rationale for further development of tailored treatments for specific pathways that orchestrate inflammatory signaling in different subtypes of these psychiatric illnesses. A distillation of the prominent developmental efforts aiming at various putative contributors to inflammatory pathology of these conditions is described in the following sections.

Oxidative Stress Blockade

In preclinical studies, oxidative stress could be suppressed by the antidepressant venlafaxine,[209,210] suggesting that this molecular pathology of depression might be a direct therapeutic target of these medications. Furthermore, supplementation of the antioxidant vitamin D could alleviate depressive symptoms in rats by modulating oxidative stress and inflammation.[211] Notably, the clinical efficacy of SSRI also appeared to be inversely correlated with the baseline level of lipid peroxidation products (F2-isoprostanes) and was monitorable by a reduction in IL-6 expression.[66,212] Altogether, these findings emphasize the therapeutic utility of targeting oxidative stress-inflammation signaling in depressive disorders. Given the close connection between oxidative stress and neuroexcitotoxicity, inhibition of this pathway might also provide fruitful outcomes for SB prevention.

Normalization of Hypothalamic–pituitary–adrenal Axis Response

Given the presence of numerous HPA abnormalities in depressed patients and the disappearance of exaggerated dexamethasone response with effectively treated depression symptoms,[213] the HPA axis has been suggested as a promising treatment target for depression treatment and SB prevention.[214,215] For example, suppression of VAP, the most upstream activator of HPA axis, has been proposed for depression, particularly in patients with confirmed HPA overactivity.[216,217] Plant-derived polyphenols with preclinical suppressive activities on HPA signaling, such as resveratrol or ferulic acid,[218–220] could be also explored to treat depression with a relatively favorable path for clinical development, given their good safety profile and high bioavailability. Notably, ferulic acid could markedly reduce inflammatory cytokine expression with a concomitant increase in GR expression. Other agents with observed coinhibitory effects on HPA signaling and inflammation, such as the retinoic acid receptor α (RARα) agonist and the antibiotic minocycline,[221] are under investigation as novel therapies for MDD.[222] Lastly, a strategy to improve negative feedback control of GR for HPA activation with the GR antagonist mifepristone has also been proposed for various psychiatric disorders, including MDD.[223–225]

Kynurenine Inhibition

Various molecular regulators of the kynurenine pathways have gained attention as promising targets for drug development in psychiatric disorders, including MDD and SB.[226] Among them, inhibitors of IDO and kynurenine monooxygenase (KMO, a key enzyme that controls the production of quinolinic acid) are at more advanced development stages. Several IDO inhibitors have been examined in clinical trials for cancer, which could be repurposed for CNS indications,[227] providing that these molecules have suitable pharmacological features that allow favorable brain penetrance. Furthermore, the recent report on the crystallized structure of human KMO has accelerated the development and physicochemical characterization of KMO inhibitors, including those of synthetic as well as natural origins.[228–230] Nevertheless, whether these inhibitors could effectively reduce the quinolinic acid synthesis and affect neuropsychiatric manifestations in MDD and SB remains to be determined.

Melatonin

Regarding melatonin, a pharmacologic agonist of its receptors, agomelatine, reportedly exhibited antidepressant properties in preclinical studies.[231–233] Specific depression trials tried to target the engagement of this molecule with particular regard to its effects on sleep and melatonin onset[234,235]). Preliminary clinical efficacy of melatonin against depression depressive symptoms has also been observed but its direct antidepressant activity and its impact on depression-associated inflammation remain to be explored in future trials.[236,237] Of importance, treatment with melatonin has been linked to increased risk of SA/SI, warranting additional caution regarding its use for psychiatric disorders.[238]

Immunotherapy

Major cytokine inhibitor therapies, including TNF-α inhibitors,[239,240] IL-12/IL-23 antagonists,[241] neutralizing IL-17A antibodies,[46] or anti–IL-6 biologics,[242] were efficacious in MDD. However, infliximab, a TNF-α inhibitor, was not efficacious in the treatment of bipolar depression and was also linked to SB.[243,244] Furthermore, neuropsychiatric complications of cytokine therapies are of significant concern with the potentiation of suicide risk and psychiatric illnesses in psoriasis patients who received the anti–IL-17RA therapy.[245] These findings suggested the importance of further immunophenotyping in different subtypes of depression as well as in patients with the distinct presentation of suicidal symptoms might be necessary to identify pathological cell subsets responsible for the production of specific inflammatory mediators in these conditions. As such, novel inflammatory cellular targets could be addressed, rather than nonspecific inhibition of cytokine signaling, which might exhibit some level of toxicity.

Anti-infectives

The use of anti-infective agents for depression dates back to the discovery of the antidepressant effect of isoniazid,[246] an antibacterial medication for tuberculosis. Recently, some anti-infective agents have been tried for the treatment of neuropsychiatric conditions. For example, minocycline has been suggested as an antiviral with concurrent antidepressant properties, potentially via its suppressive activity on inflammation.[247] Interestingly, given the bidirectional relationship between infection and depression, some antidepressants have recently been ascribed with antiviral properties against MERS and SARS-CoV-2.[248] It's also worth noting that some anti-infectives might also trigger psychiatric complications, including depression and SB. For example, the antimalaria drugs chloroquine/hydroxychloroquine have been associated with suicide.[249,250] Additionally, some antibiotics might also exert detrimental effects on mental health due to their interference with homeostatic communication between the host microbiome and the nervous system.[246] Therefore, repurposing anti-infectives for neuropsychiatric diseases, including SB and MDD, requires a cautious approach and further investigation.

Microbiome Modification

Approaches to modification, the dysregulated microbiome in MDD and SB have attracted recent attention in the scientific community, with some promising results. For example, multispecies probiotics could reduce neurobehavioral parameters associated with depression and suicidal ideation,[251] while single-species probiotic supplementation reduced depression and anxiety in PPD.[252] Results of other trials with different forms of probiotics also suggested that probiotics were efficacious in reducing depressive symptoms in patients with MDD.[253,254] Notably, the anti-inflammatory omega-3 PUFAs, which could be derived from microbes, have been shown to be effective against depressive symptoms in multiple clinical trials.[255] Collectively, these findings confirmed the therapeutic utility of targeting the microbiome-inflammation axis for the treatment of MDD, and potentially other neuropsychiatric conditions, including SB.

Other Approaches

Besides the aforementioned therapeutic strategies to suppress inflammation, several other pharmacologic agents have been found to have anti-inflammatory properties. These medications not only provided novel mechanistic insights regarding the etiology of inflammation in MDD and SB but also emphasize the potential role of inflammation as a causative factor in the development of these psychiatric illnesses. For example, some psychoactive substances, such as psilocybin,[256] might also exert anti-inflammatory activities and have been proposed as a novel therapeutic target in suicide prevention.[257] Similarly, coinhibition of depressive symptoms and inflammation was also observed with SSRI.[258] However, other studies have shown that SSRI could trigger inflammatory responses, which might explain for the increased suicide risk associated with these medication[259] and suggest a complex interplay between antidepressants and inflammatory signaling. Besides antidepressants, ketamine, an antagonist of the N-methyl-d-aspartate type of glutamate receptor and a common anesthetic drug, exhibited both antidepressants and anti-inflammatory properties.[260,261] HDAC inhibitors with anti-inflammatory features, such as vorinostat and romidepsin,[262,263] exhibited preclinical efficacy against depression and has been suggested as a promising drug target for suicide prevention.[264] Lastly, cognitive behavioral therapies (CBT), which have been used for depression treatment and suicide prevention,[265,266] also suppressed inflammation in depressed patients who were responsive to this therapy.[48,267]

SUMMARY

The inflammatory pathology of MDD and SB might result from the dysregulation of neuroendocrine signaling pathways, unrestrained activation of the immune system, and aberrant interaction of the host with pathogenic and commensal microbes. It's important to emphasize that inflammatory pathology is not unique for SB and depression, as elevated levels of inflammatory cytokines have been noted in other psychiatric diseases.[268] As such, these collective findings not only suggest the possible presence of a common inflammatory pathway of behavioral disorders but also highlight the necessity to determine the precise contribution of individual cytokine to each neuropsychiatric disease. Nevertheless, anti-inflammatory approaches for the treatment of depression and the prevention of suicide might benefit from these aforementioned insights. In this regard, an integrated and comprehensive yet pathway-specific approach to inhibit pathological inflammation is warranted to improve the effectiveness of treatment and suicide prevention in these psychiatric illnesses.

Abnormal neuroendocrine signaling, including processes related to the hypotha-lamic–pituitary–adrenal axis (HPA), melatonin production, kynurenine metabolism, and oxidative stress, dysregulated immune response of myeloid innate immune cells from peripheral tissues (monocytes, macrophages, and neutrophils) and the central nervous system (microglia) as well as adaptive immune cells (T cells), and dysbiosis of host commensals and infection from exogenous pathogens might heighten the pro-duction of inflammatory mediators in the circulation and the brain, leading to an increased risk of depression and suicide.

CONFLICTS OF INTEREST

The authors declare no conflicts of interest.

FUNDING

This work did not receive any funding from the public, commercial or not-for-profit sectors.

CLINICS CARE POINTS

- Distinct inflammatory pathology might be present in different subtypes of depression, or in suicidal ideation vs. different subtypes of suicidal behavior (SB).
- Inflammatory pathology could be monitored for diagnosis, prevention, and treatment responsiveness in these psychiatric conditions.
- Pathway-focused blockade of inflammation treatment might be useful for to improve outcomes.

REFERENCES

1. Alejos M, Vázquez-Bourgon J, Santurtún M, et al. Do patients diagnosed with a neurological disease present increased risk of suicide? Neurologia (Engl Ed). 2020. S0213-4853:30129-8.
2. Kessler RC, Berglund P, Demler O. The epidemiology of major depressive dis-order: results from the National Comorbidity Survey Replication (NCS-R). JAMA 2003;289:3095–105.
3. Menon V, Vijayakumar L. Interventions for attempted suicide. Curr Opin Psychi-atry 2022;35(5):317–23.
4. Messaoud A, Mensi R, Douki W, et al. Reduced peripheral availability of trypto-phan and increased activation of the kynurenine pathway and cortisol correlate with major depression and suicide. World J Biol Psychiatry 2019;20(9):703–11.
5. Liu Q, He H, Yang J, et al. Changes in the global burden of depression from 1990 to 2017: findings from the global burden of disease study. J Psychiatr Res 2020;126:134–40.
6. Hasler G. Pathophysiology of depression: do we have any solid evidence of in-terest to clinicians? World Psychiatry 2010;9(3):155–61.
7. Koo PC, Berger C, Kronenberg G, et al. Combined cognitive, psychomotor and electrophysiological biomarkers in major depressive disorder. Eur Arch Psychi-atry Clin Neurosci 2019;269:823–32.

8. Perna G, Alciati A, Daccò S, et al. Personalized psychiatry and depression: the role of sociodemographic and clinical variables. Psychiatry Investig 2020;17: 193–206.
9. Koolschijn PCM, van Haren NE, Lensvelt-Mulders GJ, et al. Brain volume abnormalities in major depressive disorder: A meta-analysis of magnetic resonance imaging studies. Hum Brain Mapp 2009;30:3719–35.
10. Menke A. Precision pharmacotherapy: psychiatry's future direction in preventing, diagnosing, and treating mental disorders. Pharmacogenomics Pers Med 2018;11:211–22.
11. Costanza A, Amerio A, Aguglia A, et al. When sick brain and hopelessness meet: some aspects of suicidality in the neurological patient. CNS Neurol Disord Drug Targets 2020;19(4):257–63.
12. Costanza A, D'Orta I, Perroud N, et al. Neurobiology of suicide: do biomarkers exist? Int J Legal Med 2014;128:73–82.
13. Lutz PE, Mechawar N, Turecki G. Neuropathology of suicide: recent findings and future directions. Mol Psychiatr 2017;22:395–1412.
14. Hawton KI, Casañas I, Comabella C, et al. Risk factors for suicide in individuals with depression: a systematic review. J Affect Disord 2013;147(1–3):17–28.
15. Moitra M, Santomauro D, Degenhardt L, et al. Estimating the risk of suicide associated with mental disorders: A systematic review and meta-regression analysis. J Psychiatr Res 2021;137:242–9.
16. Ribeiro JD, Huang X, Fox KR, et al. Depression and hopelessness as risk factors for suicide ideation, attempts and death: meta-analysis of longitudinal studies. Br J Psychiatry 2018;212(5):279–86.
17. Réus GZ, Titus SE, Abelaira HM. Neurochemical correlation between major depressivedisorder and neurodegenerative diseases. Life sciences 2016;158: 121–9.
18. Pandey GN, Rizavi HS, Zhang H, et al. Abnormal protein and mRNA expression of inflammatory cytokines in the prefrontal cortex of depressed individuals who died by suicide. J Psychiatry Neurosci 2018;43:376–85.
19. Costanza A, Amerio A, Aguglia A, et al. Hyper/neuroinflammation in COVID-19 and suicide etiopathogenesis: hypothesis for a nefarious collision? Neurosci Biobehav Rev 2022;136:104606.
20. Courtet P, Giner L, Seneque M, et al. Neuroinflammation in suicide: Toward a comprehensive model. World J Biol Psychiatry 2016;17:564–86.
21. Crawford B, Craig Z, Mansell G, et al. DNA methylation and inflammation marker profiles associated with a history of depression. Hum Mol Genet 2009;27(16): 2840–50.
22. Jackson NA, Jabbi M,M. Integrating biobehavioral information to predict mood disordersuiciderisk. Brain Behav Immun Health 2022;24:100495.
23. Serafini G, Parisi VM, Aguglia A, et al. A specific inflammatory profile underlying suicide risk? Systematic review of the main literature findings. Int J Environ Res Public Health 2020;17(7):2393.
24. Serafini G, Pompili M, Seretti EM, et al. The role of inflammatory cytokines in suicidal behavior: a systematic review. Eur Neuropsychopharmacol 2013;23: 1672–86.
25. Bergmans RS, Kelly KM, Mezuk B. Inflammation as a unique marker of suicide ideation distinct from depression syndrome among U.S. adults. J Affect Disord 2019;245:1052–60.

26. Bouças AP, Rheinheimer J, Lagopoulos J. Why severe COVID-19 patients are at greater risk of developing depression: a molecular perspective. Neuroscientist 2020;28(1):11–9.
27. Brundin L, Sellgren CM, Lim CK, et al. An enzyme in the kynurenine pathway that governs vulnerability to suicidal behavior by regulating excitotoxicity and neuroinflammation. Transl Psychiatry 2016;6:e865.
28. Kayser MS, Dalmau J. The emerging link between autoimmune disorders and neuropsychiatric disease. J Neuropsychiatry Clin Neurosci 2011;23:90–7.
29. Raison CL, Borisov AS, Broadwell SD, et al. Depression during pegylated interferon-alpha plus ribavirin therapy: prevalence and prediction. J Clin Psychiatry 2005;66:41–8.
30. Jabbi M, Arasappan D, Eickhoff SB, et al. Neuro-transcriptomic signatures for mood disorder morbidity and suicide mortality. J Psychiatr Res 2020;127:62–74.
31. Pantazatos SP, Huang YY, Rosoklija GB, et al. Whole-transcriptome brain expression and exon-usage profiling in major depression and suicide: evidence for altered glial, endothelial and ATPase activity. Mol Psychiatr 2017;22:760–73.
32. Barnes J, Mondelli V, Pariante CM. Genetic contributions of inflammation to depression. Neuropsychopharmacology 2017;42:81–98.
33. Bufalino C, Hepgul N, Aguglia E, et al. The role of immune genes in the association between depression and inflammation: a review of recent clinical studies. Brain Behav Immun 2013;31:31–47.
34. Dantzer R, O'Connor JC, Freund GG, et al. From inflammation to sickness and depression: when the immune system subjugates the brain. Nat Rev Neurosci 2008;9:46–56.
35. Miller AH, Maletic V, Raison CL. Inflammation and its discontents: the role of cytokines in the pathophysiology of major depression. Biol Psychiatry 2009;65(9): 732–41.
36. Crawford B, Craig Z, Mansell G, et al. DNA methylation and inflammation marker profiles associated with a history of depression. Hum Mol Genet 2009;27: 2840–5.
37. Karlovic D, Serretti A, Vrkic N, et al. Serum concentrations of CRP, IL-6, TNF-alpha and cortisol in major depressive disorder with melancholic or atypical features. Psychiatry Res 2012;198:74–80.
38. Köhler CA, Freitas TH, Maes M, et al. Peripheral cytokine and chemokine alterations in depression: a meta-analysis of 82 studies. Acta Psychiatr Scand 2017; 135:373–87.
39. Maes M, Yirmyia R, Noraberg J, et al. The inflammatory & neurodegenerative (I&ND) hypothesis of depression: leads for future research and new drug developments in depression. Metab Brain Dis 2009;24(1):27–53.
40. Hepgul N, Cattaneo A, Zunszain PA, et al. Depression pathogenesis and treatment: what can we learn from blood mRNA expression? BMC Med 2013;11:28.
41. Maes M, Stevens W, Peeters D, et al. A study on the blunted natural killer cell activity in severely depressed patients. Life Sci 1992;50:505–13.
42. Myint AM, Leonard BE, Steinbusch HW, et al. Th1, Th2, and Th3 cytokine alterations in major depression. J Affect Disord 2005;88:167–73.
43. Huang TL, Lee CT. T-helper 1/T-helper 2 cytokine imbalance and clinical phenotypes of acute-phase major depression. Psychiatry Clin Neurosci 2007;61(4): 415–20.
44. Cheng Y, Desse S, Martinez A, et al. TNFa disrupts blood brain barrier integrity to maintain prolonged depressive-like behavior in mice. Brain Behav Immun 2018;69:556-56.

45. Nadeem A, Ahmad SF, Al-Harbi NO, et al. IL-17A causes depression-like symptoms via NF-κB and p38MAPK signaling pathways in mice: Implications for psoriasis associated depression. Cytokine 2017;97:14–24.
46. Griffiths CEM, Fava M, Miller AH, et al. Impact of ixekizumab treatment on depressive symptoms and systemic inflammation in patients with moderate-to-severe psoriasis: an integrated analysis of three phase 3 clinical studies. Psychother Psychosom 2017;86(5):260–7.
47. Lee HY, Kim YK. Transforming growth factor-beta1 and major depressive disorder with and without attempted suicide: preliminary study. Psychiatry Res 2010; 178:92–6.
48. Syed SA, Beurel E, Loewenstein DA, et al. Defective inflammatory pathways in never-treated depressed patients are associated with poor treatment response. Neuron 2018;99:914–24.e3.
49. Lamers F, Milaneschi Y, de Jonge P, et al. Metabolic and inflammatory markers: associations with individual depressive-symptoms. Psychol Med 2018;48: 1102–10.
50. Li Z, Qi D, Chen J, et al. Venlafaxine inhibits the upregulation of plasma tumor necrosis factor-alpha (TNFα) in the Chinese patients with major depressive disorder: a prospective longitudinal study. Psychoneuroendocrinology 2013;38: 107–14.
51. Réus GZ, Titus SE, Abelaira HM, et al. Neurochemical correlation between major depressive disorder and neurodegenerative diseases. Life Sci 2016;158:121–9.
52. Rothermundt M, Arolt V, Fenker J, et al. Different immune patterns in melancholic and non-melancholic major depression. Eur Arch Psychiatry Clin Neurosci 2001; 251:90–7.
53. Dunjic-Kostic B, Ivkovic M, Radonjic NV, et al. Melancholic and atypical major depression–connection between cytokines, psychopathology and treatment. Prog Neuropsychopharmacol Biol Psychiatry 2013;43:1–6.
54. Black C, Miller BJ. Meta-analysis of cytokines and chemokines in suicidality: distinguishing suicidal versus nonsuicidal patients. Biol Psychiatry 2015;78:28–37.
55. Kowalczyk P, Sulejczak D, Kleczkowska P, et al. Mitochondrial oxidativestress-a causative factor and therapeutic target in many diseases. Int J Mol Sci 2021; 22(24):13384.
56. Lushchak VI, Duszenko M, Gospodaryov DV, et al. Oxidativestress and energy metabolism in the brain: midlife as a turning point. Antioxidants (Basel) 2021; 10(11):1715.
57. Ng F, Berk M, Dean O, et al. Oxidative stress in psychiatric disorders: evidence base and therapeutic implications. Int J Neuropsychopharmacol 2008 Sep; 11(6):851–76.
58. Bansal Y, Kuhad A. Mitochondrial dysfunction in depression. Curr Neuropharmacol 2016;14(6):610–8.
59. Szebeni A, Szebeni K, DiPeri TP, et al. Elevated DNA Oxidation and DNA Repair Enzyme Expression in Brain White Matter in Major Depressive Disorder. Int J Neuropsychopharmacol 2017;20(5):363–73.
60. Bal N, Acar ST, Yazici A, et al. Altered levels of malondialdehyde and Vitamin E in major depressive disorder and generalized anxiety disorder. Dusunen Adam J Psychiatry Neurol Sci 2012;25:206.
61. Maes M, De Vos N, Pioli R, et al. Lower serum vitamin E concentrations in major depression. Another marker of lowered antioxidant defenses in that illness. J Affect Disord 2000;58:241–6.

62. Maes M, Mihaylova I, Kubera M, et al. Lower whole blood glutathione peroxidase (GPX) activity in depression, but not in myalgic encephalomyelitis/chronic fatigue syndrome: another pathway that may be associated with coronary artery disease and neuroprogression in depression. Neuroendocrinol Lett 2011;32: 133–40.

63. Rybka J, Kedziora-Kornatowska K, Banaś-Lezańska P, et al. Interplay between the pro-oxidant and antioxidant systems and proinflammatory cytokine levels, in relation to iron metabolism and the erythron in depression. Free Radic Biol Med 2013;63:187–94.

64. Jiménez-Fernández S, Gurpegui M, Garrote-Rojas D, et al. Oxidativestress parameters and antioxidants in adults with unipolar or bipolar depression versus healthy controls: Systematic review and meta-analysis. J Affect Disord 2022; 314:211–21.

65. Kong Y, Liu C, Zhang C, et al. Association between serum uric acid levels and suicide attempts in adolescents and young adults with major depressive disorder: a retrospective study. Neuropsychiatr Dis Treat 2022;18:1469–77.

66. Lindqvist D, Dhabhar FS, James SJ, et al. Oxidative stress, inflammation and treatment response in major depression. Psychoneuroendocrinology 2017;76: 197–205.

67. Li Y, Song W, Tong Y, et al. Isoliquiritin ameliorates depression by suppressing NLRP3-mediated pyroptosis via miRNA-27a/SYK/NF-κB axis. J Neuroinflam 2021;18:1–23.

68. López-López AL, Jaime HB, Escobar Villanueva MDC, et al. Chronic unpredictable mild stress generates oxidative stress and systemic inflammation in rats. Physiol Behav 2016;161:15–23.

69. Wigner P, Synowiec E, Czarny P, et al. Effects of venlafaxine on the expression level and methylation status of genes involved in oxidative stress in rats exposed to a chronic mild stress. J Cell Mol Med 2020;24:5675.

70. Celikbilek A, Yesim Gocmen A, Tanik N, et al. Serum lipid peroxidation markers are correlated with those in brain samples in different stress models. Acta Neuropsychiatr 2014;26:51–7.

71. Danese A, Pariante CM, Caspi A, et al. Childhood maltreatment predicts adult inflammation in a life-course study. Proc Natl Acad Sci U S A 2007;104:1319.

72. Belvederi Murri M, Pariante C, Mondelli V, et al. HPA axis and aging in depression: systematic review and meta-analysis. Psychoneuroendocrinology 2014;41: 46–62.

73. Du X, Pang TY. Is Dysregulation of the HPA-axis a core pathophysiology mediating co-morbid depression in neurodegenerative diseases? Front Psychiatry 2015;6:32.

74. Schatzberg AF, Rothschild AJ, Langlais PJ, et al. A corticosteroid/dopamine hypothesis for psychotic depression and related states. J Psychiatr Res 1985;19: 57–64.

75. Bielajew C, Konkle A, Merali Z. The effects of chronic mild stress on male Sprague–Dawley and Long Evans rats: I. Biochemical and physiological analyses. Behav Brain Res 2002;136:583–92.

76. Davenport MD, Tiefenbacher S, Lutz CK, et al. Analysis of endogenous cortisol concentrations in the hair of rhesus macaques. Gen Comp Endocrinol 2006;147: 255–61.

77. De Andrade J, Céspedes I, Abrão R, et al. Chronic unpredictable mild stress alters an anxiety-related defensive response, Fos immunoreactivity and hippocampal adult neurogenesis. Behav Brain Res 2013;250:81–90.

78. Qin D, Rizak J, Chu X, et al. A spontaneous depressive pattern in adult female rhesus macaques. Sci Rep 2015;5:11267.
79. Zoubovsky SP, Hoseus S, Tumukuntala S, et al. Chronic psychosocial stress during pregnancy affects maternal behavior and neuroendocrine function and modulates hypothalamic CRH and nuclear steroid receptor expression. Transl Psychiatry 2020;10:6.
80. Feng X, Wang L, Yang S, et al. Maternal separation produces lasting changes in cortisol and behavior in rhesus monkeys. Proc Natl Acad Sci U S A 2011;108: 14312–7.
81. Holsboer F. The corticosteroid receptor hypothesis of depression. Neuropsychopharmacology 2000;23(5):477–501.
82. Raison CL, Miller AH. When not enough is too much: the role of insufficient glucocorticoid signaling in the pathophysiology of stress-related disorders. Am J Psychiatry 2003;160:1554–65.
83. Genis-Mendoza AD, Dionisio-García DM, Gonzalez-Castro TB, et al. Increased levels of cortisol in individuals with suicide attempt and its relation with the number of suicide attempts and depression. Front Psychiatry 2022;13:912021.
84. Dhabhar FS. Enhancing versus suppressive effects of stress on immune function: implications for immunoprotection and immunopathology. Neuroimmunomodulation 2009;16(5):300–17.
85. Alcocer-Gómez E, de Miguel M, Casas-Barquero N, et al. NLRP3 inflammasome is activated in mononuclear blood cells from patients with major depressive disorder. Brain Behav Immun 2014;36:111–7.
86. Paugh SW, Bonten EJ, Evans WE. Inflammasome-mediated glucocorticoid resistance: the receptor rheostat. Mol Cell. Oncol. 2015;3:e106594.
87. Hestad K, Alexander J, Rootwelt H, et al. The role of tryptophan dysmetabolism and quinolinic acid in depressive and neurodegenerative diseases. Biomolecules 2022;12(7):998.
88. Correia AS, Vale N. Tryptophan metabolism in depression: a narrative review with a focus on serotonin and kynurenine pathways. Int J Mol Sci 2022;23(15): 8493.
89. Moreno FA, Parkinson D, Palmer C, et al. CSF neurochemicals during tryptophan depletion in individuals with remitted depression and healthy controls. Eur Neuropsychopharmacol 2010;20(1):18–24.
90. Capuron L, Gumnick JF, Musselman DL, et al. Neurobehavioral effects of interferon-alpha in cancer patients: phenomenology and paroxetine responsiveness of symptom dimensions. Neuropsychopharmacology 2002;26(5):643–52.
91. Kohl C, Walch T, Huber R, et al. Measurement of tryptophan, kynurenine and neopterin in women with and without postpartum blues. J Affect Disord 2005; 86(2–3):135–42.
92. Swardfager W, Herrmann N, Dowlati Y, et al. Indoleamine 2,3-dioxygenase activation and depressive symptoms in patients with coronary artery disease. Psychoneuroendocrinology 2009;34(10):1560–6.
93. Serafini G, Adavastro G, Canepa G, et al. Abnormalities in kynurenine pathway metabolism in treatment-resistant depression and suicidality: a systematic review. CNS Neurol Disord Drug Targets 2017;16(4):440–5.
94. Raison CL, Dantzer R, Kelley KW, et al. CSF concentrations of brain tryptophan and kynurenines during immune stimulation with IFN-alpha: relationship to CNS immune responses and depression. Mol Psychiatry 2010;15(4):393–403.
95. O'Connor JC, André C, Wang Y, et al. Interferon-gamma and tumor necrosis factor-alpha mediate the upregulation of indoleamine 2,3-dioxygenase and the

induction of depressive-like behavior in mice in response to bacillus Calmette-Guerin. J Neurosci 2009;29(13):4200–9.

96. O'Connor JC, Lawson MA, André C, et al. Lipopolysaccharide-induced depressive-like behavior is mediated by indoleamine 2,3-dioxygenase activation in mice. Mol Psychiatry 2009;14(5):511–22.

97. O'Connor JC, André C, Wang Y, et al. Interferon-gamma and tumor necrosis factor-alpha mediate the upregulation of indoleamine 2,3-dioxygenase and the induction of depressive-like behavior in mice in response to bacillus Calmette-Guerin. J Neurosci 2009;29(13):4200–9.

98. Lugo-Huitron R, Blanco-Ayala T, Ugalde-Muniz P, et al. On the antioxidant properties of kynurenic acid: free radical scavenging activity and inhibition of oxidative stress. Neurotoxicol Teratol 2011;33:538–47.

99. Maddison DC, Giorgini F. The kynurenine pathway and neurodegenerative disease. Semin Cell Dev Biol 2015;40:134–41.

100. Steiner J, Walter M, Gos T, et al. Severe depression is associated with increased microglial quinolinic acid in subregions of the anterior cingulate gyrus: evidence for an immune-modulated glutamatergic neurotransmission? J Neuroinflammation 2011;8:94.

101. Meier TB, Drevets WC, Wurfel BE, et al. Relationship between neurotoxic kynurenine metabolites and reductions in right medial prefrontal cortical thickness in major depressive disorder. Brain Behav Immun 2016;53:39–48.

102. Melatonin in mood disorders. World J Biol Psychiatry 2006;7(3):138–51.

103. Savitz J, Drevets WC, Smith CM, et al. Putative neuroprotective and neurotoxic kynurenine pathway metabolites are associated with hippocampal and amygdalar volumes in subjects with major depressive disorder. Neuropsychopharmacology 2015;40:463–71.

104. Tanaka M, Bohár Z, Martos D, et al. Antidepressant-like effects of kynurenic acid in a modified forced swim test. Pharmacol Rep 2020;72:449–55.

105. Jovanovic F, Sudhakar A, Knezevic NN. The Kynurenine pathway and polycystic ovary syndrome: inflammation as a common denominator. Int J Tryptophan Res 2022;15. 11786469221099214.

106. Liu J, Clough SJ, Dubocovich ML. Role of the MT1 and MT2 melatonin receptors in mediating depressive- and anxiety-like behaviors in C3H/HeN mice. Genes Brain Behav 2017;16:546–53.

107. Demirkan A, Lahti J, Direk N, et al. Somatic, positive and negative domains of the Center for Epidemiological Studies Depression (CES-D) scale: a meta-analysis of genome-wide association studies. Psychol Med 2016;46:1613–23.

108. Valdes-Tovar M, Estrada-Reyes R, Solis-Chagoyan H, et al. Circadian modulation of neuroplasticity by melatonin: a target in the treatment of depression. Br J Pharmacol 2018;175:3200–8.

109. Srinivasan V, Smits M, Spence W, Lowe AD, Kayumov L, Pandi-Perumal SR, Parry B, Cardinali DP.

110. Soumier A, Banasr M, Lortet S, et al. Mechanisms contributing to the phase-dependent regulation of neurogenesis by the novel antidepressant, agomelatine, in the adult rat hippocampus. Neuropsychopharmacology 2009;34:2390–403.

111. Lee MY, Kuan YH, Chen HY, et al. Intravenous administration of melatonin reduces the intracerebral cellular inflammatory response following transient focal cerebral ischemia in rats. J Pineal Res 2007;42:297–309.

112. Silva SO, Rodrigues MR, Ximenes VF, et al. Neutrophils as a specific target for melatonin and kynuramines: Effects on cytokine release. J Neuroimmunol 2004; 156:146–52.
113. Anderson G. Linking the biological underpinnings of depression: role of mitochondria interactions with melatonin, inflammation, sirtuins, tryptophan catabolites, DNA repair and oxidative and nitrosative stress, with consequences for classification and cognition. Prog Neuropsychopharmacol Biol Psychiatry 2018;80:255–66.
114. Dominguez-Alonso A, Ramirez-Rodriguez G, Benitez-King G. Melatonin increases dendritogenesis in the hilus of hippocampal organotypic cultures. J Pineal Res 2012;52:427–36.
115. Won E, Na KS, Kim YK. Associations between melatonin, neuroinflammation, and brain alterations in depression. Int J Mol Sci 2021;23(1):305.
116. Müller N. Immunology of major depression. Neuroimmunomodulation 2014;21: 123–30.
117. Dvorakova M, Zvolský P, Herzog P, et al. Endogenous psychoses and T and B lymphocytes. Leipzig, Germany 1980;107(2):221–8.
118. Dantzer R. Cytokine, sickness behavior, and depression. Immunol Allergy Clin N Am 2009;29:247–64.
119. Smith RS. The macrophage theory of depression. Med Hypotheses 1991;35: 298–306.
120. Kronfol Z, Silva J Jr, Greden J, et al. Impaired lymphocyte function in depressive illness. Life Sci 1983;33:241–7.
121. Schleifer SJ, Keller SE, Meyerson AT, et al. Lymphocyte function in major depressive disorder. Arch Gen Psychiatry 1984;41:484–6.
122. Wu MK, Huang TL, Huang KW, et al. Association between toll-like receptor 4 expression and symptoms of major depressive disorder. Neuropsychiatr Dis Treat 2015;11:1853–7.
123. Grosse L, Carvalho LA, Birkenhager TK, et al. Circulating cytotoxic T cells and natural killer cells as potential predictors for antidepressant response in melancholic depression. Restoration of T regulatory cell populations after antidepressant therapy. Psychopharmacology (Berl.) 2016;233:1679–88.
124. Irwin M, Gillin JC. Impaired natural killer cell activity among depressed patients. Psychiatry Res 1987;20:181–2.
125. Darko DF, Lucas AH, Gillin JC, et al. Cellular immunity and the hypothalamic-pituitary axis in major affective disorder: a preliminary study. Psychiatry Res 1988;25:1–9.
126. Schiweck C, Valles-Colomer M, Arolt V, et al. Depression and suicidality: a link to premature T helper cell aging and increased Th17 cells. Brain Behav Immun 2020. https://doi.org/10.1016/j.bbi.2020.02.005.
127. Tondo L, Burrai C, Scamonatti L, et al. Comparison between clinician-rated and self-reported depressive symptoms in Italian psychiatric patients. Neuropsychobiology 1988;19:1–5.
128. Rock RB, Gekker G, Hu S, et al. Role of microglia in central nervous system infections. Clin Microbiol Rev 2004;17:942–64.
129. Cotter D, Mackay D, Landau S, et al. Reduced glial cell density and neuronal size in the anterior cingulate cortex in major depressive disorder. Arch Gen Psychiatry 2001;58:545–55.
130. Ongür D, Drevets WC, Price JL. Glial reduction in the subgenual prefrontal cortex in mood disorders. Proc Natl Acad Sci U S A 1998;95:13290–5.

131. Owen DR, Narayan N, Wells L, et al. Pro-inflammatory activation of primary microglia and macrophages increases 18 kDa translocator protein expression in rodents but not humans. J Cereb Blood Flow Metab 2017;37:2679–90.
132. Enache D, Pariante CM, Mondelli V. Markers of central inflammation in major depressive disorder: a systematic review and meta-analysis of studies examining cerebrospinal fluid, positron emission tomography and post-mortem brain tissue. Brain Behav Immun 2019;81:24.
133. Luczynski P, Whelan SO, O'Sullivan C, et al. Adult microbiota-deficient mice have distinct dendritic morphological changes: differential effects in the amygdala and hippocampus. Eur J Neurosci 2016;44(9):2654–66.
134. Jiang H, Ling Z, Zhang Y, et al. Altered fecal microbiota composition in patients with major depressive disorder. Brain Behav Immun 2015;48:186–94.
135. Zheng P, Zeng B, Zhou C, et al. Gut microbiome remodeling induces depressive-like behaviors through a pathway mediated by the host's metabolism. Mol Psychiatry 2016;21(6):786–96.
136. Zheng X, Cheng Y, Chen Y, et al. Ferulicacid improves depressive-like behavior in prenatally-stressed offspring rats via anti-inflammatory activity and HPA axis. Int J Mol Sci 2019;20(3):493.
137. Spiller R, Garsed K. Infection, inflammation, and the irritable bowel syndrome. Dig Liver Dis 2009;41(12):844–9.
138. Kelly JR, Borre Y, O' Brien C, et al. Transferring the blues: depression-associated gut microbiota induces neurobehavioural changes in the rat. J Psychiatr Res 2016;82:109–18.
139. Desbonnet L, Garrett L, Clarke G, et al. Effects of the probiotic Bifidobacterium infantis in the maternal separation model of depression. Neuroscience 2010; 170(4):1179–88.
140. Westfall S, Pasinetti GM. The gut microbiota links dietary polyphenols with management of psychiatric mood disorders. Front Neurosci 2019;13:1196.
141. Cai T, Zheng SP, Shi X, et al. Therapeutic effect of fecal microbiota transplantation on chronic unpredictable mild stress-induced depression. Front Cell Infect Microbiol 2022;12:900652.
142. Guo Y, Xie JP, Deng K, et al. Prophylactic Effects of Bifidobacterium adolescentis on Anxiety and Depression-Like Phenotypes After Chronic Stress: A Role of the Gut Microbiota-Inflammation Axis. Front Behav Neurosci 2019 Jun 18; 13:126.
143. Skonieczna-żydecka K, Grochans E, Maciejewska D, et al. Faecal short chain fatty acids profile is changed in Polish depressive women. Nutrients 2018; 10(12):1939.
144. Webster MJ. Infections, inflammation, and psychiatric illness: review of postmortem evidence. Curr Top Behav Neurosci 2022. https://doi.org/10.1007/7854_2022_362. Epub ahead of print. PMID: 35505055.
145. Horwath E. Psychiatric and neuropsychiatric manifestations of HIV infection. J Int Assoc Physicians AIDS Care (Chic) 2002;1(Suppl 1):S1–15.
146. Kirch DG. Infection and autoimmunity as etiologic factors in schizophrenia: a review and reappraisal. Schizophr Bull 1993;19(2):355–70.
147. Llach CD, Vieta E. Mind long COVID: Psychiatric sequelae of SARS-CoV-2 infection. Eur Neuropsychopharmacol 2021;49:119–21.
148. Lyketsos CG, Federman EB. Psychiatric disorders and HIV infection: impact on one another. Epidemiol Rev 1995;17(1):152–64.
149. Schwemmle M. Borna disease virus infection in psychiatric patients: are we on the right track? Lancet Infect Dis 2001;1(1):46–52.

150. Okusaga O, Yolken RH, Langenberg P, et al. Association of seropositivity for influenza and coronaviruses with history of mood disorders and suicide attempts. J Affect Disord 2011;130:220–5.
151. Yirmiya R, Rimmerman N, Reshef R. Depression as a microglial disease. Trends Neurosci 2015;38:637–58.
152. Rakofsky JJ, Dunlop BW. Nothing to sneeze at: upper respiratory infections and mood disorders. Curr Psychiatry 2019;18:29–34.
153. Zhang R, Jiang T, Li N, et al. [The negative psychology for the public in Zhejiang province during the epidemic of human H7N9 avian influenza. Zhonghua Yu Fang Yi Xue Za Zhi 2015;49:1073–9.
154. Lee SH, Shin HS, Park HY, et al. Depression as a mediator of chronic fatigue and post-traumatic stress symptoms in Middle East respiratory syndrome survivors. Psychiatry Investig 2019;16:59–64.
155. Glaser R, Robles TF, Sheridan J, et al. Mild depressive symptoms are associated with amplified and prolonged inflammatory responses after influenza virus vaccination in older adults. Arch Gen Psychiatry 2003;60:1009–14.
156. Ismael F, Bizario JCS, Battagin T, et al. Post-infection depressive, anxiety and post-traumatic stress symptoms: a prospective cohort study in patients with mild COVID-19. Prog Neuropsychopharmacol Biol Psychiatry 2021;111:110341.
157. Adams TB, Wharton CM, Quilter L, et al. The association between mental health and acute infectious illness among a national sample of 18- to 24-year-old college students. J Am Coll Health 2008;56:657–63.
158. Andersson NW, Goodwin RD, Okkels N, et al. Depression and the risk of severe infections: prospective analyses on a nationwide representative sample. Int J Epidemiol 2016;45:131–9.
159. Janssen HL, Brouwer JT, van der Mast RC, et al. Suicide associated with alfa-interferon therapy for chronic viral hepatitis. J Hepatol 1994;21(2):241–3.
160. Courtet P, Jaussent I, Genty C, et al. Increased CRP levels may be a trait marker of suicidal attempt. Eur Neuropsychopharmacol 2015;25(10):1824–31.
161. Gananança L, Oquendo MA, Tyrka AR, et al. The role of cytokines in the pathophysiology of suicidal behavior. Psychoneuroendocrinology 2016;63:296–310.
162. Vasupanrajit A, Jirakran K, Tunvirachaisakul C, et al. Suicide attempts are associated with activated immune-inflammatory, nitro-oxidative, and neurotoxic pathways: a systematic review and meta-analysis. J Affect Disord 2021;295:80–92.
163. Saiz PA, Garcia-Portilla P, Paredes B, et al. Association study of the interleukin-1 gene complex and tumor necrosis factor alpha gene with suicide attempts. Psychiatr Genet 2008;18:147–50.
164. Sowa-Kucma M, Styczen K, Siwek M, et al. Are there differences in lipid peroxidation and immune biomarkers between major depression and bipolar disorder: effects of melancholia, atypical depression, severity of illness, episode number, suicidal ideation and prior suicide attempts. Prog Neuropsychopharmacol Biol Psychiatry 2018;81:372–83.
165. Kim YK, Hong JP, Hwang JA, et al. TNF-alpha -308G>A polymorphism is associated with suicide attempts in major depressive disorder. J Affect Disord 2013;150:668–72.
166. Janelidze S, Ventorp F, Erhardt S, et al. Altered chemokine levels in the cerebrospinal fluid and plasma of suicide attempters. Psychoneuroendocrinology 2013;38:853–62.
167. Asberg M. Neurotransmitters and suicidal behavior. The evidence from cerebrospinal fluid studies. Ann N Y Acad Sci 1997;836:158–81.

168. Hernández-Díaz Y, Genis-Mendoza AD, González-Castro TB, et al. Association and genetic expression between genes involved in HPA axis and suicide behavior: a systematic review. Genes (Basel). 2021;12(10):1608.
169. Sandyk R. Awerbuch GI Nocturnal melatonin secretion in suicidal patients with multiple sclerosis. Int J Neurosci 1993;71(1–4):173–82.
170. Stanley M, Brown GM. Melatonin levels are reduced in the pineal glands of suicide victims. Psychopharmacol Bull 1988;24(3):484.
171. Steenbergen L, Sellaro R, van Hemert S, et al. A randomized controlled trial to test the effect of multispecies probiotics on cognitive reactivity to sad mood. Brain Behav Immun 2015;48:258–64.
172. Miranda O, Fan P, Qi X, et al. DeepBiomarker: identifying important lab tests from electronic medical records for the prediction of suicide-related events among PTSD patients. J Pers Med 2022 Mar 24;12(4):524.
173. Lindqvist D, Janelidze S, Hagell P, et al. Interleukin-6 is elevated in the cerebrospinal fluid of suicide attempters and related to symptom severity. Biol Psychiatry 2009;66:287–92.
174. Isung J, Aeinehband S, Mobarrez F, et al. Low vascular endothelial growth factor and interleukin-8 in cerebrospinal fluid of suicide attempters. Transl Psychiatry 2012;2:e196.
175. Isung J, Mobarrez F, Nordström P, et al. Low plasma vascular endothelial growth factor (VEGF) associated with completed suicide. World J Biol Psychiatry 2012; 13:468–73.
176. Noroozi R, Omrani MD, Ayatollahi SA, et al. Interleukin (IL)-8 polymorphisms contribute in suicide behavior. Cytokine 2018;111:28–32.
177. Janelidze S, Mattei D, Westrin A, et al. Cytokine levels in the blood may distinguish suicide attempters from depressed patients. Brain Behav Immun 2011;25: 335–9.
178. Nässberger L, Träskman-Bendz L. Increased soluble interleukin-2 receptor concentrations in suicide attempters. Acta Psychiatr Scand 1993;88:48–52.
179. Conejero I, Jaussent I, Cazals A, et al. Association between baseline pro-inflammatory cytokines and brain activation during social exclusion in patients with vulnerability to suicide and depressive disorder. Psychoneuroendocrinology 2019;99:236–42.
180. Bay-Richter C, Linderholm KR, Lim CK, et al. A role for inflammatory metabolites as modulators of the glutamate N-methyl-D-aspartate receptor in depression and suicidality. Brain Behav Immun 2015;43:110–7.
181. Sublette ME, Galfalvy HC, Fuchs D, et al. Plasma kynurenine levels are elevated in suicide attempters with major depressive disorder. Brain Behav Immun 2011; 25:1272–8.
182. Knowles EEM, Curran JE, Göring HHH, et al. Family-based analyses reveal novel genetic overlap between cytokine interleukin-8 and risk for suicide attempt. Brain Behav Immun 2019;80:292–9.
183. Melhem NM, Munroe S, Marsland A, et al. Blunted HPA axis activity prior to suicide attempt and increased inflammation in attempters. Psychoneuroendocrinology 2017;77:284–94.
184. Vasupanrajit A, Jirakran K, Tunvirachaisakul C, et al. Inflammation and nitro-oxidativestress in current suicidal attempts and current suicidalideation: a systematic review and meta-analysis. Mol Psychiatry 2022;27(3):1350–61.
185. Keaton SA, Madaj ZB, Heilman P, et al. An inflammatory profile linked to increased suicide risk. J Affect Disord 2019;247:57–65.

186. Grudet C, Malm J, Westrin A, et al. Suicidal patients are deficient in vitamin D, associated with a pro-inflammatory status in the blood. Psychoneuroendocrinology 2014;50:210–9.
187. Ohlsson L, Gustafsson A, Lavant E, et al. Leaky gut biomarkers in depression and suicidal behavior. Acta Psychiatr Scand 2019;139:185–93.
188. O'Donovan A, Rush G, Hoatam G, et al. Suicidal ideation is associated with elevated inflammation in patients with major depressive disorder. Depress Anxiety 2013;30:307–14.
189. Kim YK, Hong JP, Hwang JA, et al. TNF-alpha -308G>A polymorphism is associated with suicide attempts in major depressive disorder. J Affect Disord 2013; 150:668–72.
190. Coryell W, Wilcox H, Evans SJ, et al. Aggression, impulsivity and inflammatory markers as risk factors for suicidal behavior. J Psychiatr Res 2018;106:38–42.
191. Kim YK, Lee SW, Kim SH, et al. Differences in cytokines between non-suicidal patients and suicidal patients in major depression. Prog Neuropsychopharmacol Biol Psychiatry 2008;32(2):356–61.
192. Gabbay V, Klein RG, Alonso CM, et al. Immune system dysregulation in adolescent major depressive disorder. J Affect Disord 2009;115(1–2):177–82.
193. Mendlovic S, Mozes E, Eilat E, et al. Immune activation in non-treated suicidal major depression. Immunol Lett 1999;67:105–8.
194. Grassi-Oliveira R, Brieztke E, Teixeira A, et al. Peripheral chemokine levels in women with recurrent major depression with suicidal ideation. Br J Psychiatry 2012;34:71–5.
195. Wang Q, Roy B, Turecki G, et al. Role of complex epi-genetic switching in tumor necrosis factor-alpha upregulation in the prefrontal cortexof suicide subjects. Am J Psychiatry 2018;175:262–74.
196. Schiavone S, Neri M, Mhillaj E, et al. The NADPH oxidase NOX2 as a novel biomarker for suicidality: evidence from human post mortem brain samples. Transl Psychiatry 2016;6:e813.
197. Tonelli LH, Stiller J, Rujescu D, et al. Elevated cytokine expression in the orbitofrontal cortex of victims of suicide. Acta Psychiatr Scand 2008;117:198–206.
198. Pandey GN, Rizavi HS, Ren X, et al. Region-specific alterations in glucocorticoid receptor expression in the postmortem brain of teenage suicide victims. Psychoneuroendocrinology 2013;38:2628–39.
199. Gonçalves de Andrade E, González Ibáñez F, Tremblay MÈ. Microglia as a hub for suicide neuropathology: future investigation and prevention targets. Front Cell Neurosci 2022;16:839396.
200. Torres-Platas SG, Cruceanu C, Chen GG, et al. Evidence for increased microglial priming and macrophage recruitment in the dorsal anterior cingulate white matter of depressed suicides. Brain Behav Immun 2014;42:50–9.
201. Janelidze S, Ventorp F, Erhardt S, et al. Altered chemokine levels in the cerebrospinal fluid and plasma of suicide attempters. Psychoneuroendocrinology 2013; 38:853–62.
202. Hennings JM, Ising M, Uhr M, et al. Effects of weariness of life, suicide ideations and suicide attempt on HPA axis regulation in depression. Psychoneuroendocrinology 2021;131:105286.
203. Chandley MJ, Szebeni A, Szebeni K, et al. Markers of elevated oxidativestress in oligodendrocytes captured from the brainstem and occipital cortex in major depressive disorder and suicide. Prog Neuropsychopharmacol Biol Psychiatry 2022;117:110559.

204. Vargas HO, Nunes SO, Pizzo de Castro M, et al. Oxidative stress and lowered total antioxidant status are associated with a history of suicide attempts. J Affect Disord 2013;150:923–30.

205. Köhler-Forsberg O, N Lydholm C, Hjorthøj C, Nordentoft M, et al. Efficacy of anti-inflammatory treatment on major depressive disorder or depressive symptoms: meta-analysis of clinical trials. Acta Psychiatr Scand 2019;139:404–19.

206. Beurel E, Toups M, Nemeroff CB. The Bidirectional Relationship of Depression and Inflammation: Double Trouble. Neuron 2020;107(2):234–56.

207. Eyre HA, Air T, Proctor S, et al. A critical review of the efficacy of non-steroidal anti-inflammatory drugs in depression. Prog Neuropsychopharmacol Biol Psychiatry 2015;57:11.

208. Lehrer S, Rheinstein PH. Nonsteroidal anti-inflammatory drugs (NSAIDs) reduce suicidal ideation and depression. Discov Med 2019;28(154):205–12.

209. Eren I, Naziroğlu M, Demirdaş A, et al. Venlafaxine modulates depression-induced oxidative stress in brain and medulla of rat. Neurochem Res 2007;32: 497–505.

210. Wigner P, Synowiec E, Czarny P, et al. Effects of venlafaxine on the expression level and methylation status of genes involved in oxidative stress in rats exposed to a chronic mild stress. J Cell Mol Med 2020;24:5675.

211. Bakhtiari-Dovvombaygi H, Izadi S, Zare Moghaddam M, et al. Beneficial effects of vitamin D on anxiety and depression-like behaviors induced by unpredictablechronic mild stress by suppression of brain oxidative stressand neuroinflammation in rats. Naunyn Schmiedebergs Arch Pharmacol 2021;394(4):655–67.

212. Steenkamp LR, Hough CM, Reus VI, et al. Severity of anxiety- but not depression- is associated with oxidative stress in Major Depressive Disorder. J Affect Disord 2017;219:193–200.

213. Ising M, Horstmann S, Kloiber S, et al. Combined dexamethasone/corticotropin releasing hormone test predicts treatment response in major depression - a potential biomarker? Biol Psychiatry 2007;62(1):47–54.

214. Berardelli I, Serafini G, Cortese N, et al. The involvement of hypothalamus-pituitary-adrenal (HPA) axis in suicide risk. Brain Sci 2020 Sep 21;10(9):653.

215. Pompili M, Serafini G, Innamorati M, et al. The hypothalamic-pituitary-adrenal axis and serotonin abnormalities: a selective overview for the implications of suicide prevention. Eur Arch Psychiatry Clin Neurosci 2010;260(8):583–600.

216. Chaki S. Vasopressin V1B Receptor Antagonists as Potential Antidepressants. Int J Neuropsychopharmacol 2021;24:450–63.

217. Iijima M, Yoshimizu T, Shimazaki T, et al. Antidepressant and anxiolytic profiles of newly synthesized arginine vasopressin V1Breceptor antagonists: TASP0233278 and TASP0390325. Br J Pharmacol 2014;171:3511–25.

218. Ge J-F, Peng L, Cheng J-Q, et al. Antidepressant-like effect of resveratrol: Involvement of antioxidant effect and peripheral regulation on HPA axis. Pharmacol Biochem Behav 2013;114–115:64–9.

219. Yang X-H, Song S-Q, Xu Y. Resveratrol ameliorates chronic unpredictable mild stress-induced depression-like behavior: Involvement of the HPA axis, inflammatory markers, BDNF, and Wnt/β-catenin pathway in rats. Neuropsychiatr Dis Treat 2017;13:2727–36.

220. Zheng P, Zeng B, Zhou C, et al. Gut microbiome remodeling induces depressive-like behaviors through a pathway mediated by the host's metabolism. Mol Psychiatry 2016;21(6):786–96.

221. Majidi J, Kosari-Nasab M, Salari A-A. Developmental minocycline treatment reverses the effects of neonatal immune activation on anxiety- and depression-like

behaviors, hippocampal inflammation, and HPA axis activity in adult mice. Brain Res Bull 2016;120:1–13.
222. Ke Q, Li R, Cai L, et al. Ro41-5253, a selective antagonist of retinoic acid receptor α, ameliorates chronic unpredictable mild stress-induced depressive-like behaviors in rats: Involvement of regulating HPA axis and improving hippocampal neuronal deficits. Brain Res Bull 2019;146:302–9.
223. Howland RH. Mifepristone as a therapeutic agent in psychiatry. J Psychosoc Nurs Ment Health Serv 2013;51:11–4.
224. Huang TL, Lee CT. T-helper 1/T-helper 2 cytokine imbalance and clinical phenotypes of acute-phase major depression. Psychiatry Clin Neurosci 2007 Aug; 61(4):415–20.
225. Isingrini E, Desmidt T, Belzung C, et al. Endothelial dysfunction: a potential therapeutic target for geriatric depression and brain amyloid deposition in Alzheimer's disease? Curr Opin Investig Drugs 2009;10:46–55, 2007.
226. Hughes TD, Güner OF, Iradukunda EC, et al. The Kynurenine Pathway and Kynurenine 3-Monooxygenase Inhibitors. Molecules 2022;27(1):273.
227. Guo Y, Liu Y, Wu W, et al. Indoleamine 2,3-dioxygenase (Ido) inhibitors and their nanomedicines for cancer immunotherapy. Biomaterials 2021;276:121018.
228. Feng Y, Bowden BF, Kapoor V. Ianthellamide A, a selective kynurenine-3-hydroxylase inhibitor from the Australian marine sponge Ianthella quadrangulata. Bioorg Med Chem Lett 2012;22(10):3398–401.
229. Kim HT, Na BK, Chung J, et al. Structural Basis for Inhibitor-Induced Hydrogen Peroxide Production by Kynurenine 3-Monooxygenase. Cell Chem. Biol. 2018; 25:426–38.
230. Röver S, Cesura AM, Huguenin P, et al. Synthesis and biochemical evaluation of N-(4-phenylthiazol-2- yl)benzenesulfonamides as high-affinity inhibitors of kynurenine 3-hydroxylase. J Med Chem 1997;40:4378–85.
231. Detanico BC, Piato AL, Freitas JJ, et al. Antidepressant-like effects of melatonin in the mouse chronic mild stress model. Eur J Pharmacol 2009;607:121–5.
232. Mantovani M, Pertile R, Calixto JB, et al. Melatonin exerts an antidepressant-like effect in the tail suspension test in mice: Evidence for involvement of N-methyl-D-aspartate receptors and the L-arginine-nitric oxide pathway. Neurosci Lett 2003;343:1–4.
233. Raghavendra V, Kaur G, Kulkarni SK. Anti-depressant action of melatonin in chronic forced swimming-induced behavioral despair in mice, role of peripheral benzodiazepine receptor modulation. Eur Neuropsychopharmacol 2000;10: 473–81.
234. Norman TR, Olver JS. Agomelatine for depression: expanding the horizons? Expert Opin Pharmacother 2019;20:647–56.
235. Wang XQ, Wang DQ, Bao YP, et al. Preliminary Study on Changes of Sleep EEG power and plasmamelatonin in male patients with majordepressivedisorder after 8 weeks treatment. Front Psychiatry 2021;12:736318.
236. Garzon C, Guerrero JM, Aramburu O, et al. Effect of melatonin administration on sleep, behavioral disorders and hypnotic drug discontinuation in the elderly: A randomized, double-blind, placebo-controlled study. Aging Clin Exp Res 2009; 21:38–42.
237. Madsen MT, Isbrand A, Andersen UO, et al. The effect of melatonin on depressive symptoms, anxiety, circadian and sleep disturbances in patients after acute coronary syndrome (MEDACIS): Study protocol for a randomized controlled trial. Trials 2017;18:81.

238. Høier NK, Madsen T, Spira AP, et al. Associations between treatment with melatonin and suicidal behavior: a nationwide cohort study. J Clin Sleep Med 2022; 18(10):2451–8.

239. Raison CL, Rutherford RE, Woolwine BJ, et al. A randomized controlled trial of the tumor necrosis factor antagonist infliximab for treatment-resistant depression: the role of baseline inflammatory biomarkers. JAMA Psychiatry 2013;70: 31–41.

240. Tyring S, Bagel J, Lynde C, et al. Patient-reported outcomes in moderate-to-severe plaque psoriasis with scalp involvement: results from a randomized, double-blind, placebo-controlled study of etanercept. J Eur Acad Dermatol Venereol 2013;27:125–8.

241. Langley RG, Feldman SR, Han C, et al. Ustekinumab significantly improves symptoms of anxiety, depression, and skin-related quality of life in patients with moderate-to-severe psoriasis: Results from a randomized, double-blind, placebo-controlled phase III trial. J Am Acad Dermatol 2010;63:457–65.

242. Sun Y, Wang D, Salvadore G, et al. The effects of interleukin-6 neutralizing antibodies on symptoms of depressed mood and anhedonia in patients with rheumatoid arthritis and multicentric Castleman's disease. Brain Behav Immun 2017; 66:156–64.

243. McIntyre RS, Subramaniapillai M, Lee Y, et al. Efficacy of adjunctive infliximab vs placebo in the treatment of adults with Bipolar I/II depression: a randomized clinical trial. JAMA Psychiatry 2019;76(8):783–90.

244. Shayowitz M, Bressler M, Ricardo AP, et al. Infliximab-induced depression and suicidal behavior in adolescent with crohn's disease: case report and review of literature. Pediatr Qual Saf 2019;4(6):e229.

245. Lebwohl MG, Papp KA, Marangell LB, et al. Psychiatric adverse events during treatment with brodalumab: analysis of psoriasis clinical trials. J Am Acad Dermatol 2018;78:81–9.e5.

246. Dinan K, Dinan T. Antibiotics and mental health: The good, the bad and the ugly. J Intern Med 2022. https://doi.org/10.1111/joim.13543. Epub ahead of print. PMID: 35819136.

247. Kacal MJ. Is minocycline effective for treating depression? J Am Acad Physician Assist 2022;35(6):13–4.

248. Kutkat O, Moatasim Y, Al-Karmalawy AA, et al. Robust antiviral activity of commonly prescribed antidepressants against emerging coronaviruses: in vitro and in silico drug repurposing studies. Sci Rep 2022;12(1):12920.

249. Costanza A, Placenti V, Amerio A, et al. Chloroquine/hydroxychloroquine use and suicide risk: hypotheses for confluent etiopathogenetic mechanisms? Behav Sci (Basel) 2021 Nov 7;11(11):154.

250. Hamm BS, Rosenthal LJ. Psychiatric aspects of chloroquine and hydroxychloroquine treatment in the wake of coronavirus disease-2019: psychopharmacological interactions and neuropsychiatric sequelae. Psychosomatics 2020; 61(6):597–606.

251. Steenbergen L, Sellaro R, van Hemert S, et al. A randomized controlled trial to test the effect of multispecies probiotics on cognitive reactivity to sad mood. Brain Behav Immun 2015;48:258–26.

252. Slykerman RF, Hood F, Wickens K, et al. Effect of Lactobacillus rhamnosus HN001 in pregnancy on postpartum symptoms of depression and anxiety: a randomised double-blind placebo-controlled trial. EBioMedicine 2017;24: 159–65.

253. Akkasheh G, Kashani-Poor Z, Tajabadi-Ebrahimi M, et al. Clinical and metabolic response to probiotic administration in patients with major depressive disorder: a randomized, double-blind, placebo-controlled trial. Nutrition 2016;32(3): 315–20.
254. Kazemi A, Noorbala AA, Azam K, et al. Effect of probiotic and prebiotic vs placebo on psychological outcomes in patients with major depressive disorder: a randomized clinical trial. Clin Nutr 2019;38(2):522–8.
255. Shah AM, Yang W, Mohamed H, et al. Microbes: a hidden treasure of polyunsaturated fatty acids. Front Nutr 2022 Mar 17;9:827837.
256. Goldberg SB, Pace BT, Nicholas CR, et al. The experimental effects of psilocybin on symptoms of anxiety and depression: a meta-analysis. Psychiatry Res 2020;284:112749.
257. Strumila R, Nobile B, Korsakova L, et al. Psilocybin, a Naturally Occurring Indoleamine Compound, Could Be Useful to Prevent Suicidal Behaviors. Pharmaceuticals (Basel) 2021;14(12):1213.
258. Wang L, Wang R, Liu L, et al. Effects of SSRIs on peripheral inflammatory markers in patients with major depressive disorder: A systematic review and meta-analysis. Brain Behav Immun 2019;79:24–38.
259. O'Donnell C, Demler TL, Trigoboff E. Selective Serotonin Reuptake Inhibitors (SSRIs) and Their Effect on Patient Aggression in Adult Patients in a State Psychiatric Facility: A Retrospective Analysis. Innov Clin Neurosci 2022; 19(1–3):33–8.
260. Murrough JW, Iosifescu DV, Chang LC, et al. Antidepressant efficacy of ketamine in treatment-resistant major depression: a two-site randomized controlled trial. Am J Psychiatry 2013;170:1134–42.
261. Yang Y, Song Y, Zhang X, et al. Ketamine relieves depression-like behaviors induced by chronic postsurgical pain in rats through anti-inflammatory, antioxidant effects and regulating BDNF expression. Psychopharmacology 2020; 237:1657–69.
262. Chen S, Sang N. Histone deacetylase inhibitors: the epigenetic therapeutics that repress hypoxia-inducible factors. J Biomed Biotechnol 2010;2011:197946.
263. Peng X, Huang M, Zhao W, et al. RAGE mediates airway inflammation via the HDAC1 pathway in a toluene diisocyanate-induced murine asthma model. BMC Pulm Med 2022;22(1):61.
264. Emanuele E. The histone deacetylase inhibitor FK228 may have therapeutic usefulness to prevent suicidal behaviour via upregulation of the guanosine triphosphatase Rap-1. Med Hypotheses 2007;68(2):451–2.
265. Li SH, Achilles MR, Werner-Seidler A, et al. Appropriate use and operationalization of adherence to digital cognitive behavioral therapy for depression and anxiety in youth: systematic review. JMIR Ment Health 2022;9(8):e37640.
266. Núñez D, Gaete J, Meza D, et al. Testing the effectiveness of a blended intervention to reduce suicidalideation among school adolescents in chile: a protocol for a cluster randomized controlled trial. Int J Environ Res Public Health 2022; 19(7):3947.
267. Shields GS, Spahr CM, Slavich GM. Psychosocial Interventions and immune system function: a systematic review and meta-analysis of randomized clinical trials. JAMA Psychiatry 2020;77:1031–43.
268. Goldsmith DR, Rapaport MH, Miller BJ. A meta-analysis of blood cytokine network alterations in psychiatric patients: comparisons between schizophrenia, bipolar disorder and depression. Mol Psychiatry 2016;21:1696–709.

Fire and Darkness: On the Assessment and Management of Bipolar Disorder

Katerina Nikolitch, MD, CM, MSc[a,b], Gayatri Saraf, MD[a],
Marco Solmi, MD, PhD[a,c,e], Kurt Kroenke, MD[d],
Jess G. Fiedorowicz, MD, PhD[a,c],*

KEYWORDS

- Bipolar disorder • Psychopharmacology • Diagnosis • Treatment • Primary care

KEY POINTS

- Bipolar disorder is a chronic remitting and relapsing illness, defined by (hypo)manic syndromes but most frequently presenting in its depressive phase.
- There is significant heterogeneity in presentation and course. Bipolar I and bipolar II disorder subtypes both carry significant morbidity.
- Owing to the low prevalence of bipolar disorder, diagnostic scales are of little use in screening, but a step-based approach of progressive questioning can be effective.
- Collateral information obtained from patients' proxies is vital to correctly diagnosing bipolar disorder.
- The best approach to treatment and management involves an integrated system of pharmacotherapy, psychoeducation, and psychosocial interventions, as well as addressing comorbidities and monitoring course with measurement-based care.

INTRODUCTION
Prevalence

Bipolar disorder (BD) is a condition characterized by recurrent mood episodes and narrowly defined affects just more than 2% of the population in the United States National Comorbidity Services and 1% of the population from the World Health

[a] Department of Psychiatry, The University of Ottawa, The Ottawa Hospital, Ottawa Hospital Research Institute, 501 Smyth Road, Box 400, Ottawa, ON K1H 8L6, Canada; [b] Institute for Mental Health Research, Ottawa, Ontario, Canada; [c] School of Epidemiology and Public Health, The University of Ottawa, Ottawa, Ontario, Canada; [d] Indiana University School of Medicine and Regenstrief Institute, 1101 W 10th St, Indianapolis, IN 46202, USA; [e] Department of Child and Adolescent Psychiatry, Charité Universitätsmedizin, Berlin, Germany
* Corresponding author. Department of Psychiatry, The University of Ottawa, The Ottawa Hospital, Ottawa Hospital Research Institute, Ottawa, Ontario, Canada.
E-mail address: jfiedorowicz@toh.ca

Med Clin N Am 107 (2023) 31–60
https://doi.org/10.1016/j.mcna.2022.04.002
0025-7125/23/© 2022 Elsevier Inc. All rights reserved.

medical.theclinics.com

Organization Mental Health Surveys.[1,2] Despite significant geographic variation, the overall estimated prevalence has remained stable over the last 30 years.[3] It affects men and women equally and has a mean age of onset between the ages of 18 and 23 years.[1,2,4] The prevalence is higher in Native Americans and lower in Black, Hispanic, and Asian/Pacific Islander Americans, compared with White Americans.[5]

Defining Features

Although there is evidence that mood disorders may broadly share some genetic predisposition,[6] the distinction of bipolar from unipolar disorders has been well-validated, as has the distinct subtype of bipolar II disorder (BD II).[7,8] Hypomania and mania are distinct and defining syndromes in BD, and treatment for these mood states tends to be acute. In recent decades, it has become more apparent that the treatment of bipolar depression is not equivalent to the treatment of unipolar major depression, and antidepressants may have adverse effects on mood stability.[9] This has led many to question the application of treatments for unipolar major depression to BD or treatments for bipolar I disorder (BD I) to BD II.

IMPACT

According to the World Health Organization, BD is the fourth leading cause of disability in young people worldwide.[10] BD also carries considerable medical comorbidity and has been associated with approximately twice the expected mortality in representative samples.[11] As a result, those with BD have a life expectancy that is approximately 10 to 20 years shorter than the general population.[12,13]

BIPOLAR SUBTYPES AND COURSE OF ILLNESS

Although BD exists on a spectrum, there are sufficient differences in the phenomenology, course of illness, and response to treatment to warrant the identification of at least 2 separate phenotypes. BD I is defined by the presence of extreme mood elevation episodes or manias and, usually, although not always,[14] a course of illness characterized by episodes of major depression. BD II is defined by less severe episodes of mood elevation than mania, termed hypomania, which are associated with an unequivocal and uncharacteristic change, although not necessarily a decline in function, and occur in those with a history of major depressive episodes.

Depressive syndromes rather than mood elevation syndromes predominate in the course of illness for both BD I and BD II. BD I differs from BD II based on more than the mere threshold for mania. Individuals with BD II are more likely to suffer a course of chronic depression[15] (**Fig. 1**). See **Box 1** for a summary of clinical differences between BD I and BD II.

Genetics

BD is highly heritable, with twin and adoption studies indicating 60% to 85% heritability.[16,17] Genome-wide association studies have identified multiple loci that collectively can explain approximately 20% of BD heritability.[18] The largest genome-wide association studies to date (including >40,000 cases and 370,000 controls)[19] implicates 15 genes, including potential treatment targets such as HTR6, MCHR1, DCLK3, and FURIN. Many of the identified genes have been linked to schizophrenia, especially BD I, and major depressive disorder (MDD), particularly BD II, indicating at least a partially a common genetic pathway for these disorders.

% TIME SPENT IN EACH PHASE

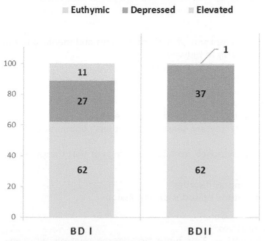

Fig. 1. Mean time spent in dmood states for BD I and BD II.

ASSESSMENT
Diagnostic and Nosologic Challenges

BD can be difficult to diagnose owing to the high frequency of depressive episodes, the patients' inability to accurately recall and report manic symptoms, and syndromic overlap with other diagnostic categories. It is both over- and underdiagnosed,[20] depending on patient populations. BD is most frequently missed in patients who present with depressive episodes and who perceive emergent manic or hypomanic symptoms as a return to baseline, as well as in those who present with a primarily psychotic syndrome at evaluation. Another group in which BD can be missed is youth and children in whom behavioral symptoms are seen as part of attention-deficit hyperactivity disorder (ADHD).[21] The misdiagnosis of non-BD conditions as BD is most frequent in patients with borderline personality disorder, impulse control disorder, and post-traumatic stress disorder, as well as in patients with history of substance use disorder.[22]

Box 1
Comparative impairment in BD I and BD II[15,106–109]

Impairment in BD I (compared with BD II)
• Higher number of elevated (manic and hypomanic) episodes
• Longer periods of disability and complete disruption of occupational function

Impairment in BD II (compared with BD I)
• Chronic depression
• Higher number of depressive episodes
• Higher number of any type of affective episode
• More likely comorbid anxiety and/or personality disorder

Similarly impaired in BD I and BD II
• Incidence of suicide attempts
• Interepisode neurocognitive function

Box 2
Characteristics suggesting bipolar, rather than unipolar, depression[31-35]:

Clinical features
- Psychosis
- Mixed symptoms (i.e., symptoms of both depression and mania simultaneously or in rapid sequence without recovery in between)
- Hypersomnia and psychomotor retardation
- Hyperphagia and/or weight gain
- Diurnal mood variation or lability
- Mood worse in the morning
- Less likely to report initial insomnia or diminished libido
- Interpersonal sensitivity (overly sensitive to others' opinions and rejection; feelings of inferiority)
- Derealization (feeling detached from surroundings or that things are unreal or artificial)

Course
- Early age of onset of mood disorder
- Greater number of lifetime episodes of depression

Family history
- BD in first-degree relatives
- Family loading, defined as 3 or more first-degree relatives with any affective disorder (especially in children and adolescents)

When and How to Screen

The goal of screening is to identify BD, including individuals who are not displaying the defining features of illness ([hypo]mania).

An accurate and timely diagnosis is important to treat and prevent affective episodes, as well as improve cognitive and functional outcomes. Owing to the low prevalence of BD, administering self-report screening measures such as the Mood Disorder Questionnaire[23] or the Bipolar Spectrum Diagnostic Scale[24] in all patients can be used to rule out but not to rule in BD, owing to most scales low specificity, and prior probability plays a much larger role in identifying positive cases.[25]

There are 4 groups of patients with an increased probability of being diagnosed with BD: (1) patients with MDD, particularly those with certain presentations (**Box 2**), (2) patients with a family history of BD or schizophrenia, (3) patients with medical conditions known to have a higher prevalence of BD (migraine,[26] multiple sclerosis,[27] hidradenitis suppurativa,[28] and chronic obstructive pulmonary disease[29]), and (4) patients diagnosed with a psychiatric disorder known to be highly comorbid with or to obscure symptoms of BD (see Differential diagnosis and comorbidity). Patients belonging to 1 or more of these groups can be screened by initial interviewing of both patient and, if possible, their spouse, partner, or family of origin. Alternatively, high-probability patients can be screened with the Rapid Mood Screener, a novel self-report screening instruments with acceptable sensitivity and specificity[30] (**Fig. 2**).

Box 2 summarizes the characteristics that suggest bipolar, rather than unipolar, depression.[31-35] They are neither necessary nor sufficient for diagnosing BD, but their presence can increase clinical suspicion.

Assessment

The goal of assessment is to systematically follow-up on a positive screen for BD. As with other psychiatric disorders, there is no decisive test for BD. The best approach lies in eliciting either a history of past (hypo)manic episode or recognizing one when

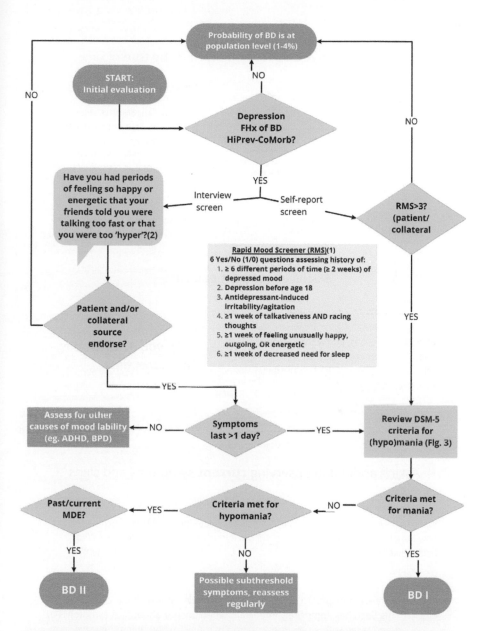

FHx = Family history; HiPrev-CoMorb = High-prevalence comorbidity; RMS = Rapid Mood Screener; MDE= major depressive episode; ADHD= attention-deficit hyperactivity disorder; BPD= borderline personality disorder; BD I= bipolar I disorder; BD II= bipolar II disorder

1. McIntyre RS, Patel MD, Masand PS, et al. The Rapid Mood Screener (RMS): a novel and pragmatic screener for bipolar I disorder. Current Medical Research and Opinion. 2021/01/02 2021;37(1):135-144. doi:10.1080/03007995.2020.1860358
2. Carlat DJ. The psychiatric review of symptoms: a screening tool for family physicians. Am Fam Physician. Nov 1 1998;58(7):1617-24.

Fig. 2. Screening and assessment of BD in primary care. DSM, *Diagnostic and Statistical Manual of Mental Disorders*; FHx, family history; MDE, major depressive episode; RMS, rapid Mood Screener.

A

Criterion A: all of the below must be true

Distinct ✔
period

✔
Most of the day,
nearly every day

Abnormally and ✔
persistently elevated,
expansive, or irritable
mood

✔
Abnormally and
persistently increased
activity or energy

⟳ At least

1 week (mania) -
unless
hospitalized

—— OR, 4 days
(hypomania)

Notes for the clinician:

- Since August 2015, increased activity does not have to be goal-directed.
- Mood and activity must be abnormal as compared to the patient's euthymic state: some patients misconstrue a normalization of their mood as "abnormal", particularly if the depressive episode has lasted a long time

Asking about **past** episodes

Was there a time in your life when, for at least a few days, you were feeling so happy or energetic that your friends told you were talking too fast or that you were too 'hyper'?

⋯▷ Can you describe this period of time?

Asking about and observing **current** symptoms and signs

You seem exuberant - how long have you been feeling like this?

Is this amount of activity usual for you/your loved one?

Have you/they felt like this before? What happened then?

- It is always helpful to interview family, friends, spouse, etc.
- This becomes immensely important when unsure about past symptoms or when faced with a new presentation of manic/hypomanic symptoms

Fig. 3. (*A*) Interview aide for BD I and BD II from the *Diagnostic and Statistical Manual of Mental Disorders*, fifth edition criteria. (*B*) Interview aide for BD I and BD II from the *Diagnostic and Statistical Manual of Mental Disorders*, fifth edition criteria. (*C*) Interview aide for the diagnosis of BD I and BD II.

it presents. Patients sometimes misunderstand or misreport symptoms, and may not recognize symptoms as pathologic.

Upon a positive screen, review the criteria for past or current (hypo)manic (**Fig. 3**). It is important, whenever possible, to obtain collateral information from those close to

B

Criterion B: at least 3 of the following
(at least 4 if mood is only irritable)

Must
- be during the same period
- represent a <u>noticeable</u> change from usual behaviour
- be present to a <u>significant</u> degree

↑ activity/ agitation

↑ self-esteem/ grandiose

pressure to keep talking

flight of ideas/ racing thoughts

activities with painful consequences

↓ need for sleep

distractible

- Decreased need for sleep should not be confused with insomnia, which is an inability to fall or stay asleep despite a desire to sleep.

Asking about past episodes

Did you do things you later regretted? What kinds of things?

Did others tell you to slow down? Were you talking unusually fast/too much?

Was it hard to make sense of all your ideas and thoughts?

Asking about and observing current symptoms and signs

How many hours are you sleeping these days? Do you feel tired?

Do you feel that you have special powers or that you are special in some way?

Observe

- Thought process and distractibility
- Is it possible to interrupt the patient?
- Behaviour can be inappropriate (overly familiar), agitated

Ask family/spouse:
Is this unusual? Are you concerned?

Fig. 3. (continued)

the patient (family, spouse, friends, roommates, etc), particularly about how different symptoms are from the patient's baseline functioning.

Differential Diagnosis and Comorbidity

BD is one of the most comorbid psychiatric disorders,[36] with up to 65%[37] patients with BD having 1 or several additional psychiatric disorders,[38] most of which precede the

C

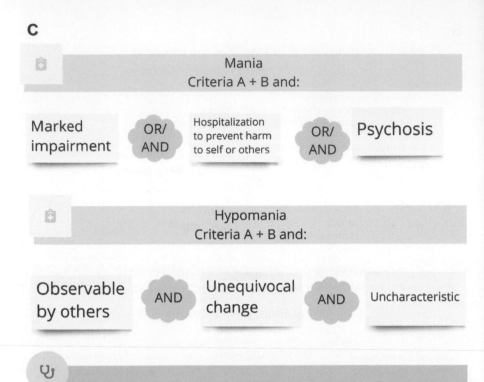

Mania
Criteria A + B and:

| Marked impairment | OR/ AND | Hospitalization to prevent harm to self or others | OR/ AND | Psychosis |

Hypomania
Criteria A + B and:

| Observable by others | AND | Unequivocal change | AND | Uncharacteristic |

- The diagnosis of BD I requires a history of at least one manic episode

- BD II requires at least one hypomanic and one major depressive episode

- Hypomania is common in BD I but is not required for diagnosis

- In both manic and hypomanic episodes, the symptoms should not be due to substance use or another medical condition

- If a full manic switch occurs during antidepressant treatment AND persists fully beyond the physiological effects of the treatment, it is sufficient for BD I diagnosis

Fig. 3. (*continued*)

diagnosis of BD.[36] The most common comorbidities are anxiety disorder, substance use disorder, and personality disorders.

Comorbid diagnoses in BD are strongly associated with a more severe course of illness and poorer response to treatment.[39] The mean delay between illness onset and diagnosis of BD is 5 to 10 years.[40] This delay is often the result of many BD

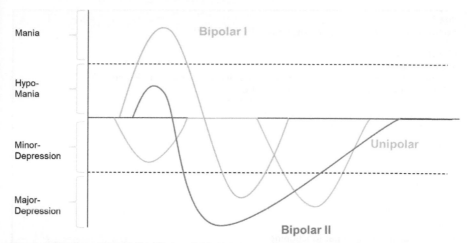

Mania

Hypo-
Mania

Minor-
Depression

Major-
Depression

Bipolar I

Unipolar

Bipolar II

Fig. 4. Affective episodes in BD I and BD II compared with unipolar depression.

symptoms presenting as a part of a different diagnosis. Decreased sleep, restlessness, agitation, and impulsivity can be seen as symptoms of (hypo)mania and lead to misdiagnosis and the undertreatment of the comorbid syndromes. Conversely, genuine symptoms of (hypo)mania may be misattributed to a pre-existent psychiatric disorder. It is important to follow the criteria for (hypo)mania when assessing, and to screen for comorbid disorders in all patients with BD.

Most clinicians find borderline personality disorder, MDD, and ADHD most difficult to distinguish from BD.[41] Establishing a timeline of symptoms and a baseline of functioning can be helpful (**Fig. 4**). Neurodevelopmental syndromes, personality disorders, and generalized anxiety disorder tend to have a longitudinal, fluctuating but generally unremitting course, as opposed to the clearly defined and recognizable episodes in BD.

Markers of Severity and Prognosis in Bipolar Disorder

As discussed elsewhere in this article, the differences between the bipolar subtypes are well-recognized. Within each subtype, there is tremendous individual variability in course of illness, as highlighted more than a century ago in the life charts assembled by the team of Emil Kraepelin.[42–44] It is the severity and burden of affective symptoms that drive disability and impacts function, rather than the BD subtype, with the exception of less functional impairment and at times even improvement in function during hypomania in BD II, compared with BD I.[45] Prospective studies suggest that the course of illness tends to be generally stable over time, with some increase in depressive symptoms in younger adults over subsequent decades and no change in manic symptom burden.[46]

Variables Associated with Poor Outcomes

Several, often correlated, variables have been associated with a more persistent or severe course of illness in BD (**Box 3**). Early identification and treatment[47] and adherence to medications[48] are associated with better outcomes.

The use of antidepressant medications is controversial; in some studies, it seems to point to a decreased time to recurrence and increased rapid cycling,[49] whereas others consider it safe under certain conditions, that is, in combination with mood stabilizers or anticonvulsants in certain categories of patients.[50]

Box 3
Factors associated with worse outcomes[a,8,48,58–61,110–122]

Clinical course
- Earlier age of onset[b]
- Preponderance of depressive episodes in the first 2 years after index episode
- Mixed features of manic or depressive episodes
- Intraepisode cycling between depression and mania
- Persistent affective symptoms or episodes
- Presence of psychotic symptoms

Co-occurring
- Both anxiety symptoms and anxiety disorders
- Alcohol and substance abuse
- Smoking
- ADHD
- Cognitive impairment

Premorbid
- Poorer socio-occupational functioning
- History of childhood trauma

[a]Worse outcomes may include more suicide attempts, more chronic or severe depressive symptoms, higher rate of comorbid disorders and symptoms, more frequent hospitalizations, and poorer occupational functioning, etc.

[b]Also associated with delayed diagnosis and treatment, further complicating prognosis[123]

Suicide Risk and Assessment

BD is estimated to convey the highest risk of suicide of all the mental disorders. In community samples, approximately one-quarter of those with BD have a history of suicide attempts, with higher estimates in clinical samples, including the large STEP-BD trial, where 36% of patients had a history of a suicide attempt.[51,52] People with BD are 10 to 30 times as likely to die by suicide as expected from general population estimates.[53] In a recent meta-analysis, male sex and a first-degree family history of suicide are associated with suicide deaths in BD. Female sex, early age of onset, first or most recent episode depressed, co-occurring anxiety, substance use, or borderline personality disorder, and first-degree family history of suicide were associated with suicide attempts.[53] There do not seem to be differences by BD subtype (ie, I vs II) and risk.[53,54]

The assessment of suicide risk can be a daunting task for the primary care clinician and has been previously comprehensively reviewed in this journal.[55] Those in need of a formal suicide risk assessment may be identified on screening, for instance, through the use of common instruments for measurement-based care such as the Patient Health Questionnaire 9[56] or the Columbia Suicide Severity Rating Scale.[57] Where such screening is not done routinely, screening should be considered for changes in mood, anxiety or distress, and sleep complaints; in those with unpredictable or impulsive behavior; in those who have had a sudden change in life circumstances; and in those who have an escalated alcohol or other drug use. It should also be considered for those who are not adhering to treatment recommendations, are increasing their use of health care services, or have to be convinced by family or a friend to access such services when needed.[55] The presence of suicidal ideation or other concerns on screening warrants a risk assessment.

When an individual has been identified at risk, a formal suicide risk assessment should occur. The risk assessment identifies risk and protective factors and estimates the overall level or risk to direct management with a focus on modifiable risk factors. A

Box 4
Factors associated with relapse[49,62,63]

Clinical
- Number of prior episodes
- Interepisode residual mood symptoms
- Inconsistent adherence to medication

Psychological
- Introverted and obsessive personality pattern (likely mediating response to stress)
- Sleep reduction in response to stress

Social and environmental
- Stressful life events
- Lack of social support
- High expressed emotion (criticism) in family members (for depressive episode recurrence)
- Transmeridian travel and other circadian disruption
- Rotating shift work

---

review of general risk and protective factors extends beyond the scope of this review and can be found elsewhere.[55] Mood or anxiety syndromes are potentially modifiable risk factors specific to BD. Other co-occurring syndromes or substance use may also be targets for intervention. With regard to mood state, those who experience mixed states have more suicide attempts. This factor seems to be due not to the mixed states themselves, but rather their association with a course of illness characterized by more persistent depressive symptoms. Thus, depressive symptoms are the primary syndrome that drives suicide risk in BD.[58-61]

Relapse Recognition in Patients with a Known Diagnosis of Bipolar Disorder

In patients with known diagnosis of BD, once acute episode remission has been achieved, a focus on relapse prevention is crucial. BD is a highly recurrent illness, even in patients receiving high-quality, consistent care.[62] Factors associated with relapse are summarized in **Box 4** (for an overview of factors associated with poor long-term outcomes in general, see **Box 3**).[49,62,63]

Individuals may be sensitive to particular factors and this tends to be stable over the course of individual illness, which aids in the early identification and treatment of recurrence.[64-67]

Teaching patients and their proxies to recognize and address the factors that have previously precipitated particular types of mood episodes can be valuable,[68] as can establishing the sequence of symptoms leading up to each type of episode,[69] as well as how likely the patient is to recognize the symptom when it occurs.[65] Early warning signs can trigger a predetermined action plan, including coping strategies for early symptoms, as well as a motivation for the patient to act. For a system like this to work, the patient needs to have quick access to a health care provider who is familiar with the patient's symptoms and treatment history. A pitfall to be considered is that occasionally patients may become overly reliant on the early warning system and prefer it over taking medications, which should be addressed with psychoeducation and cognitive–behavioral techniques.[65]

MANAGEMENT

The goals of treatment are (1) full and early remission from acute episodes, (2) relapse prevention and delay, and (3) interepisode maintenance and support of emotional and cognitive function.

Table 1
CANMAT 2018[70] recommendations for adjunctive psychosocial interventions in BD[a]

Intervention	Definition and Setting	Depression	Maintenance
Psychoeducation	Focus on education on early detection of prodromes of relapse, stress management, problem solving, stigma and insight, medication adherence, and healthy lifestyle (substances, exercise, sleep). Aims to develop tailored coping strategies. Setting: Individual or groups	Insufficient evidence	First-line
Cognitive–behavioral therapy	Focuses on cognitive and related behavioral alterations that maintain depressive symptoms and facilitate relapses. Setting: Individual or groups	Second-line	Second-line
FFT	FFT involves patient and family, focusing on communication styles between patients and their families or marital relationships, aiming to improve relationship functioning. Setting: Individual and family	Second-line	Second-line
IPSRT	IPSRT addresses on interpersonal role transition, role dispute, and interpersonal functioning, with a specific focus on regulation of social and sleep rhythms. Setting: Individual or group	Third-line	Third-line
Peer support	Peer-groups or one-on-one support. Duration: Setting: Group	Insufficient evidence	Third-line

Abbreviations: FFT, family-focused therapy; IPSRT, interpersonal and social rhythm therapy.
[a] Insufficient evidence is available on cognitive and functional remediation, dialectical behavioral therapy, family/caregiver intervention, mindfulness-based cognitive therapy, online interventions.

Table 2
Mechanism of action, usual dose range, formulations, main safety issues and clinical monitoring of main medications used for BD[124]

Medication	Mechanism of Action	Dose-Range	Available Formulations	Safety	Baseline and Monitoring Essentials
Lithium	Second messengers, transcriptional/post-transcriptional changes	Serum level 0.6–1.0 mEq/L	Oral (also XR)	Thyroid, renal toxicity, consider risk–benefit in pregnancy	ECG, weight, lithium levels, TSH, creatinine.
Aripiprazole	Dopamine receptor partial agonist	15–30 mg 7.5 mg each 300–400 mg	Oral Intramuscular acute LAI q4w	Weight gain, dyslipidemia, diabetes, gambling/impulse control	ECG, weight, glucose, lipids
Olanzapine	Dopamine and serotonin receptor antagonist	20–40 mg 10 mg each 150–405 mg	Oral Intramuscular acute LAI q2–4w	Weight gain, dyslipidemia, diabetes, syncope/hypotension with benzodiazepines if both intramuscular	ECG, weight, glucose, lipids, prolactin
Asenapine	Dopamine, serotonin, noradrenaline receptor antagonist	10–20 mg	Oral	Weight gain, dyslipidemia, diabetes, hypotension	ECG, weight, glucose, lipids, prolactin
Valproic acid	Glutamate, voltage-gated sodium channel blocker	Serum level 45–125 μg/mL 15–20 mg/kg	Oral, intravenous	Weight gain, liver toxicity, skin reaction with eosinophilia, polycystic ovaries, avoid in pregnancy (teratogen)	Weight, valproic acid levels, liver function
Risperidone	Dopamine, serotonin, noradrenaline receptor antagonist	2–8 mg 12.5–50 mg	Oral LA q2w	Weight gain, dyslipidemia, diabetes, tardive dyskinesia, hyperprolactinemia	ECG, prolactin
Paliperidone	Dopamine and serotonin receptor antagonist	6–12 mg 39–819 mg	Oral LAI q4–12w	Weight gain, dyslipidemia, diabetes, tardive dyskinesia	ECG, prolactin

(continued on next page)

Table 2
(continued)

Medication	Mechanism of Action	Dose-Range	Available Formulations	Safety	Baseline and Monitoring Essentials
Quetiapine	Dopamine and serotonin receptor antagonist	400–800 mg	Oral (also XR)	Weight gain, dyslipidemia, diabetes	ECG, weight, glucose, lipids
Cariprazine	Dopamine, serotonin, noradrenaline receptor antagonist/partial agonist	3–6 mg	Oral	Weight gain, dyslipidemia, diabetes	ECG
Ziprasidone	Dopamine and serotonin receptor antagonist	80–160 mg 20 mg each	Oral Intramuscular acute	Hypotension	ECG
Carbamazepine	Glutamate, voltage-gated sodium channel blocker	400–1200 mg	Oral	Drug–drug interaction, liver toxicity, anemia/leukopenia, syndrome of inappropriate antidiuretic hormone, Stevens–Johnson syndrome	Liver function, CBC
Lamotrigine	Glutamate, voltage-gated sodium channel blocker	200–400 mg	Oral	Skin reaction with eosinophilia	—
Haloperidol	Dopamine receptor antagonist	1–40 mg 5 mg each 50–100 mg	Oral Intramuscular acute LAI q2–4w	Tardive dyskinesia	ECG
Lurasidone	Dopamine and serotonin receptor antagonist	40–160 mg	Oral	—	—

Abbreviations: CBC, complete blood count; ECG, electrocardiogram; LAI, long-acting injectable antipsychotic; TSH, thyroid stimulating hormone; XR, extended release.

Table 3
Pharmacologic treatment of mania[a]

Medication	Level of Evidence[b]	Response vs Placebo RR (95% CI)	Symptom Reduction vs Placebo SMD (95% CI)
First-line monotherapy			
Lithium (Li)	1	1.45 (1.28 to 1.65)	−0.35 (−0.48 to −0.22)
Quetiapine	1	1.55 (1.32 to 1.83)	−0.38 (−0.54 to −0.21)
Divalproex (DVP)	1	1.42 (1.19 to 1.71)	−0.22 (−0.37 to −0.06)
Asenapine	1	1.28 (1.05 to 1.56)	−0.31 (−0.51 to −0.12)
Aripiprazole	1	1.53 (1.33 to 1.76)	−0.36 (−0.50 to −0.22)
Paliperidone[c]	1	1.39 (1.10 to 1.76)	−0.38 (−0.62 to −0.13)
Risperidone	1	1.69 (1.41 to 2.02)	−0.60 (−0.77 to −0.43)
Cariprazine	1	1.56 (1.26 to 1.92)	−0.50 (−0.71 to −0.29)
First-line combination therapy			
Quetiapine + Li/DVP	1	Not included in network meta-analyses[125,126]	
Risperidone + Li/DVP	1		
Aripiprazole + Li/DVP	2		
Asenapine + Li/DVP	2		
Second-line therapies			
Olanzapine	1	1.59 (1.40 to 1.80)	−0.49 (−0.61 to −0.37)
Carbamazepine	1	1.90 (1.41 to 2.57)	−0.58 (−0.84 to −0.32)
Olanzapine + Li/DVP	1		
Ziprasidone	1		−0.34 (−0.56 to −0.12)
Haloperidol[d]	1	1.64 (1.43 to 1.88)	−0.61 (−0.75 to −0.47)
Li + DVP	3		
ECT	3		

Abbreviations: Adj, adjunctive therapy; CI, confidence interval; DVP, divalproex; LAI, long-acting injection; Li, LITHIUM; NA, not applicable (level of evidence not examined by CANMAT 2018); RR, relative risk.

The relative risk (RR) is statistically significant if 95% CI does not include 1: *Response*: RR > 1 indicates the degree to which the response rate to the medication is greater than placebo; *Prevention*: RR < 1 indicates lower relapse rate in medication, compared with placebo; *Symptom reduction*: a larger standardized mean difference (SMD) indicates a greater treatment effect size (where 0.2, 0.5, and 0.8 represent a small, moderate, and large treatment effect, respectively). A negative SMD for the effect size means treatment effect is greater for medication than for placebo.

[a] CANMAT 2018[70] recommendations and relative magnitude of effects from network meta-analyses,[125–127,129]

[b] *Level of evidence (LE)*[70]: 1 = Meta-analysis with narrow confidence interval or replicated double-blind (DB) (randomized controlled trial (RCT) that includes a placebo or active control comparison ($n \geq 30$ in each active treatment arm); 2 = Meta-analysis with wide confidence interval or 1 DB RCT with placebo or active control comparison condition ($n \geq 30$ in each active treatment arm); 3 = At least 1 DB RCT with placebo or active control comparison condition ($n = 10$–29 in each active treatment arm) or health system administrative data; 4 = Uncontrolled trial (anecdotal reports (or expert opinion.

[c] Daily dose of >6 mg.

[d] There is risk of switching to (hypo)mania. All-cause discontinuation for all medications was similar to or lower than placebo.

There are multiple clinical practice guidelines for the evaluation and treatment of BD. The most recent guidelines in North America are the ones released by the Canadian

Table 4
Pharmacologic treatment of acute depression in BD I[a]

Medication	Level of evidence[b,c]	Response vs Placebo RR (95% CI)[75,127]
First-line therapies		
Quetiapine	1	2.09 (1.74–1.82)
Lurasidone + Li/DVP	1	
Lithium	2	1.28 (0.86–1.92)
Lamotrigine	2	1.53 (1.23–1.90)
Lurasidone	2	2.58 (1.67–3.81)
Lamotrigine (adj)	2	1.43 (1.00–2.04)
Second-line therapies		
Divalproex	2	2.94 (1.33–6.46)
SSRIs/bupropion[d] (adj)	1	
Fluoxetine[d]		1.51 (1.11–2.06)
Sertraline[d]		1.61 (0.51–5.05)
Paroxetine[d]		1.31 (0.70–2.44)
Citalopram[d]		1.28 (0.73–2.25)
Bupropion[d]		1.30 (0.42–4.00)
Cariprazine	1	1.47 (1.17–1.82)
Olanzapine + fluoxetine[d]	2	2.57 (1.93–3.41)
ECT[d]	4	

Abbreviations: Adj, adjunctive therapy; CI, confidence interval; DVP, divalproex; LAI, long-acting injection; Li, lithium; NA, not applicable (level of evidence not examined by CANMAT 2018); RR, relative risk.

The relative risk (RR) is statistically significant if the 95% CI does not include 1: *Response*: RR > 1 indicates the degree to which the response rate to the medication is greater than placebo; *Prevention*: RR < 1 indicates lower relapse rate in medication, compared with placebo; *Symptom reduction*: a larger standardized mean difference (SMD) indicates a greater treatment effect size (where 0.2, 0.5, and 0.8 represent a small, moderate, and large treatment effect, respectively. A negative SMD for effect size means treatment effect is greater for medication than for placebo.

[a] CANMAT 2018[70] recommendations and relative magnitude of effects from network meta-analyses.[125–127,129]

[b] *Level of evidence (LE)*[70]: 1 = Meta-analysis with narrow confidence interval or replicated double-blind (DB) (randomized controlled trial (RCT) that includes a placebo or active control comparison (n ≥ 30 in each active treatment arm); 2 = Meta-analysis with wide confidence interval or 1 DB RCT with placebo or active control comparison condition (n ≥ 30 in each active treatment arm); 3 = At least 1 DB RCT with placebo or active control comparison condition (n = 10–29 in each active treatment arm) or health system administrative data; 4 = Uncontrolled trial (anecdotal reports (or expert opinion.

[c] Daily dose of >6 mg.

[d] There is risk of switching to (hypo)mania. All-cause discontinuation for all medications was similar to or lower than placebo.

Network for Mood and Anxiety Treatments (CANMAT) and International Society for Bipolar Disorders in 2018,[70] which we summarize in this section.

Psychosocial Interventions

Psychosocial interventions recommended refer to adjunctive use in the prevention of recurrence of either polarity or as an augmentation in the treatment of depressive symptoms. A recent network meta-analysis[71] suggests that skill-based manualized

Table 5
Pharmacologic treatment for relapse prevention in BD I[a]

Medication	Prevention of Any Episode[128] RR (95% CI) - LE[b]	Prevention of Mania[128] RR (95% CI) - LE[b]	Prevention of Depressive Episode[128] RR, 95% CI - LE[b]
First-line therapies			
Li	0.63 (0.54–0.73) - 1	0.54 (0.45–0.66) - 1	0.79 (0.66–0.95) - 1
Quetiapine	0.53 (0.41–0.67) - 1	0.56 (0.44–0.71) - 1	0.48 (0.36–0.63) - 1
DVP	0.63 (0.49–0.83) - 1	0.64 (0.48–0.86) - 3	0.85 (0.60–1.21) - 2
Lamotrigine	0.76 (0.63–0.93) - 1	0.89 (0.65–1.22) - 2	0.71 (0.55–0.93) - 1
Asenapine	0.26 (0.13–0.52) - 2	0.21 (0.08–0.53) - 2	0.39 (0.14–1.07) - 2
Quetiapine + Li/DVP	1	1	1
Aripiprazole + Li/DVP	For DVP combination: 0.29 (0.11–0.75) - 2	2	0.27 (0.08–0.99) - NA
Aripiprazole	0.62 (0.38–1.00) - 2	0.42 (0.21–0.84) - 2	0.90 (0.42–1.94) - NA
Aripiprazole LAI	2	0.30 (0.17–0.55) - 2	1.06 (0.58–1.96) - NA
Second-line therapies			
Olanzapine	0.50 (0.40–0.63) - 1	0.35 (0.27–0.45) - 1	0.74 (0.56–0.98) - 1
Risperidone LAI	0.64 (0.48–0.84) - 1	0.37 (0.27–0.51) - 1	1.29 (0.86–1.93) - NA
Risperidone LAI (adj)	2	2	3
Carbamazepine	0.68 (0.44–1.06) - 2	2.07 (0.26–16.66) - 2	2.73 (0.64–11.38) - 2
Paliperidone[c,d]	0.84 (0.58–1.21) - 2	2	1.31 (0.80–2.16) - NA
Lurasidone + Li/DVP	3	4	2
Ziprasidone + Li/DVP	2	2	NA

Abbreviations: Adj, adjunctive therapy; CI, confidence interval; DVP, divalproex; LAI, long-acting injection; Li, lithium; NA, not applicable (level of evidence not examined by CANMAT 2018); RR relative risk.

The relative risk (RR) is statistically significant if the 95% CI does not include 1: *Response*: RR > 1 indicates the degree to which the response rate to the medication is greater than placebo. *Prevention*: RR < 1 indicates lower relapse rate in medication, compared with placebo. *Symptom reduction*: A larger standardized mean difference (SMD) indicates a greater treatment effect size (where 0.2 (0.5 (and 0.8 represent small (moderate (and large treatment effects (respectively. Negative SMD for effect size means treatment effect is greater for medication than for placebo.

[a] CANMAT 2018[70] recommendations and relative magnitude of effects from network meta-analyses[125–127,129].

[b] *Level of evidence (LE)*[70]: 1 = Meta-analysis with narrow confidence interval or replicated double-blind (DB) (randomized controlled trial (RCT) that includes a placebo or active control comparison (n ≥ 30 in each active treatment arm); 2 = Meta-analysis with wide confidence interval or 1 DB RCT with placebo or active control comparison condition (n ≥ 30 in each active treatment arm); 3 = At least 1 DB RCT with placebo or active control comparison condition (n = 10–29 in each active treatment arm) or health system administrative data; 4 = Uncontrolled trial (anecdotal reports (or expert opinion.

[c] Daily dose of >6 mg.

[d] There is risk of switching to (hypo)mania. All-cause discontinuation for all medications was similar to or lower than placebo.

psychotherapies, such as cognitive–behavioral therapy, can improve depressive symptoms and decrease recurrence, in combination with pharmacotherapy. Psycho-education, with active illness management skills practice, in group and family format may be superior in prevention of relapse, compared with the same intervention in individual format.[71] See **Table 1** for CANMAT recommendations for adjunctive psychosocial interventions.

Pharmacologic Interventions

Some key clinical insights on medications indicated from CANMAT for BD are listed in **Table 2**. The CANMAT recommendations for the pharmacologic treatment recommendations for BDI are in **Tables 3–5** and for BD II in **Table 6**. For BD I, efficacy and discontinuation risk estimates from network meta-analyses are displayed as well.

We present a critical selection of pharmacologic options merging CANMAT recommendations and effect sizes of network meta-analyses (which pool direct and indirect comparisons from RCTs). In BD I, among the first-line treatments, risperidone has the greatest efficacy for mania, lurasidone for bipolar depression, asenapine to prevent recurrence of any episodes and manic episodes, and aripiprazole in combination with valproate to prevent depressive episodes. Lithium as well is among the most effective first-line treatments for mania and the prevention of recurrence. These and additional first-line options in order of decreasing efficacy are summarized in **Table 7**. Currently, there is no role for antidepressants in the first-line treatment of bipolar depression.

Although the CANMAT recommendations for the treatment of BD II and BD I depressive episode differ, in clinical practice an initial BD II diagnosis can change to BD I, and a clear distinction is not always possible if collateral information is missing. When the differential diagnosis is not clear, the guidelines for BD I can be followed. Hypomania in BD II does not always warrant treatment, because it can be self-limiting and even productive. Treatment recommendations for hypomania are based on the lowest level of evidence (Level 4; see **Tables 3–5** for legend).[70]

The Psychopharmacology Algorithm Project can be used in conjunction with this review to guide treatment decisions in BD[72,73]: https://psychopharm.mobi/.

Neurostimulation and Other Nonpharmacological and Biological Treatments

There is little literature overall on the effectiveness and outcomes of neurostimulation in BD. The available evidence suggests that electroconvulsive treatment (ECT) can be an effective treatment option in patients with mania who are refractory to pharmacotherapy.[74,75] Notable safety issues include cognitive side effects and treatment-emergent affective switch.[76,77]

It is safest to discontinue lithium before commencing ECT, because it can increase the risk of post-ECT delirium, and promptly reintroduced afterward. Anticonvulsants should also be tapered off before ECT to prevent incomplete seizures.[74] Light therapy and repetitive transcranial magnetic stimulation are effective for bipolar depression, with a small effect size, but overall good safety and tolerability.[78–80]

Complementary and Alternative Medicine Approaches

Complementary and alternative medicine (CAM) use is highly prevalent among patients with BD.[81] These include oral (herbs and supplements), physical (aromatherapy, acupuncture, massage, yoga), and cognitive (meditation, prayer, visualization and relaxation) treatments. Physical and psychological CAMs are generally safe and can have a true or subjective placebo-like effect[81] on different outcomes, also depending on the patient's cultural community. However, the vast majority of oral CAMs are not effective and can have interactions that affect evidence-based medications' safety and efficacy.[82] Some CAM treatments have been studied in MDD but not in BD and use in bipolar depression can carry a risk of treatment-emergent affective switch (eg, St. John's Wort or S-adenosyl-L-methionine). Weight loss supplements often contain ephedra or similar compounds, which can affect the sleep–wake cycle and trigger manic episodes. While two prior meta-analyses were conflicting, the most

Table 6
CANMAT 2018 pharmacotherapy recommendations for the treatment of BD II

Treatment Phase	First Line	Second Line	Third Line
Acute hypomania (level 4 evidence available only)	Lithium Divalproex Second-generation antipsychotics N-acetyl cysteine		
BD II depression	Quetiapine	Lithium Lamotrigine Electroconvulsive therapy[a] Sertraline[a] Venlafaxine[a]	Divalproex Ziprasidone Tranylcypromine Fluoxetine[a] Agomelatine (adj) Bupropion (adj)[a] Eicosapentanoic acid Ketamine N-acetyl cysteine Pramipexole[a] Thyroid hormones
Maintenance	Quetiapine Lithium Lamotrigine	Venlafaxine[a]	Carbamazepine Divalproex Escitalopram[a] Fluoxetine[a] Risperidone

[a] Increased risk of treatment-emergent affective switch , particularly in patients with mixed features, history of antidepressant-induced hypomania or rapid cycling.

recent meta-analysis of omega-3 fatty acids for treatment of bipolar depression suggested a small benefit.[83] The only other oral CAM supported by meta-analytic evidence is N-acetyl cysteine, with a small effect size on functioning.[84] Overall, no CAM can replace any first-line pharmacologic or psychosocial treatment for BD. In counseling patients who wish to use CAM, the clinician should maintain a nonjudgmental stance, encourage an open dialogue, and use the therapeutic rapport to inform the patient about the potential benefits and risks of psychosocial CAM and the low benefit-to-risk ratio of oral CAM.

For a database of supplement–allopathic medicine interactions, see https://supp.ai/.

POPULATIONS OF SPECIAL INTEREST
Children and Adolescents

BD has an onset before the age of 21 years in approximately 60% of individuals.[85] In childhood and adolescence, its presentation may be more difficult to recognize because of predominance of mixed and rapid cycling syndromes, lack of a clear report of mood symptoms, short-lasting (hypo)manic symptoms, overlap with other childhood disorders such as ADHD, and the presence of irritability and temper outbursts that taint the clinical picture.[86]

The general principles that apply to treatment of adults should be used in children and adolescents, but with special consideration to comorbidities, especially ADHD, emphasis on lifestyle intervention including that for substance use, and sensitivity to the metabolic side effects of medication(s).

Older Age

Late-onset BD may often be related to a neurologic or physical comorbidity.[87] Depressive symptoms and cognitive impairment may be more pronounced in late-life BD, and

Table 7
First-line medication options by phase of treatment, in order of decreasing efficacy[13,14,70,75,125–12771]

Phase	Medication
Mania	Risperidone Cariprazine, quetiapine, aripiprazole, lithium, divalproex, paliperidone, asenapine
BD I depression	Lurasidone Quetiapine, lamotrigine
Prevention of mania	Asenapine
Prevention of bipolar depression	Aripiprazole + divalproex
Prevention of both manic and depressive episodes	Asenapine Lithium Quetiapine Aripiprazole + lithium/divalproex

a structured cognitive assessment should be used to quantify this impairment. Owing to higher medical comorbidity and aging-related changes, clinicians need to be sensitive to drug interactions, adverse effects, and the need for frequent monitoring.

In general, even though there is a dearth of data on efficacy, treatments that have shown to be efficacious in BD, also work for older adults. Lithium (0.80–.99 mEq/L) was found superior to valproate (80–99 μg/mL) in the treatment of older adults (>60 years old) with mania in the GERI-BD study.[88] Owing to higher propensity for adverse effects with mood stabilizers and antipsychotics in older age, which may be started at a low dose and increased gradually.[70]

Pregnancy and Breastfeeding

Because BD starts in early adulthood, females are at risk for episodes throughout their reproductive years. The management of BD in pregnancy and postpartum needs complex shared decision-making accounting for the teratogenicity of medications, passage of drug across placenta and breastmilk, neonatal complications such as withdrawal, and changes in drug metabolism in pregnancy and lactation. Treatment in this population is often complicated and limited by the lack of long-term data owing to the ethical concerns and feasibility of carrying out randomized, controlled trials.

Psychotropic drugs during pregnancy and breastfeeding

Both pregnancy and the postpartum period constitute time for an increased risk of the recurrence of mood episodes, and this risk is very high after treatment discontinuation.[89,90] The CANMAT and International Society for Bipolar Disorders guidelines recommend that, wherever possible, medication use be avoided in the first trimester. If that is not feasible, monotherapy at a minimum effective dose is recommended. One or more drugs may be stopped before conception if the patient has been clinically stable for 4 to 6 months and is at a low risk for relapse.[70] Owing to changes in drug metabolism in the second and third trimesters, higher doses of drugs may be needed.

Owing to the risk of neural tube defects, avoid the use of carbamazepine and valproate in women in the reproductive age group' switch to an alternate medication if possible in those who are already on these drugs, ensure effective contraception during the cross-over, and start folic acid supplementation. The risk with lithium is higher

---

Box 5
Principles of treatment in pregnant and reproductive-age patients with BD

- A discussion about pregnancy needs to be held with every woman in reproductive age group. Does she plan to conceive, and if so, when? What does she already know about medication use during pregnancy and breastfeeding? Does she plan to breastfeed?

- Document the method of contraception and date of last menstrual period.

- Start treatment with the knowledge that there is always a likelihood for unplanned pregnancy, even if the patient does not plan to conceive in the near future.

- It is also important to closely monitor patients for therapeutic level, side effects and to avoid polypharmacy as much as possible.

- If breastfeeding, enlist measures such as expressed milk, timing medication and feeds optimally to minimize transfer of medications to the infant.

---

for first trimester or higher dose exposure, necessitating appropriate dose adjustments for patients on lithium who wish to conceive.[91]

For mild to moderate postpartum depression, evidence-based psychotherapies are valuable adjuncts to medications in pregnancy and postpartum, especially in women who have psychosocial stressors that may worsen the illness course.[92]

There is evidence favoring lithium, antipsychotics, and benzodiazepines for postpartum mania[93] and for quetiapine, lithium, lamotrigine, and lurasidone in postpartum depression. However, lithium use may be complicated by concerns with breastfeeding and infant level monitoring.[94] In general, quetiapine and olanzapine are the preferred antipsychotics during postpartum, owing to low secretion in breast milk. Some resources to aid shared decision-making with the patient include the US Food and Drug Administration Pregnancy and Lactation Labeling Final Rule and the Drugs and Lactation Database (LactMed) by the National Library of Medicine: https://www.ncbi.nlm.nih.gov/books/NBK501922/.

Finally, ECT has been recommended as a safe and efficacious treatment for severe mood episodes and suicidality during the pregnancy and in the postpartum period.[95] See **Box 5** for general principles in approaching BD in pregnant and reproductive-age women.

FOLLOW-UP AND MONITORING WITH MEASUREMENT-BASED CARE

The significant gap between outcomes achieved in randomized controlled trials and in real-world clinical practice has led to an increasing emphasis and a gradual shift toward measurement-based care. Measurement-based care consists of the systematic use of symptom rating scales to track symptom frequency and severity, side effect burden, and adherence to optimize clinical outcomes by detecting nonresponse.[96] In the context of BD, this is important, because mood symptoms can fluctuate between and within an episode.[43]

The choice of a rating scale depends on various factors such as ease of administration, presenting problem and brevity.[97] Some of the widely used, validated and reliable clinician-rated measures in studies include Young Mania Rating Scale, Hamilton Depression Rating Scale-17, Quick Inventory of Depressive Symptomatology, and the Montgomery–Åsberg Depression Rating Scale.[98] A newer but perhaps more accessible scale is the Patient Mania Questionnaire 9,[99] a self-report scale for the monitoring of mania symptoms, with high internal, test–retest, and concurrent validity, as well as sensitivity to change, suggesting high promise in monitoring and treating BD in primary care. With the length and response set of the Patient Mania Questionnaire 9 modeled after the Patient Health Questionnaire 9, the 2 measures can be used together to monitor manic and depressive symptoms, respectively.

Assessing Cognition

Patients with BD often have cognitive impairment in the domains of attention and processing speeds, as well as memory and executive functioning, both during acute episodes and interepisodically, on average less severe than those seen in schizophrenia.[100–104] Cognitive screening can help to detect those at risk for cognitive impairment, track cognitive symptoms over time, and guide treatment selection. Currently, there are no approved treatment for this indication. Mitigation strategies include referral to a neuropsychologist, assessment for causes of these deficits, using compensatory measures such as reminders and alarms, and lifestyle modifications.[105]

When to Refer for Help

Patients with complex symptom presentations where a diagnosis is unclear, as well as those with treatment-resistant episodes, suicidality, frequent hospitalizations, or persistent interepisodic symptoms, children and adolescents, those who are planning pregnancy, pregnant, or breastfeeding, and those needing ECT are appropriate for referral to a psychiatrist for diagnostic clarification and treatment or treatment recommendations. Involving other specialized care (neurology, endocrinology, addictions services, etc) is also appropriate for addressing complex comorbid conditions.

SUMMARY

BD is characterized by recurrent mood episodes, affecting 1% to 2% of the population. Although its defining features are manic and hypomanic episodes, it is predominantly characterized by depressive syndromes. Diagnosis can be challenging owing to symptom overlap with other disorders. Two distinct subtypes warrant different treatment: BD II is defined by less severe episodes of mood elevation than mania, termed hypomania, and occur in those with history of MDD. BD I and BD II subtypes differ also in the ratio of elevated to depressed episodes and co-occurrence of comorbidities but not in overall severity, risk of suicide attempt, or neurocognitive impairment. Treatment goals include early and complete remission of acute episodes and relapse prevention between episodes. The CANMAT 2018 guidelines are the most recent North American clinical guidelines for the treatment of BD. Anticonvulsant and antipsychotic medications are the mainstay of pharmacologic treatment in both acute and maintenance phases. Psychosocial interventions, in combination with pharmacotherapy, are recommended for the prevention of relapse and to help address depressive symptoms. Antidepressants are not recommended in the first-line treatment of bipolar depression, which warrants more careful treatment. Patients with complex presentations, treatment-resistant patients, and populations of special interest, such as children and youth, older adults, and pregnant and breastfeeding people, should be referred to a psychiatrist where possible.

CLINICS CARE POINTS

- BD can be differentiated from ADHD, personality disorders, and anxiety disorders by its relapsing and remitting course and distinct sustained affective changes during episodes.
- Screen all patients who present with depression, have family history of BD, or a comorbid medical or psychiatric disorder with known high prevalence of BD.

- Involve patient proxies in the assessment and obtain collateral information whenever possible.
- Avoid antidepressants in the treatment of bipolar depression.
- Refer patients with difficult-to-treat BD to a specialist.

ACKNOWLEDGEMENT

JGF was funded through US National Institute of Mental Health 5R01-MH111578-05 (PI Magnotta).

DISCLOSURE

MS received honoraria/has been a consultant for Angelini, Lundbeck, Otsuka. All other authors have no conflicts to disclosure. JGF work was funded through the U.S. National Institute of Mental Health (R01MH111578).

REFERENCES

1. Merikangas KR, Akiskal HS, Angst J, et al. Lifetime and 12-month prevalence of bipolar spectrum disorder in the National Comorbidity Survey replication. Arch Gen Psychiatry 2007;64(5):543–52.
2. Merikangas KR, Jin R, He JP, et al. Prevalence and correlates of bipolar spectrum disorder in the world mental health survey initiative. Arch Gen Psychiatry 2011;68(3):241–51.
3. Moreira ALR, Van Meter A, Genzlinger J, et al. Review and meta-analysis of epidemiologic studies of adult bipolar disorder. Meta-analysis research support, Non-U.S. Gov't. J Clin Psychiatry 2017;78(9):e1259–69.
4. Rowland TA, Marwaha S. Epidemiology and risk factors for bipolar disorder. Ther Adv Psychopharmacol 2018;8(9):251–69.
5. Blanco C, Compton WM, Saha TD, et al. Epidemiology of DSM-5 bipolar I disorder: results from the National Epidemiologic Survey on Alcohol and Related Conditions - III. Research Support, N.I.H., Intramural. J Psychiatr Res 2017; 84:310–7.
6. Liu Y, Blackwood DH, Caesar S, et al. Meta-analysis of genome-wide association data of bipolar disorder and major depressive disorder. Letter Meta-Analysis Research Support, Non-U.S. Gov't. Mol Psychiatry 2011;16(1):2–4.
7. Coryell W, Endicott J, Reich T, et al. A family study of bipolar II disorder. Br J Psychiatry 1984;145:49–54.
8. Coryell W, Keller M, Endicott J, et al. Bipolar II illness: course and outcome over a five-year period. Psychol Med 1989;19(1):129–41.
9. Fornaro M, Anastasia A, Novello S, et al. Incidence, prevalence and clinical correlates of antidepressant-emergent mania in bipolar depression: a systematic review and meta-analysis. Meta-Analysis Systematic Review. Bipolar Disord 2018;20(3):195–227.
10. Gore FM, Bloem PJ, Patton GC, et al. Global burden of disease in young people aged 10-24 years: a systematic analysis. Lancet 2011;377(9783):2093–102. https://doi.org/10.1016/S0140-6736(11)60512-6.
11. Weiner M, Warren L, Fiedorowicz JG. Cardiovascular morbidity and mortality in bipolar disorder. Research Support, N.I.H., Extramural Research Support, Non-U.S. Gov't. Ann Clin Psychiatry 2011;23(1):40–7.

12. Laursen TM. Life expectancy among persons with schizophrenia or bipolar affective disorder. Schizophr Res 2011;131(1–3):101–4.

13. Nordentoft M, Wahlbeck K, Hällgren J, et al. Excess mortality, causes of death and life expectancy in 270,770 patients with recent onset of mental disorders in Denmark, Finland and Sweden. PLoS One 2013;8(1):e55176.

14. Solomon DA, Leon AC, Endicott J, et al. Unipolar mania over the course of a 20-year follow-up study. Comparative Study Research Support, U.S. Gov't, P.H.S. Am J Psychiatry 2003;160(11):2049–51.

15. Fiedorowicz JG, Solomon DA, Endicott J, et al. Manic/hypomanic symptom burden and cardiovascular mortality in bipolar disorder. Psychosom Med 2009;71(6):598–606.

16. Smoller JW, Finn CT. Family, twin, and adoption studies of bipolar disorder. Am J Med Genet C Semin Med Genet 2003;123c(1):48–58.

17. Johansson V, Kuja-Halkola R, Cannon TD, et al. A population-based heritability estimate of bipolar disorder – in a Swedish twin sample. Psychiatry Res 2019; 278:180–7.

18. Fabbri C. The role of genetics in bipolar disorder. In: Young AH, Juruena MF, editors. Bipolar disorder: from neuroscience to treatment. Switzerland: Springer International Publishing; 2021. p. 41–60.

19. Mullins N, Forstner AJ, O'Connell KS, et al. Genome-wide association study of more than 40,000 bipolar disorder cases provides new insights into the underlying biology. Nat Genet 2021;53(6):817–29.

20. Cegla-Schvartzman F, Ovejero S, Lopez-Castroma J, et al. Diagnostic stability in bipolar disorder: a follow-up study in 130,000 patient-years. Research Support, Non-U.S. Gov't. J Clin Psychiatry 2021;82(6):14.

21. Chilakamarri JK, Filkowski MM, Ghaemi SN. Misdiagnosis of bipolar disorder in children and adolescents: a comparison with ADHD and major depressive disorder. Ann Clin Psychiatry 2011;23(1):25–9.

22. Zimmerman M, Ruggero CJ, Chelminski I, et al. Psychiatric diagnoses in patients previously overdiagnosed with bipolar disorder. J Clin Psychiatry 2010; 71(1):26–31.

23. Hirschfeld RMA, Williams JBW, Spitzer RL, et al. Development and validation of a screening instrument for bipolar spectrum disorder: the Mood Disorder Questionnaire. Am J Psychiatry 2000;157(11):1873–5.

24. Nassir Ghaemi S, Miller CJ, Berv DA, et al. Sensitivity and specificity of a new bipolar spectrum diagnostic scale. J Affect Disord 2005;84(2–3):273–7.

25. Phelps JR, Ghaemi SN. Improving the diagnosis of bipolar disorder: predictive value of screening tests. J Affective Disord 2006;92(2):141–8.

26. Kivilcim Y, Altintas M, Domac FM, et al. Screening for bipolar disorder among migraineurs: the impact of migraine–bipolar disorder comorbidity on disease characteristics. Neuropsychiatr Dis Treat 2017;13:631–41.

27. Joseph B, Nandakumar AL, Ahmed AT, et al. Prevalence of bipolar disorder in multiple sclerosis: a systematic review and meta-analysis. Meta-Analysis Research Support, Non-U.S. Gov't Review Systematic Review. Evidence-Based Ment Health 2021;24(2):88–94.

28. Tzur Bitan D, Berzin D, Cohen A. Hidradenitis suppurativa and bipolar disorders: a population-based study. Dermatology 2020;236(4):298–304.

29. Su VY-F, Hu L-Y, Yeh C-M, et al. Chronic obstructive pulmonary disease associated with increased risk of bipolar disorder. Chronic Respir Dis 2017;14(2): 151–60.

30. McIntyre RS, I MD, Masand PS, et al. The Rapid Mood Screener (RMS): a novel and pragmatic screener for bipolar I disorder. Curr Med Res Opin 2021;37(1): 135–44.
31. Manning JS. Tools to improve differential diagnosis of bipolar disorder in primary care. Prim Care Companion J Clin Psychiatry 2010;12(Suppl 1):17–22.
32. Mitchell PB, Malhi GS. Bipolar depression: phenomenological overview and clinical characteristics. Bipolar Disord 2004;6(6):530–9.
33. Motovsky B, Pecenak J. Psychopathological characteristics of bipolar and unipolar depression - potential indicators of bipolarity. Psychiatr Danub 2013; 25(1):34–9.
34. Nakamura K, Iga J, Matsumoto N, et al. Risk of bipolar disorder and psychotic features in patients initially hospitalised with severe depression. Acta Neuropsychiatrica 2015;27(2):113–8.
35. Perlis RH, Brown E, Baker RW, et al. Clinical features of bipolar depression versus major depressive disorder in large multicenter trials. Am J Psychiatry 2006;163(2):225–31.
36. Loftus J, Scott J, Vorspan F, et al. Psychiatric comorbidities in bipolar disorders: an examination of the prevalence and chronology of onset according to sex and bipolar subtype. Research Support, Non-U.S. Gov't. J Affective Disord 2020; 267:258–63.
37. McElroy SL, Altshuler LL, Suppes T, et al. Axis I psychiatric comorbidity and its relationship to historical illness variables in 288 patients with bipolar disorder. Am J Psychiatry 2001;158(3):420–6.
38. Kessler RC, Chiu WT, Demler O, et al. Prevalence, severity, and comorbidity of 12-month DSM-IV disorders in the National Comorbidity Survey Replication. Arch Gen Psychiatry 2005;62(6):617.
39. Eisner LR, Johnson SL, Youngstrom EA, et al. Simplifying profiles of comorbidity in bipolar disorder. J Affective Disord 2017;220.102–7.
40. Berk M, Dodd S, Callaly P, et al. History of illness prior to a diagnosis of bipolar disorder or schizoaffective disorder. J Affect Disord 2007;103(1–3):181–6.
41. McIntyre RS, Zimmerman M, Goldberg JF, et al. Differential diagnosis of major depressive disorder versus bipolar disorder: current status and best clinical practices. J Clin Psychiatry 2019;80(3). https://doi.org/10.4088/JCP. ot18043ah2.
42. Kraepelin E. Manic-depressive insanity and paranoia. 1976. TbRMBi. Thoemmes Press; 1920.
43. Judd LL, Akiskal HS, Schettler PJ, et al. The long-term natural history of the weekly symptomatic status of bipolar I disorder. Arch Gen Psychiatry 2002; 59(6):530–7.
44. Judd LL, Akiskal HS, Schettler PJ, et al. A prospective investigation of the natural history of the long-term weekly symptomatic status of bipolar II disorder. Arch Gen Psychiatry 2003;60(3):261–9.
45. Judd LL, Akiskal HS, Schettler PJ, et al. Psychosocial disability in the course of bipolar I and II disorders: a prospective, comparative, longitudinal study. Arch Gen Psychiatry 2005;62(12):1322–30.
46. Coryell W, Fiedorowicz J, Solomon D, et al. Age transitions in the course of bipolar I disorder. Psychol Med 2009;39(8):1247–52.
47. Ketter TA, Houston JP, Adams DH, et al. Differential efficacy of olanzapine and lithium in preventing manic or mixed recurrence in patients with bipolar I disorder based on number of previous manic or mixed episodes. J Clin Psychiatry 2006;67(1):95–101.

48. Tsai SM, Chen C, Kuo C, et al. 15-year outcome of treated bipolar disorder. J Affect Disord 2001;63(1–3):215–20.

49. Etain B, Bellivier F, Olié E, et al. Clinical predictors of recurrences in bipolar disorders type 1 and 2: a FACE-BD longitudinal study. J Psychiatr Res 2021;134: 129–37.

50. Pacchiarotti I, Bond DJ, Baldessarini RJ, et al. The International Society for Bipolar Disorders (ISBD) Task Force report on antidepressant use in bipolar disorders. Am J Psychiatry 2013;170(11):1249–62.

51. Schaffer A, Isometsä ET, Tondo L, et al. Epidemiology, neurobiology and pharmacological interventions related to suicide deaths and suicide attempts in bipolar disorder: Part I of a report of the International Society for Bipolar Disorders Task Force on suicide in bipolar disorder. Aust N Z J Psychiatry 2015;49(9):785–802.

52. Dennehy EB, Marangell LB, Allen MH, et al. Suicide and suicide attempts in the Systematic Treatment Enhancement Program for Bipolar Disorder (STEP-BD). J Affect Disord 2011;133(3):423–7.

53. Schaffer A, Isometsä ET, Tondo L, et al. International Society for Bipolar Disorders Task Force on Suicide: meta-analyses and meta-regression of correlates of suicide attempts and suicide deaths in bipolar disorder. Bipolar Disord 2015;17(1):1–16.

54. Novick DM, Swartz HA, Frank E. Suicide attempts in bipolar I and bipolar II disorder: a review and meta-analysis of the evidence. Bipolar Disord 2010; 12(1):1–9.

55. Weber AN, Michail M, Thompson A, et al. Psychiatric emergencies: assessing and managing suicidal ideation. Med Clin North Am 2017;101(3):553–71.

56. Kroenke K, Spitzer RL, Williams JB. The PHQ-9: validity of a brief depression severity measure. J Gen Intern Med 2001;16(9):606–13.

57. Posner K, Brown GK, Stanley B, et al. The Columbia-Suicide Severity Rating Scale: initial validity and internal consistency findings from three multisite studies with adolescents and adults. Am J Psychiatry 2011;168(12):1266–77.

58. Fiedorowicz JG, Persons JE, Assari S, et al. Depressive symptoms carry an increased risk for suicidal ideation and behavior in bipolar disorder without any additional contribution of mixed symptoms. J Affect Disord 2019;246: 775–82.

59. Fiedorowicz JG, Persons JE, Assari S, et al. Moderators of the association between depressive, manic, and mixed mood symptoms and suicidal ideation and behavior: an analysis of the National Network of Depression Centers Mood Outcomes Program. J Affect Disord 2021;281:623–30.

60. Persons JE, Coryell WH, Solomon DA, et al. Mixed state and suicide: Is the effect of mixed state on suicidal behavior more than the sum of its parts? Bipolar Disord 2018;20(1):35–41.

61. Persons JE, Lodder P, Coryell WH, et al. Symptoms of mania and anxiety do not contribute to suicidal ideation or behavior in the presence of bipolar depression. Psychiatry Res 2022;307:114296.

62. Altman S, Haeri S, Cohen LJ, et al. Predictors of relapse in bipolar disorder: a review. J Psychiatr Practice® 2006;12(5):269–82.

63. Inder ML, Crowe MT, Porter R. Effect of transmeridian travel and jetlag on mood disorders: evidence and implications. Aust N Z J Psychiatry 2016;50(3):220–7.

64. Keitner GI, Solomon DA, Ryan CE, et al. Prodromal and residual symptoms in bipolar I disorder. Compr Psychiatry 1996;37(5):362–7.

65. Morriss R. The early warning symptom intervention for patients with bipolar affective disorder. Adv Psychiatr Treat 2004;10(1):18–26.
66. Sahoo MK, Chakrabarti S, Kulhara P. Detection of prodromal symptoms of relapse in mania and unipolar depression by relatives and patients. Indian J Med Res 2012;135(2):177–83.
67. Smith JA, Tarrier N. Prodromal symptoms in manic depressive psychosis. Soc Psychiatry Psychiatr Epidemiol 1992;27(5):245–8.
68. Perry A, Tarrier N, Morriss R, et al. Randomised controlled trial of efficacy of teaching patients with bipolar disorder to identify early symptoms of relapse and obtain treatment. BMJ 1999;318(7177):149–53.
69. Young MA, Grabler P. Rapidity of symptom onset in depression. Psychiatry Res 1985;16(4):309–15.
70. Yatham LN, Kennedy SH, Parikh SV, et al. Canadian Network for Mood and Anxiety Treatments (CANMAT) and International Society for Bipolar Disorders (ISBD) 2018 guidelines for the management of patients with bipolar disorder. Bipolar Disord 2018;20(2):97–170.
71. Miklowitz DJ, Efthimiou O, Furukawa TA, et al. Adjunctive psychotherapy for bipolar disorder: a systematic review and component network meta-analysis. JAMA Psychiatry 2021;78(2):141–50.
72. Mohammad O, Osser DN. The psychopharmacology algorithm project at the Harvard South Shore Program: an algorithm for acute mania. Harv Rev Psychiatry 2014;22(5):274–94.
73. Wang D, Osser DN. The Psychopharmacology Algorithm Project at the Harvard South Shore Program: an update on bipolar depression. Bipolar Disord 2020; 22(5):472–89.
74. Loo C, Katalinic N, Mitchell PB, et al. Physical treatments for bipolar disorder: A review of electroconvulsive therapy, stereotactic surgery and other brain stimulation techniques. J Affective Disord 2011;132(1):1–13.
75. Bahji A, Hawken ER, Sepehry AA, et al. ECT beyond unipolar major depression: systematic review and meta-analysis of electroconvulsive therapy in bipolar depression. Acta Psychiatr Scand 2019;139(3):214–26.
76. Angst J, Angst K, Baruffol I, et al. ECT-induced and drug-induced hypomania. Convulsive therapy; 1992.
77. Henry C, Sorbara F, Lacoste J, et al. Antidepressant-induced mania in bipolar patients: identification of risk factors. J Clin Psychiatry 2001;62(4):911.
78. Tee MMK, Au CH. A systematic review and meta-analysis of randomized sham-controlled trials of repetitive transcranial magnetic stimulation for bipolar disorder. Psychiatr Q 2020;91(4):1225–47.
79. Lam RW, Teng MY, Jung YE, et al. Light therapy for patients with bipolar depression: systematic review and meta-analysis of randomized controlled trials. Can J Psychiatry 2020;65(5):290–300.
80. Konstantinou G, Hui J, Ortiz A, et al. Repetitive transcranial magnetic stimulation (rTMS) in bipolar disorder: a systematic review. Bipolar Disord 2021. https://doi.org/10.1111/bdi.13099.
81. Kilbourne AM, Copeland LA, Zeber JE, et al. Determinants of complementary and alternative medicine use by patients with bipolar disorder. Psychopharmacol Bull 2007;40(3):104–15.
82. Andreescu C, Mulsant BH, Emanuel JE. Complementary and alternative medicine in the treatment of bipolar disorder — a review of the evidence. J Affective Disord 2008;110(1):16–26.

83. Kisho T, Sakuma K, Okuya M, et al. Omega-3 fatty acids for treating residual depressive symptoms in adult patients with bipolar disorder: A systematic review and meta-analysis of double-blind randomized, placebo-controlled trials. Bipolar Disord 2021;23(7):730–1.

84. Firth J, Teasdale SB, Allott K, et al. The efficacy and safety of nutrient supplements in the treatment of mental disorders: a meta-review of meta-analyses of randomized controlled trials. World Psychiatry 2019;18(3):308–24.

85. Duffy A. The early course of bipolar disorder in youth at familial risk. J Can Acad Child Adolesc Psychiatry 2009;18(3):200–5.

86. Grande I, Berk M, Birmaher B, et al. Bipolar disorder. Lancet 2016;387(10027): 1561–72.

87. Subramaniam H, Dennis MS, Byrne EJ. The role of vascular risk factors in late onset bipolar disorder. Int J Geriatr Psychiatry 2007;22(8):733–7.

88. Young RC, Mulsant BH, Sajatovic M, et al. GERI-BD: a randomized double-blind controlled trial of lithium and divalproex in the treatment of mania in older patients with bipolar disorder. Am J Psychiatry 2017;174(11):1086–93.

89. Wesseloo R, Kamperman AM, Munk-Olsen T, et al. Risk of postpartum relapse in bipolar disorder and postpartum psychosis: a systematic review and meta-analysis. Am J Psychiatry 2016;173(2):117–27.

90. Salim M, Sharma V, Anderson KK. Recurrence of bipolar disorder during pregnancy: a systematic review. Arch Womens Ment Health 2018;21(4):475–9.

91. Fornaro M, Maritan E, Ferranti R, et al. Lithium exposure during pregnancy and the postpartum period: a systematic review and meta-analysis of safety and efficacy outcomes. Am J Psychiatry 2020;177(1):76–92.

92. Epstein RA, Moore KM, Bobo WV. Treatment of bipolar disorders during pregnancy: maternal and fetal safety and challenges. Drug Healthc Patient Saf 2015;7:7–29.

93. Bergink V, Burgerhout KM, Koorengevel KM, et al. Treatment of psychosis and mania in the postpartum period. Am J Psychiatry 2015;172(2):115–23.

94. Sharma V, Bergink V, Berk M, et al. Childbirth and prevention of bipolar disorder: an opportunity for change. Lancet Psychiatry 2019;6(9):786–92.

95. Khan SJ, Fersh ME, Ernst C, et al. Bipolar disorder in pregnancy and postpartum: principles of management. Curr Psychiatry Rep 2016;18(2):13.

96. Harding KJ, Rush AJ, Arbuckle M, et al. Measurement-based care in psychiatric practice: a policy framework for implementation. J Clin Psychiatry 2011;72(8): 1136–43.

97. Cerimele JM, Goldberg SB, Miller CJ, et al. Systematic review of symptom assessment measures for use in measurement-based care of bipolar disorders. Psychiatr Serv 2019;70(5):396–408.

98. Davidson J, Turnbull CD, Strickland R, et al. The Montgomery-Åsberg Depression Scale: reliability and validity. Acta Psychiatrica Scand 1986;73(5):544–8.

99. Cerimele JM, Russo J, Bauer AM, et al. The Patient Mania Questionnaire (PMQ-9): a brief scale for assessing and monitoring manic symptoms. J Gen Intern Med 2021. https://doi.org/10.1007/s11606-021-06947-7.

100. Torres IJ, Boudreau VG, Yatham LN. Neuropsychological functioning in euthymic bipolar disorder: a meta-analysis. Acta Psychiatr Scand Suppl 2007;(434):17–26.

101. Lima F, Rabelo-da-Ponte FD, Bucker J, et al. Identifying cognitive subgroups in bipolar disorder: a cluster analysis. J Affect Disord 2019;246:252–61.

102. Jensen JH, Knorr U, Vinberg M, et al. Discrete neurocognitive subgroups in fully or partially remitted bipolar disorder: associations with functional abilities. J Affect Disord 2016;205:378–86.
103. Chakrabarty T, Torres IJ, Su WW, et al. Cognitive subgroups in first episode bipolar I disorder: Relation to clinical and brain volumetric variables. Acta Psychiatr Scand 2021;143(2):151–61.
104. Burdick KE, Russo M, Frangou S, et al. Empirical evidence for discrete neurocognitive subgroups in bipolar disorder: clinical implications. Psychol Med 2014;44(14):3083–96.
105. Miskowiak KW, Burdick KE, Martinez-Aran A, et al. Assessing and addressing cognitive impairment in bipolar disorder: the International Society for Bipolar Disorders Targeting Cognition Task Force recommendations for clinicians. Bipolar Disord 2018;20(3):184–94.
106. Judd LL, Schettler PJ, Solomon DA, et al. Psychosocial disability and work role function compared across the long-term course of bipolar I, bipolar II and unipolar major depressive disorders. J affective Disord 2008;108(1–2):49–58.
107. Judd LL, Akiskal HS, Schettler PJ, et al. The comparative clinical phenotype and long term longitudinal episode course of bipolar I and II: a clinical spectrum or distinct disorders? J affective Disord 2003;73(1–2):19–32.
108. Pallaskorpi S, Suominen K, Ketokivi M, et al. Incidence and predictors of suicide attempts in bipolar I and II disorders: a 5-year follow-up study. Bipolar Disord. 2017;19(1):13-22.
109. King S, Stone JM, Cleare A, et al. A systematic review on neuropsychological function in bipolar disorders type I and II and subthreshold bipolar disorders—something to think about. CNS Spectrums 2019;24(1):127–43.
110. Joslyn C, Hawes DJ, Hunt C, et al. Is age of onset associated with severity, prognosis, and clinical features in bipolar disorder? A meta-analytic review. Bipolar Disord 2016;18(5):389–403.
111. Yapıcı Eser H, Taşkıran AS, Ertınmaz B, et al. Anxiety disorders comorbidity in pediatric bipolar disorder: a meta-analysis and meta-regression study. Acta Psychiatr Scand 2020;141(4):327–39.
112. Cirone C, Secci I, Favole I, et al. What do we know about the long-term course of early onset bipolar disorder? A review of the current evidence. Brain Sci 2021; 11(3). https://doi.org/10.3390/brainsci11030341.
113. Tozzi F, Manchia M, Galwey NW, et al. Admixture analysis of age at onset in bipolar disorder. Psychiatry Res 2011;185(1–2):27–32.
114. Coryell W, Fiedorowicz J, Leon AC, et al. Age of onset and the prospectively observed course of illness in bipolar disorder. J affective Disord 2013; 146(1):34–8.
115. Coryell W, Solomon DA, Fiedorowicz JG, et al. Anxiety and outcome in bipolar disorder. Am J Psychiatry 2009;166(11):1238–43.
116. Otto MW, Simon NM, Wisniewski SR, et al. Prospective 12-month course of bipolar disorder in out-patients with and without comorbid anxiety disorders. Br J Psychiatry 2006;189:20–5.
117. Mazza M, Mandelli L, Di Nicola M, et al. Clinical features, response to treatment and functional outcome of bipolar disorder patients with and without co-occurring substance use disorder: 1-year follow-up. J Affect Disord 2009; 115(1–2):27–35.
118. Baethge C, Baldessarini RJ, Khalsa HM, et al. Substance abuse in first-episode bipolar I disorder: indications for early intervention. Am J Psychiatry 2005; 162(5):1008–10.

119. Strakowski SM, Keck PE, McElroy SL, et al. Twelve-month outcome after a first hospitalization for affective psychosis. Arch Gen Psychiatry 1998;55(1):49–55.

120. Perlis RH, Delbello MP, Miyahara S, et al. Revisiting depressive-prone bipolar disorder: polarity of initial mood episode and disease course among bipolar I systematic treatment enhancement program for bipolar disorder participants. Biol Psychiatry 2005;58(7):549–53.

121. Treuer T, Tohen M. Predicting the course and outcome of bipolar disorder: a review. Eur Psychiatry 2010;25(6):328–33.

122. Farias CA, Cardoso TA, Mondin TC, et al. Clinical outcomes and childhood trauma in bipolar disorder: a community sample of young adults. Research Support, Non-U.S. Gov't. Psychiatry Res 2019;275:228–32.

123. Post RM, Altshuler LL, Kupka R, et al. Double jeopardy in the United States: early onset bipolar disorder and treatment delay. Psychiatry Res 2020;292: 113274.

124. Stahl S. In: G, Meghan M, editors. Stahl's Essential Psychopharmacology Prescriber's guide. New York: Cambridge University Press; 2014.

125. Kishi T, Ikuta T, Matsuda Y, et al. Pharmacological treatment for bipolar mania: a systematic review and network meta-analysis of double-blind randomized controlled trials. Mol Psychiatry 2021;1–9.

126. Miura T, Noma H, Furukawa TA, et al. Comparative efficacy and tolerability of pharmacological treatments in the maintenance treatment of bipolar disorder: a systematic review and network meta-analysis. Lancet Psychiatry 2014;1(5): 351–9.

127. Kadakia A, Dembek C, Heller V, et al. Efficacy and tolerability of atypical antipsychotics for acute bipolar depression: a network meta-analysis. BMC Psychiatry 2021;21(1):1–16.

128. Kishi T, Ikuta T, Matsuda Y, et al. Mood stabilizers and/or antipsychotics for bipolar disorder in the maintenance phase: a systematic review and network meta-analysis of randomized controlled trials. Mol Psychiatry 2021;26(8): 4146–57.

129. Bahji A, Ermacora D, Stephenson C, et al. Comparative efficacy and tolerability of pharmacological treatments for the treatment of acute bipolar depression: a systematic review and network meta-analysis. J affective Disord 2020;269: 154–84.

Schizophrenia: One Name, Many Different Manifestations

Justin Faden, DO[a],*, Leslie Citrome, MD, MPH[b,1]

KEYWORDS

- Schizophrenia • Antipsychotics • Psychopharmacology • Neuropathophysiology
- Psychosis • Dopamine • First episode psychosis

KEY POINTS

- Schizophrenia is a disabling syndrome associated with functional impairment, social isolation, and a decreased life-expectancy.
- Characteristic symptoms include a range of positive, negative, and cognitive psychopathology, with no pathognomonic presentation.
- The etiology of schizophrenia is diverse, and likely includes genetic and environmental risk factors involving distinct neurotransmitters and neurocircuits.
- The pharmacologic treatment of schizophrenia currently consists of postsynaptic dopamine D2 receptor antagonists and can be enhanced by supportive psychosocial interventions.
- New pharmacologic treatments for schizophrenia targeting nondopaminergic receptors are in clinical development.

INTRODUCTION

Schizophrenia is a chronic and debilitating condition with a global prevalence of approximately 1% varying by location and diagnostic criterion.[1,2] The average age of onset is in late adolescence to early twenties in men, and slightly later in women. However, determining the age of onset depends on the recognized symptom, with changes in personality and cognition often occurring before frank psychosis.[3,4] Schizophrenia is associated with considerable morbidity, and is considered one of the top 20 causes of global disability, and the top cause during its acute phase.[5,6]

Although there are effective pharmacologic and supportive psychosocial treatments for schizophrenia, most patients will have an incomplete response to treatment and have residual symptoms.[7] There is often a stepwise decline, especially after episodes of symptom exacerbation, whereby the time to treatment response is variable and

[a] Lewis Katz School of Medicine at Temple University, 100 East Lehigh Avenue, Suite 305B, Philadelphia, PA 19125, USA; [b] New York Medical College, Valhalla, NY, USA
[1] Present address: 11 Medical Park Drive, Suite 102, Pomona, NY 10970.
* Corresponding author.
E-mail address: Justin.Faden@tuhs.temple.edu

Med Clin N Am 107 (2023) 61–72
https://doi.org/10.1016/j.mcna.2022.05.005
0025-7125/23/© 2022 Elsevier Inc. All rights reserved.

medical.theclinics.com

can take longer to occur after each schizophrenia relapse.[8] Consequently, a key aspect of treatment is enhancing medication adherence and limiting relapse. Continuous treatment has been shown to be more efficacious than intermittent treatment (pharmacologic treatment only being restarted during the first manifestation of acute symptoms).[9]

Schizophrenia is associated with multiple psychosocial sequelae and low rates of functional recovery. Individuals with schizophrenia have high rates of unemployment, homelessness, incarceration, divorce/being unmarried, social isolation, and a decreased overall quality of life.[7] They also report high rates of shame and experiencing stigma.[10] Moreover, the caregivers of those with schizophrenia also report subjective and objective increases in burden and decreases in quality of life.[7,11] Stigmatization and social isolation can also extend to the caregivers which can further exacerbate family burden and reduced quality of life.

Patients diagnosed with schizophrenia have a 2.08 times increased risk of mortality compared with the general population.[12] The life expectancy for individuals with schizophrenia is approximately 15 years less than the general population with the most common cause of death being cardiovascular disease.[13] Individuals with schizophrenia have poor physical health along with low rates of health care utilization, sedentary lifestyles, high rates of nicotine dependence, alcohol use, metabolic syndrome, and obesity.[14] Furthermore, antipsychotic medications, the cornerstone of treatment of schizophrenia, can precipitate and exacerbate metabolic syndrome and weight gain, though studies have also shown that antipsychotic naïve individuals with schizophrenia can also have impaired lipid and glucose regulation. Nearly 1/3 of individuals with schizophrenia will attempt suicide, and 5% will die by suicide.[7,15] Young individuals are at the greatest risk for suicide, with rates 10 times higher than that of the general US population (Standardized mortality ratio: 10.19; 95% confidence interval (CI): 9.29–11.18).[15]

DIAGNOSIS

The diagnosis of schizophrenia is reached after satisfying the criteria in the Diagnostic and Statistical Manual of Mental Disorders (DSM-5-TR).[16] Individuals must have 2 or more of the following symptoms: delusions, hallucinations, disorganized speech, disorganized behavior, and negative symptoms (eg, avolition, anhedonia). Symptoms should be present for at least 1 month, with continuous signs of disturbance for at least 6 months (or less if successfully treated). Additionally, symptoms must be associated with functional impairment.[16] Although the diagnosis can be made using standardized interviewing or scales, such as the Structured Clinical Interview for DSM-5 (SCID-5), clinicians typically assess for schizophrenia by obtaining a comprehensive history, including family history, speaking with collateral sources of information, and conducting a mental status examination.[17,18] Although psychotic symptoms typically result in the patient first receiving medical attention and may be the most concerning and obvious, any symptom can predominate.

Another method of conceptualizing schizophrenia is as a constellation of symptoms with 3 primary domains: (1) positive (eg, delusions, hallucinations, disorganized thought process), (2) negative (eg, apathy, affective flattening, social isolation, anhedonia), and (3) cognitive (eg, memory, executive function). Schizophrenia is heterogeneous. There is no pathognomonic presentation and individual symptoms vary. However, despite a myriad of distinct symptom presentations, pharmacologic treatment is fairly uniform consisting of antipsychotic medications.

Although psychotic symptoms may be the most apparent, they are often preceded by negative and cognitive symptoms in a period known as the psychosis prodrome. The duration of the prodrome varies and can last for months to years, typically characterized by subtle and gradual changes in behavior, personality, and functioning.[19] However, in other cases, the onset of psychosis can occur abruptly in otherwise highly functioning individuals. Characterizing symptoms is important as positive symptoms are much more amenable to treatment than negative and cognitive symptoms.

At present, there is no blood test for schizophrenia, and as such, schizophrenia is a diagnosis of exclusion. Not all psychosis is schizophrenia, and alternative organic and psychiatric etiologies must be ruled out before a diagnosis of schizophrenia can be reached.[20] A partial list of conditions that can present with symptoms of psychosis is listed in **Table 1**.

ETIOLOGY

The etiology of schizophrenia is unclear and there any many different hypotheses. However, it is likely multifactorial, and as schizophrenia is a heterogeneous condition with different presentations, it is likely that there is more than one cause. Schizophrenia is likely an umbrella concept with multiple distinct conditions and subtypes.[21]

Genetics Versus Environment

Evidence from family, twin, and adoption studies have identified a strong genetic predisposition toward schizophrenia, with heritability ranging from 64% to 81%.[22] Moreover, psychiatric disorders are polygenic, and the family of those with schizophrenia also has an increased risk for manifesting other psychiatric conditions, such as bipolar disorder, major depressive disorder, ADHD, and autism spectrum disorder.[23] Genome-wide association studies have identified that approximately 1/3 of the genetic risk for schizophrenia could be attributed to common genetic variation in over 100 distinct loci which individually contribute small genetic effects.[23,24] Although inheritance is the greatest risk factor, only 1/3 of individuals with schizophrenia have a family history of it. Environmental factors also likely contribute, including male sex, greater paternal age, obstetric and prenatal complications, adverse childhood events,

Table 1 Selected psychiatric and medical causes of psychosis	
Psychiatric Conditions	**Medical Conditions**
Schizoaffective disorder	Delirium
Bipolar disorder	Dementia
Major depressive disorder	Substance abuse
Postpartum depression	Thyroid disorder
Brief psychotic episode	Systemic lupus erythematosus
Schizophreniform disorder	Temporal lobe epilepsy
Delusional disorder	Brain tumor
Obsessive-compulsive disorder	Anti-NMDA receptor encephalitis
Body dysmorphic disorder	Acute intermittent porphyria
Schizotypal personality disorder	Wilson's disease
Borderline personality disorder	Neurosyphilis
Autism spectrum disorder	Vitamin deficiency
	Cushing syndrome
	HIV
	Parkinsons disease
	Multiple sclerosis
	Medication induced
	Traumatic brain injury
	Huntington disease
	Sepsis

immigration, being born or raised in urban areas, and being born in the late-winter to early-spring. Infections have also shown an increased risk, suggesting that the immune system may play a role in the pathogenesis of schizophrenia.[25,26]

Pathophysiology

Historically it was felt that dopaminergic dysfunction resulted in the symptoms of schizophrenia; however, it is likely more complex involving multiple neurotransmitter systems including dopamine, serotonin, and glutamate.

Antipsychotic medications function, in part, by blocking postsynaptic dopamine D2 receptors in the striatum, leading to the hypothesis that dopamine neurotransmitter dysfunction at that location is central to the pathogenesis of schizophrenia. Individuals at: (1) high risk to develop schizophrenia, (2) are in their prodromal phase, (3) are in their first episode of psychosis (FEP), and (4) with chronic schizophrenia have an increased striatal presynaptic dopamine synthesis capacity relative to those without schizophrenia.[27] Administration of dopamimetic agents, such as cocaine and amphetamine, and dopamine precursors such as levodopa, can mimic the positive symptoms of schizophrenia. However, the dopamine hypothesis of schizophrenia is incomplete and does not account for all presentations. Substances that also mimic schizophrenia symptoms are N-methyl-D-aspartate (NMDA) glutamate receptor antagonists, such as dextromethorphan, ketamine, and phencyclidine (PCP), giving credence to the hypofunctioning NMDA receptor hypothesis for schizophrenia, which suggests psychosis is the result of hypofunctioning NMDA receptors on GABA interneurons. Moreover, PCP and ketamine also mimic the negative and cognitive symptoms of schizophrenia, rather than just the positive. Anterior cingulate cortex proton magnetic resonance spectroscopy (^{1}H-MRS) studies and postmortem studies have identified glutamatergic abnormalities in individuals with schizophrenia.[25,28] The hypofunctioning NMDA receptor hypothesis of schizophrenia does not negate the role of dopamine dysfunction in schizophrenia. Dopaminergic hyperactivity is a downstream consequence of glutaminergic dysfunction, resulting in increased dopamine release in the mesolimbic pathway.[29]

In addition to antagonizing dopamine D2 receptors, second-generation antipsychotics (SGAs) also antagonize serotonin 5-HT2a receptors. Overactive 5-HT2a receptors and excess serotonin can result in psychotic symptoms, similar to the psychomimetic effects of 5-HT2a agonists such as LSD and psilocybin. A possible mechanism is that excess serotonin results in the downstream release of glutamate to the ventral tegmental area (VTA), and, analogous to NMDA receptor agonists, causes a further downstream release of mesolimbic dopamine.[29] To support the role of excess serotonin causing psychotic symptoms, pimavanserin, a serotonin 5-HT2a/5-HT2c antagonist/inverse agonist without affinity to the dopamine D2 receptor, treats Parkinson's disease psychosis and is being investigated as a treatment of schizophrenia and Alzheimer's disease psychosis.[30]

Although "all roads may eventually lead to dopamine," there are likely many distinct and interconnected neurotransmitter pathways involving dopamine, glutamate, and serotonin which can result in the symptoms of schizophrenia. It is unlikely that one neurotransmitter is responsible for all schizophrenia presentations, and schizophrenia remains a heterogeneous disorder. Parsing out the etiology of these pathways and individualizing treatment will be a goal of future treatments.

NEUROBIOLOGY OF SCHIZOPHRENIA

No single area of the brain is likely to account for all symptoms of schizophrenia, and several imaging modalities, such as MRI, magnetic resonance spectroscopy (MRS), positron emission tomography (PET), functional MRI (fMRI), diffusion tensor imaging (DTI), arterial spin labeling (ASL), and neurite orientation dispersion and density imaging (NODDI), among others, have consistently identified abnormalities in brain structure, function, connectivity, and chemistry.[31] Abnormalities are diffuse but are more pronounced in the cortex and subcortical brain regions. Moreover, the origins of these abnormalities have been suggested to occur during early brain development as well as around the time of psychosis onset.[31] Multiple structural abnormalities in schizophrenia have been identified, including (1) smaller hippocampal volumes followed by a smaller amygdala, thalamus, nucleus acumbens, and overall intracranial volume, (2) larger pallidum and lateral ventricle volumes, (3) widespread cortical thinning, (4) gray matter alterations in frontal, temporal, and cingulate cortices, and (5) abnormalities in white matter connections leading to inefficient communication between functional brain regions.[31–33] Additionally, these changes, including decreases in overall brain tissue and gray matter density, may worsen during each psychotic exacerbation. Differences in brain perfusion and metabolism have also been noted in those with schizophrenia in comparison to controls. Individuals with schizophrenia have decreased cerebral blood flow, along with distinct areas of hypoactivation, hyperactivation, and abnormal resting-state brain activity.[31,34] Despite the myriad of reproducible findings, after neuroimaging has ruled out an organic etiology for schizophrenia symptoms, there are few clinical implications for neuroimaging findings at this time. However, neuroimaging has been suggested as an objective biomarker that could one day assist with diagnostic uncertainty and treatment decisions.[35] Biomarkers could also help to predict the risk for developing psychosis in someone that is in their prodromal phase or is at a high risk to develop schizophrenia. Biomarker targets include gray matter loss, NMDA receptor dysconnectivity in the excitatory/inhibitory balance resulting in altered functional network architecture, dopamine hyperactivity, NMDA hypofunction, hippocampal hyperactivity, and autoimmune or neuroinflammation dysregulation.[35]

TREATMENT
Pharmacologic

Efficacy
The mainstay of pharmacologic treatment of schizophrenia consists of first-generation antipsychotic (FGA) and second-generation antipsychotic (SGA) medications. An example of a commonly used FGA is haloperidol, and an example of a commonly used SGA is risperidone. Most antipsychotics are now available as generic medications. Antipsychotic medications have efficacy in treating the positive symptoms of schizophrenia, however, they are less effective at treating negative and cognitive symptoms.[36] Most of the evidence supports continuous treatment with antipsychotic medications as opposed to intermittent treatment which is discontinued on symptomatic remission, though there is debate about this and large studies have attempted to evaluate this question.[37] A meta-analysis of 20 studies showed that the long-term mortality rate is lower in patients with schizophrenia treated with antipsychotic medications in comparison to those who did not use antipsychotic medications.[38] These results were consistent with a nationwide, register-based cohort study of 62,250 patients with schizophrenia, which found long-term antipsychotic use reduced morbidity and all-cause mortality.[39] When factoring in the adverse effects of antipsychotic medications, a critical appraisal of the literature still found that chronic antipsychotic use has a favorable benefit-to-risk ratio, with insufficient evidence to support significant dosage reduction in stabilized patients.[14]

Network meta-analyses of clinical trials of the available antipsychotic medications have established a hierarchy of efficacy: clozapine being superior to olanzapine, risperidone, and amisulpride [not available in US], and in turn potentially superior to all other antipsychotics.[40–42] However, differences in effect size for efficacy outcomes are generally small. Larger differences among the antipsychotics are noted for tolerability outcomes such as drug-induced Parkinsonism, akathisia, sedation/somnolence, weight gain, prolactin elevation, and ECG QTc prolongation. The American Psychiatric Association (APA) Practice Guideline for Schizophrenia recommends routine monitoring for efficacy and tolerability issues, especially early in the course of treatment when an individual is more prone to metabolic, anticholinergic, and motoric side effects.[18]

Considerations regarding the first episode of schizophrenia

Evidence exists that a prolonged duration of untreated psychosis in a person with first-episode psychosis (FEP) is associated lower rates of recovery and a worse response to treatment.[43–45] Fortunately, FEP has a high rate of response to treatment regardless of which antipsychotic medication is selected. In a meta-analysis of antipsychotic medications for the treatment of FEP, few clinically significant differences were found between individual medications. However, haloperidol had higher rates of all-cause discontinuation and was considered to be a suboptimal treatment.[46] SGAs are preferred. Given a similar response to treatment, medication should be selected based on the side-effect profile and dosed conservatively to enhance treatment adherence.

Treatment-refractory schizophrenia

Nearly one-third of individuals with schizophrenia will have an insufficient response to treatment and are considered to have treatment-refractory schizophrenia (TRS).[47] The reasons for this are multifactorial and could be secondary to underlying neurotransmitter abnormalities or different pathophysiological pathways. Before diagnosing a patient with TRS, rule out alternative etiologies, such as pharmacokinetic or pharmacodynamic failures including nonadherence with treatment, active substance abuse, drug–drug interactions, inadequate prior treatments, and subtherapeutic antipsychotic serum levels.[48] A trial of a long-acting injectable antipsychotic will help rule-out "pseudo-resistance" caused by covert nonadherence to oral antipsychotic treatment.[47] After a diagnosis is confirmed, the cornerstone of treatment is clozapine. Clozapine has consistently shown to be the most efficacious antipsychotic for treating TRS, and in addition has potent anti-suicidal and anti-aggressive properties.18 Clozapine dosage and serum level should be optimized, and treatment should persist for at least 12 weeks before deeming treatment failure.[47] Additional guidance is offered regarding safe and optimal titration.[49] If a patient is unable to tolerate clozapine or they show an inadequate response, alternative strategies include: high dose olanzapine, antipsychotic combination therapy, adjunctive medication including mood stabilizers, antidepressants, NMDA receptor modulators, neuromodulation, and psychotherapy, among others.[50,51]

Nonadherence

Despite high morbidity and mortality associated with medication nonadherence, rates of treatment adherence are low in people with schizophrenia. A review of naturalistic studies found rates of nonadherence ranging from approximately 11% to 60%, and another study showed that within 10 days of hospital discharge, up to 25% of patients with schizophrenia were nonadherent.[52,53] Strategies to enhance and monitor adherence include, but are not limited to: psychoeducation, psychotherapy, pill counts, checking medication serum levels, involving support system to remind or administer medicine, and phone or email reminder systems. Another option is the use of long-acting injectable antipsychotics (LAIs). Although LAIs are typically considered for those with a history of nonadherence, many patients prefer to receive LAIs. The most recent APA schizophrenia practice guideline reflects this, recommending "that patients receive treatment with an LAI if they prefer such treatment or if they have a history of poor or uncertain adherence."[18] Most of the evidence support LAIs in reducing rates of relapse and hospitalization and have also yielded positive results for individuals with FEP or early phase schizophrenia.[54,55] LAIs eliminate the need for daily oral medication and ensures stable serum levels, and using LAIs earlier in the disease course could improve the continuity of treatment.[56] There are several available LAIs with dosing frequency ranging from 2 weeks to 6 months.

New treatments
Despite schizophrenia having many different illness presentations, pharmacologic treatment is fairly uniform consisting today of dopamine receptor antagonists or partial agonists. Negative and cognitive symptoms are typically refractory to existing treatment unless these symptoms are secondary to positive symptoms. However, treatments with alternative mechanisms of action that do not block postsynaptic dopamine receptors are currently in phase 3 of clinical development. These include ulotaront, a trace amine-associated receptor 1 (TAAR1) agonist, and xanomeline-trospium, an M1 and M4 muscarinic cholinergic receptor agonist.[57,58] A glycine transport inhibitor (BI 425809) targeting the NMDA receptor is also being studied for cognitive impairment associated with schizophrenia.[59]

Psychosocial Interventions

In addition to pharmacotherapy, psychosocial treatments are also an integral component of the treatment of schizophrenia and can improve quality of life. This is especially relevant for negative and cognitive symptoms, which are less responsive to pharmacotherapy. Psychosocial interventions can work in tandem with pharmacologic treatments, and can synergistically alleviate symptoms and increase functioning. Psychosocial interventions include, but are not limited to: cognitive remediation and cognitive behavioral therapy, vocational rehabilitation, social skills training, family therapy, individual and family psychoeducation, assertive community treatment (ACT), and case management (also to assist with housing).[60] Psychosocial interventions can start before illness onset in high-risk individuals and may result in improvements in functioning and reduced or delayed risk of transitioning to psychosis.[61] A meta-analysis of psychosocial interventions for relapse prevention in schizophrenia identified family interventions, patient and family psychoeducation, and cognitive behavioral therapy as being especially effective in limiting relapse.[62] However, despite improved outcomes, psychosocial interventions are not available in all regions.

SUMMARY

Schizophrenia is a heterogeneous condition with many different symptomatic presentations. Its etiology is unclear, but likely includes complex genetic and environmental factors. There are multiple different neurotransmitters involved including dopamine, glutamate, and serotonin. It is likely that schizophrenia is an umbrella concept with several different neurobiological causes, and what we consider to be schizophrenia may be several distinct conditions. There are numerous brain changes associated with schizophrenia, including gray matter atrophy and white matter changes. Neuroimaging and neurotransmitter studies could help identify future biomarkers to individualize and guide care. The current medication treatment of schizophrenia consists of dopamine antagonists, which are reasonably effective at treating the positive symptoms of schizophrenia, but have limited efficacy at treating cognitive and negative symptoms. Common antipsychotic side-effects include metabolic disturbances and movement disorders, and judicious antipsychotic medication selection is warranted. Nondopaminergic medications targeting serotonin, muscarinic, and NMDA receptors are currently under investigation. Psychosocial treatment can be effective in combination with pharmacotherapy and is used to increase overall functioning and patient quality of life. There is a need for new medications with novel mechanisms of action and further research into the diverse etiologies of schizophrenia. Care should be individualized with a focus on improving and maintaining patient quality of life.

CLINICS CARE POINTS

- Individuals with schizophrenia have high rates of unemployment, homelessness, social isolation, and stigma. They can also have low self-esteem.
- The life expectancy for those with schizophrenia is 15 to 20 years less than the general population with high rates of cardiovascular disease; regular follow-up with a primary care provider is recommended.
- Prolonged periods of untreated psychosis are associated with a worse overall prognosis.
- Positive symptoms of schizophrenia are more responsive to treatment than negative and cognitive symptoms.
- A goal of treatment is to enhance medication adherence and limit symptomatic relapse. Continuous treatment with antipsychotic medication is more effective than intermittent treatment. A strategy that has been shown to improve long-term outcomes is long-acting injectable antipsychotics.
- Individuals in their first episode of psychosis have a high rate of response to treatment regardless of which antipsychotic medication is selected. Initial medication selection should be guided by medication side-effect profiles.
- Psychosocial interventions, such as psychotherapy, vocational rehabilitation, and cognitive remediation, can augment treatment response and increase patient overall functioning.

DISCLOSURE

J. Faden: No conflicts of interest. L. Citrome: Consultant: AbbVie/Allergan, Acadia, Adamas, Alkermes, Angelini, Astellas, Avanir, Axsome, BioXcel, Boehringer Ingelheim, Cadent Therapeutics, Eisai, Enteris BioPharma, HLS Therapeutics, Impel, Intra-Cellular Therapies, Janssen, Karuna, Lundbeck, Lyndra, Medavante-ProPhase, Merck, Neurocrine, Novartis, Noven, Otsuka, Ovid, Relmada, Reviva, Sage, Sunovion, Supernus, Teva, University of Arizona, and one-off ad hoc consulting for individuals/entities conducting marketing, commercial, or scientific scoping research; Speaker: AbbVie/Allergan, Acadia, Alkermes, Angelini, Eisai, Intra-Cellular Therapies, Janssen, Lundbeck, Neurocrine, Noven, Otsuka, Sage, Sunovion, Takeda, Teva, and CME activities organized by medical education companies such as Medscape, NACCME, NEI, Vindico, and Universities and Professional Organizations/Societies; Stocks (small number of shares of common stock): Bristol-Myers Squibb, Eli Lilly, J & J, Merck, Pfizer purchased greater than 10 years ago, stock options: Reviva; Royalties: Wiley (Editor-in-Chief, International Journal of Clinical Practice, through end 2019), UpToDate (reviewer), Springer Healthcare (book), Elsevier (Topic Editor, Psychiatry, Clinical Therapeutics).

REFERENCES

1. McGrath J, Saha S, Chant D, et al. Schizophrenia: a concise overview of incidence, prevalence, and mortality. Epidemiol Rev 2008;30:67–76.
2. Moreno-Küstner B, Martín C, Pastor L. Prevalence of psychotic disorders and its association with methodological issues. A systematic review and meta-analyses. PLoS One 2018;13(4):e0195687.
3. Kahn RS, Sommer IE. The neurobiology and treatment of first-episode schizophrenia. Mol Psychiatry 2015;20(1):84–97.
4. Häfner H, Maurer K, Löffler W, et al. The epidemiology of early schizophrenia. Influence of age and gender on onset and early course. Br J Psychiatry Suppl 1994;(23):29–38.
5. GBD 2017 Disease and Injury Incidence and Prevalence Collaborators. Global, regional, and national incidence, prevalence, and years lived with disability for 354 diseases and injuries for 195 countries and territories, 1990-2017: a systematic analysis for the Global Burden of Disease Study 2017. Lancet 2018; 392(10159):1789–858.
6. Salomon JA, Vos T, Hogan DR, et al. Common values in assessing health outcomes from disease and injury: disability weights measurement study for the Global Burden of Disease Study 2010. Lancet 2012;380(9859):2129–43.
7. Tandon R, Nasrallah HA, Keshavan MS. Schizophrenia, "just the facts" 4. Clinical features and conceptualization. Schizophr Res 2009;110(1–3):1–23.
8. Lieberman JA, Alvir JM, Koreen A, et al. Psychobiologic correlates of treatment response in schizophrenia. Neuropsychopharmacology 1996;14(3 Suppl): 13S–21S.
9. Kane JM, Correll CU. Optimizing Treatment Choices to Improve Adherence and Outcomes in Schizophrenia. J Clin Psychiatry 2019;80(5). IN18031AH1C.
10. Gerlinger G, Hauser M, De Hert M, et al. Personal stigma in schizophrenia spectrum disorders: a systematic review of prevalence rates, correlates, impact and interventions. World Psychiatry 2013;12(2):155–64.
11. Rhee TG, Rosenheck RA. Does improvement in symptoms and quality of life in chronic schizophrenia reduce family caregiver burden? Psychiatry Res 2019; 271:402–4.
12. Hayes JF, Marston L, Walters K, et al. Mortality gap for people with bipolar disorder and schizophrenia: UK-based cohort study 2000-2014. Br J Psychiatry 2017; 211(3):175–81.
13. Hjorthøj C, Stürup AE, McGrath JJ, et al. Years of potential life lost and life expectancy in schizophrenia: a systematic review and meta-analysis. Lancet Psychiatry 2017;4(4):295–301.
14. Correll CU, Rubio JM, Kane JM. What is the risk-benefit ratio of long-term antipsychotic treatment in people with schizophrenia? World Psychiatry 2018;17(2): 149–60.
15. Olfson M, Stroup TS, Huang C, et al. Suicide Risk in Medicare Patients With Schizophrenia Across the Life Span. JAMA Psychiatry 2021;78(8):876–85.
16. American Psychiatric Association. Diagnostic and statistical manual of mental disorders. 5th Edition, Text Revision (DSM-5-TR). Arlington (VA): American Psychiatric Publishing; 2022.
17. First M, Williams J, Karg R, et al. Structured clinical Interview for DSM-5 disorders, clinician version (SCID-5-CV). Arlington (VA): American Psychiatric Association; 2016.

18. Keepers GA, Fochtmann LJ, Anzia JM, et al. The American Psychiatric Association Practice Guideline for the Treatment of Patients With Schizophrenia. Am J Psychiatry 2020;177(9):868–72.
19. Lieberman JA, Perkins D, Belger A, et al. The early stages of schizophrenia: speculations on pathogenesis, pathophysiology, and therapeutic approaches. Biol Psychiatry 2001;50(11):884–97.
20. Citrome L. Differential diagnosis of psychosis. A brief guide for the primary care physician. Postgrad Med 1989;85(4):273–4, 279-280.
21. Farooq S, Agid O, Foussias G, et al. Using treatment response to subtype schizophrenia: proposal for a new paradigm in classification. Schizophr Bull 2013;39(6): 1169–72.
22. Tiwari AK, Zai CC, Müller DJ, et al. Genetics in schizophrenia: where are we and what next? Dialogues Clin Neurosci 2010;12(3):289–303.
23. Sullivan PF, Agrawal A, Bulik CM, et al. Psychiatric Genomics: An Update and an Agenda. Am J Psychiatry 2018;175(1):15–27.
24. Schizophrenia Working Group of the Psychiatric Genomics Consortium. Biological insights from 108 schizophrenia-associated genetic loci. Nature 2014; 511(7510):421–7.
25. Kahn RS, Sommer IE, Murray RM, et al. Schizophrenia. Nat Rev Dis Primers 2015; 1:15067.
26. Robinson N, Bergen SE. Environmental Risk Factors for Schizophrenia and Bipolar Disorder and Their Relationship to Genetic Risk: Current Knowledge and Future Directions. Front Genet 2021;12:686666.
27. Howes OD, Murray RM. Schizophrenia: an integrated sociodevelopmental-cognitive model. Lancet 2014;383(9929):1677–87.
28. Demjaha A, Egerton A, Murray RM, et al. Antipsychotic treatment resistance in schizophrenia associated with elevated glutamate levels but normal dopamine function. Biol Psychiatry 2014;75(5):e11–3.
29. Stahl SM. Beyond the dopamine hypothesis of schizophrenia to three neural networks of psychosis: dopamine, serotonin, and glutamate. CNS Spectr 2018; 23(3):187–91.
30. Tariot PN, Cummings JL, Soto-Martin ME, et al. Trial of Pimavanserin in Dementia-Related Psychosis. N Engl J Med 2021;385(4):309–19.
31. Keshavan MS, Collin G, Guimond S, et al. Neuroimaging in Schizophrenia. Neuroimaging Clin N Am 2020;30(1):73–83.
32. van Erp TGM, Hibar DP, Rasmussen JM, et al. Subcortical brain volume abnormalities in 2028 individuals with schizophrenia and 2540 healthy controls via the ENIGMA consortium. Mol Psychiatry 2016;21(4):585.
33. van Erp TGM, Walton E, Hibar DP, et al. Cortical Brain Abnormalities in 4474 Individuals With Schizophrenia and 5098 Control Subjects via the Enhancing Neuro Imaging Genetics Through Meta Analysis (ENIGMA) Consortium. Biol Psychiatry 2018;84(9):644–54.
34. Kühn S, Gallinat J. Resting-state brain activity in schizophrenia and major depression: a quantitative meta-analysis. Schizophr Bull 2013;39(2):358–65.
35. Kraguljac NV, McDonald WM, Widge AS, et al. Neuroimaging Biomarkers in Schizophrenia. Am J Psychiatry 2021;178(6):509–21.
36. Owen MJ, Sawa A, Mortensen PB. Schizophrenia. Lancet 2016;388(10039): 86–97.
37. Davidson M. The debate regarding maintenance treatment with antipsychotic drugs in schizophrenia. Dialogues Clin Neurosci 2018;20(3):215–21.

38. Vermeulen J, van Rooijen G, Doedens P, et al. Antipsychotic medication and long-term mortality risk in patients with schizophrenia; a systematic review and meta-analysis. Psychol Med 2017;47(13):2217–28.
39. Taipale H, Tanskanen A, Mehtälä J, et al. 20-year follow-up study of physical morbidity and mortality in relationship to antipsychotic treatment in a nationwide cohort of 62,250 patients with schizophrenia (FIN20). World Psychiatry 2020; 19(1):61–8.
40. Leucht S, Corves C, Arbter D, et al. Second-generation versus first-generation antipsychotic drugs for schizophrenia: a meta-analysis. Lancet 2009;373(9657): 31–41.
41. Leucht S, Cipriani A, Spineli L, et al. Comparative efficacy and tolerability of 15 antipsychotic drugs in schizophrenia: a multiple-treatments meta-analysis. Lancet 2013;382(9896):951–62.
42. Huhn M, Nikolakopoulou A, Schneider-Thoma J, et al. Comparative efficacy and tolerability of 32 oral antipsychotics for the acute treatment of adults with multi-episode schizophrenia: a systematic review and network meta-analysis. Lancet 2019;394(10202):939–51.
43. Levi L, Bar Haim M, Burshtein S, et al. Duration of untreated psychosis and response to treatment: an analysis of response in the OPTiMiSE cohort. Eur Neuropsychopharmacol 2020;32:131–5.
44. O'Keeffe D, Kinsella A, Waddington JL, et al. 20-Year Prospective, Sequential Follow-Up Study of Heterogeneity in Associations of Duration of Untreated Psychosis With Symptoms, Functioning, and Quality of Life Following First-Episode Psychosis. Am J Psychiatry 2022;179(4):288–97.
45. Malla A. Reducing Duration of Untreated Psychosis: The Neglected Dimension of Early Intervention Services. Am J Psychiatry 2022;179(4):259–61.
46. Zhu Y, Krause M, Huhn M, et al. Antipsychotic drugs for the acute treatment of patients with a first episode of schizophrenia: a systematic review with pairwise and network meta-analyses. Lancet Psychiatry 2017;4(9):694–705.
47. Howes OD, McCutcheon R, Agid O, et al. Treatment-Resistant Schizophrenia: Treatment Response and Resistance in Psychosis (TRRIP) Working Group Consensus Guidelines on Diagnosis and Terminology. Am J Psychiatry 2017; 174(3):216–29.
48. Faden J, Citrome L. Resistance is not futile: treatment-refractory schizophrenia - overview, evaluation and treatment. Expert Opin Pharmacother 2019;20(1): 11–24.
49. de Leon J, Schoretsanitis G, Smith RL, et al. An International Adult Guideline for Making Clozapine Titration Safer by Using Six Ancestry-Based Personalized Dosing Titrations, CRP, and Clozapine Levels. Pharmacopsychiatry 2022;55(2): 73–86.
50. Correll CU, Rubio JM, Inczedy-Farkas G, et al. Efficacy of 42 Pharmacologic Co-treatment Strategies Added to Antipsychotic Monotherapy in Schizophrenia: Systematic Overview and Quality Appraisal of the Meta-analytic Evidence. JAMA Psychiatry 2017;74(7):675–84.
51. Wagner E, Kane JM, Correll CU, et al. Clozapine Combination and Augmentation Strategies in Patients With Schizophrenia -Recommendations From an International Expert Survey Among the Treatment Response and Resistance in Psychosis (TRRIP) Working Group. Schizophr Bull 2020;46(6):1459–70.
52. Kane JM, Kishimoto T, Correll CU. Non-adherence to medication in patients with psychotic disorders: epidemiology, contributing factors and management strategies. World Psychiatry 2013;12(3):216–26.

53. Leucht S, Heres S. Epidemiology, clinical consequences, and psychosocial treatment of nonadherence in schizophrenia. J Clin Psychiatry 2006;67(Suppl 5):3–8.
54. Kishimoto T, Hagi K, Kurokawa S, et al. Long-acting injectable versus oral antipsychotics for the maintenance treatment of schizophrenia: a systematic review and comparative meta-analysis of randomised, cohort, and pre-post studies. Lancet Psychiatry 2021;8(5):387–404.
55. Tiihonen J, Haukka J, Taylor M, et al. A nationwide cohort study of oral and depot antipsychotics after first hospitalization for schizophrenia. Am J Psychiatry 2011; 168(6):603–9.
56. Rubio JM, Taipale H, Tanskanen A, et al. Long-term Continuity of Antipsychotic Treatment for Schizophrenia: A Nationwide Study. Schizophr Bull 2021;47(6): 1611–20.
57. Koblan KS, Kent J, Hopkins SC, et al. A Non-D2-Receptor-Binding Drug for the Treatment of Schizophrenia. N Engl J Med 2020;382(16):1497–506.
58. Brannan SK, Sawchak S, Miller AC, et al. Muscarinic Cholinergic Receptor Agonist and Peripheral Antagonist for Schizophrenia. N Engl J Med 2021; 384(8):717–26.
59. Fleischhacker WW, Podhorna J, Gröschl M, et al. Efficacy and safety of the novel glycine transporter inhibitor BI 425809 once daily in patients with schizophrenia: a double-blind, randomised, placebo-controlled phase 2 study. Lancet Psychiatry 2021;8(3):191–201.
60. Tandon R, Nasrallah HA, Keshavan MS. Schizophrenia, "just the facts" 5. Treatment and prevention. Past, present, and future. Schizophr Res 2010; 122(1–3):1–23.
61. Janssen H, Maat A, Slot MIE, et al. Efficacy of psychological interventions in young individuals at ultra-high risk for psychosis: A naturalistic study. Early Interv Psychiatry 2021;15(4):1019–27.
62. Bighelli I, Rodolico A, García-Mieres H, et al. Psychosocial and psychological interventions for relapse prevention in schizophrenia: a systematic review and network meta-analysis. Lancet Psychiatry 2021;8(11):969–80.

Microbiome in Anxiety and Other Psychiatric Disorders

Norman M. Spivak, BS[a,b,1,*], Jonathan Haroon, BS[b,1], Andrew Swenson[b,1], Scott A. Turnbull, DO[c], Nolan Dang, BS[b], Matthew Ganeles[d], Collin Price, MD[b], Margaret Distler, MD, PhD[b], Erika Nurmi, MD, PhD[b], Helen Lavretsky, MD, MS[b], Alexander Bystritsky, MD, PhD[b]

KEYWORDS

• Microbiome • Anxiety • Gut–brain axis • PANS

KEY POINTS

- Imbalances in the gut microbiome can cause psychiatric illness.
- Treatment of psychiatric illness using standard-of-care medication can lead to changes in the microbiome.
- Microbiota changes can be seen in medical conditions associated with psychiatric illness without the presence of the psychiatric illness itself.

INTRODUCTION

One of the exciting new avenues of exploration into psychopathophysiology is the recent interest to understand better the "Gut-Brain Axis," coined by Carabotti and colleagues in 2015.[1] Their laboratory elucidated the causal factors that link the gut microbiome to psychiatric well-being. PubMed queries for literature including "gut microbiome" and "depression" return 342 results in 2021 alone, compared with 2013, when only 8 articles were published on this subject matter. Similar Pubmed trends are also observable with "microbiome" and "OCD" or "anxiety." General trends from these studies seem to point out that loss of gut diversity or overgrowth of a group of bacteria plays a role in psychiatric illness. Understanding the effect gut dysbiosis plays in the psychopathophysiology of psychiatric illness will help to improve patient care and control a growing epidemic in America. In 2019%, 5% of the world more than

[a] UCLA-Caltech Medical Scientist Training Program; [b] Department of Psychiatry and Biobehavioral Sciences, DGSOM, UCLA, 300 UCLA Medical Plaza, Suite 2200, Los Angeles, CA 90095, USA; [c] Department of Internal Medicine, Kirk Kerkorian SOM, UNLV, 4505 South Maryland Parkway, Las Vegas, NV 89154, USA; [d] Department of Molecular, Cell and Developmental Biology, UCLA, 300 UCLA Medical Plaza, Suite 2200, Los Angeles, CA 90095, USA
[1] These authors contributed equally.
* Corresponding author. UCLA-Caltech Medical Scientist Training Program.
E-mail address: nspivak@mednet.ucla.edu
Twitter: @normanspivak (N.M.S.)

Med Clin N Am 107 (2023) 73–83
https://doi.org/10.1016/j.mcna.2022.08.010
0025-7125/23/© 2022 Elsevier Inc. All rights reserved.

20 years old (roughly 256,172,153.49 people) suffered from a depressive disorder with similar levels for Anxiety disorders (4.78%).[2] These numbers have likely increased due to the recent and ongoing COVID-19 pandemic.

Furthermore, many recent clinical studies have indicated how changes in the gut microbiota can modulate communication between the gut and brain in a bidirectional manner adding further impetus to study the role of gut microbiota health in psychiatric conditions.

Current psychotropic treatments for psychiatric disorders such as antidepressants, antipsychotics, and anxiolytics have shown to have antibacterial effects, potentially exacerbating microbiome dysbiosis and altering the intended pharmacologic effects of the medication.[3] Although many psychotropics shape the gut microbiome in a specific way, it is still yet to be known to what extent these compositional shifts will affect the mental well-being of the host.[4] This potentially counter-productive aspect of psychotropic treatment of patients with depression and anxiety highlights how important this study area is to better inform the type and dosage of antipsychotics.

This literature review summarizes findings in brain–gut interaction in major depressive disorder, generalized anxiety disorder, obsessive-compulsive disorder, and briefly PANDAS/PANS.

DISCUSSION

With the advent of brain imaging technology in the 80s, the bidirectional link between the gut–brain axis was fully recognized for its role in homeostatic processes in health and disease. More recently, the gut–brain axis (GBA) has become a hot topic because the microbiota has come into the spotlight as a critical regulator.[5] This vital role the microbiota played in the GBA was elucidated through 5 key findings. The first finding that initiated interest in this area of study was germ-free mice. Luczynski and colleagues found that exposure to microorganisms during development was necessary for typical stress responsivity, anxiety-like behavior, sociability, and cognition.[6] The second finding focused on how specific strains of bacteria influenced behavior. This study was followed by human studies that opened the door for the potential translatability of these animal studies.[7] Thirdly, in 2010 a study on the outbreak of acute bacterial gastroenteritis was associated with an increased incidence of irritable bowel syndrome.[8] The fourth finding was in preclinical studies; after antibiotic administration, long-lasting organizational effects in the brain, spinal cord, and the enteric nervous system were found.[9] The last piece of the puzzle was a culmination of the data from all these studies contrasted against the fact that hepatic encephalopathy could be treated using antibiotics that targeted the microbiota in humans.[10]

Since the inception of the microbiota–gut–brain axis (MGBA) concept, a flurry of studies has ensued looking to elucidate the mechanisms underpinning the MGBA. Among these studies on inflammatory bowel disease and irritable bowel syndrome, psychiatric disorders have been associated with the restructuring of the gut microbiome.[10] More recently, the microbiome has been implicated in psychiatric disorders such as anxiety,[11] depression,[12] obsessive-compulsive disorder (OCD), and pediatric acute-onset neuropsychiatric syndrome (PANS).[13]

DEPRESSION AND THE MICROBIOME

Major depressive disorder is characterized by either anhedonia or depressed mood lasting for more than 14 days with comorbid changes in sleep, appetite, weight, fatigue, or suicidal ideation.[14] Clinically, depression has been associated with the dysregulation of the hypothalamic–pituitary–adrenal (HPA) axis.[15] Conversely, with the normalization of the HPA axis, improvements in MDD symptoms are seen.[16] A landmark study by Sudo and colleagues showed the direct link between microbiota and HPA function; when under stressed conditions, the administration of probiotics was able to normalize basal CORT levels.[17] These findings clearly implicated the gut microbiome in HPA axis and set the stage for a greater understanding between the gut microbiome and the onset of depression.

Continuing, depression has been shown to have a marked neuroinflammatory process in the brain.[18] Thus, it is not beyond the expectation that patients with inflammatory bowel conditions can have comorbid psychiatric conditions. For example, Limbana and colleagues showed that greater than 20% of patients with inflammatory bowel disease (IBD) have depressed mood and insomnia,[12] and 80% of all patients with IBD have some form of psychiatric comorbidities.[19] Further examination of the gut microbiome in IBD patients with depression and IBD patients without depression revealed that the depressed group mainly had Firmicutes, Bacteroides, and Actinobacteria in the gut.[20–22] Depression has also been shown to increase the permeability of the gut barrier, which allows bacteria previously contained in the gut to seep into circulation, causing inflammation and leading to a condition called "leaky gut."[23] With healthier diets that include foods high in dietary fiber and low levels of saturated fat, gut microbiota health was shown to improve while decreasing the risk of depression.[23] Furthermore, in a large epidemiologic study in the United Kingdom, it was found that a single course of antibiotics can induce dysbiosis of gut microbiota and was associated with a 20% increase in depression.[24]

Although much data have been collected on the distinct composition of the depressed microbiome, the causal mechanism of the microbiome in the development of major depressive disorder (MDD) was not clear until recently. In 2016, 2 animal studies presented independent, comparable, and distinct evidence of the causal role of the microbiome in MDD through microbiome transplantation experiments from humans to animals. In these animal experiments, rats and mice received fecal transplants from humans with MDD. After fecal microbiome transplantation from MDD volunteers, increased levels of inflammation, anhedonia-like (quantified through sucrose preference test), and anxiety-like behavior (measured by open field test and elevated plus maze test) were displayed in comparison to the mice and rats that received fecal microbiome transplantation from healthy volunteers.[25,26] While these are only animal studies, these behavioral findings support the implication of microbiome health in MDD. General trends have emerged in human and animal trials associating increases in depressive-like behavior with alpha diversity and increases in the relative abundance of certain microbes with the proinflammatory state.

A further advancement toward elucidating the effect of microbiome dysbiosis was made in 2022. A study by Lee and colleagues examined the bidirectional relationship interactions between the brain and gut as applied to aging and aging-related depression. Previous studies have demonstrated that gray matter volume (GMV) loss in the limbic region on MRI has been widely observed in patients with depression.[27,28] Thus, the study set out to see if there was a correlation between gut microbiome composition and loss of GMV in the limbic system. 16 subjects were enrolled in the study and underwent T1-MRI imaging of the brain with GMV analysis of the limbic system (specifically the hippocampus, amygdala, nucleus accumbens) and stool sample collection and analysis. They found a significant correlation between GMV loss and a loss of fecal microbiota alpha diversity. In addition, fecal microbiome composition predicted treatment response and remission of geriatric depression, with 7 genera being highly predictive of depression remission. Of these, the enrichment of *Faecalibacterium*, *Agathobacter*, and *Roseburia* were most significant.

By examining the effect of different diets on the gut, Dinan and colleagues found that incorporating increased consumption of fiber and fish into diets resulted in abundant bacteria with anti-inflammatory properties.[29] This diet adjustment, similar to a large portion of the well-studied Mediterranean diet, has been shown to increase the number of microbes in the guts while also shortening episodes of depression.[30,31]

Thus, these experimental findings lend credence to the idea that specific microbiota changes are pathognomonic for major depressive disorder.

ANXIETY AND THE MICROBIOME

General Anxiety Disorder is characterized by decreased social and occupational function. Current treatments combine psychotherapy with pharmacotherapy to address the symptoms of anxiety. In recent years, a growing amount of literature has indicated that gut microbiota plays a role in regulating brain function and that dysbiosis of the gut microbiota is associated with anxiety. In a meta-analysis by Yang and colleagues, 67% of participants with anxiety also had IBS, suggesting the involvement of dysbiosis in the onset of anxiety.[13] The current hypothesis is that the microbiota provides essential inflammatory mediators in the immune system, which is why long-term dysbiosis, seen in conditions such as IBS, can lead to chronic immune activation, brain dysfunction, and anxiety disorders.[32,33]

As previously mentioned in the section on depression, the gut microbiota's impact on the HPA axis is highly implicated in these changes in brain function.[17] Anxiety and situational fear influence typical GI functions, negatively affecting the intestinal microbiome.[34] In patients with GAD, Jiang and colleagues found a lower prevalence of Faecalibacterium, Eubacterium rectale, Lachnospira, Butyricicoccus, and Sutterella, all-important producers of short-chain fatty acids (SCFA).[35] SCFAs are linked to the facilitation of the pro-inflammatory response with resultant neural feedback loops.[36] These pro-inflammatory cytokines are essential because their role in the inhibition of the enzyme tetrahydrobiopterin, which plays a critical role in synthesizing dopamine, serotonin, and norepinephrine.[18] This decrease in bacteria necessary for SCFA production is the crux of the monoamine hypothesis for anxiety and depression. These increases in inflammatory mediators are also correlated to increased levels of cortisol.[37] Both, increased cortisol and proinflammatory state lead to increased intestinal permeability and subsequently neural inflammation.

Although there have been many studies confirming the association between dysbiosis and anxiety, there have yet to be conclusive results on the effectiveness of targeting the microbiota for the treatment of anxiety in humans. The difficulty in studying the direct link between anxiety and the microbiome was the chronic diseases comorbid with anxiety symptoms. Despite this, in the limited studies on healthy individuals, there was a strong correlation between the modulation of the gut microbiome and the alleviation of anxiety symptoms.[38–40] More conclusive evidence was found in animal studies showing how anxiety-like behavior in germ-free mice could be regulated by the modulation of the gut microbiome. These findings combined with the data collected from healthy participants suggest translatability of the findings from animals studies and that the microbiota will be an effective treatment target for anxiety.[41–43]

OBSESSIVE-COMPULSIVE DISORDER AND THE MICROBIOME

Obsessive-compulsive disorder (OCD) involves intrusive (obsessions) and/or intrusive thoughts that are paired with compensatory actions to relieve the resulting mental burden (compulsions). OCD can be debilitating, and early diagnosis and treatment are vital. There are limited treatment methods for OCD, so the potential for a new pharmacologic target is desired. The current standard treatment is serotonin reuptake inhibitors. Although SRIs are adequate, with a favorable side effect profile, about 50% of patients respond incompletely.[44]

Many current studies surrounding the gut–brain axis and the microbiome are regarding anxiety and mood. For OCD specifically, there has been speculation about the role that the microbiota–gut–brain axis might play in the development of OCD; however, all these studies have only examined the association between OCD and gut dysbiosis. There is only one study by Turna and colleagues directly studying the role of gut dysbiosis on OCD. Their study compared 21 nondepressed, medication-free patients with OCD and 22 age- and sex-matched nonpsychiatric community controls.[45] Using Illumina to sequence and analyze the microbiota, Turna and colleagues found that compared with controls, the OCD group had lower species richness, evenness, and relative abundance of three butyrate-producing genera (Oscillospira, Odoribacter, and Anaerostipes). The results from this study further lend credence to gut dysbiosis and the resulting inflammation associated with OCD.

In another study, Rees and colleagues suggested that the connection between OCD and the GBA lay in the hypothalamus–pituitary–adrenal (HPA) axis.[46] This implication of the HPA axis in OCD was supported by the association of a hyperactive HPA axis and OCD. In pregnant women, there is a marked increase in HPA axis activity associated with the onset of OCD.[47–49] Other stressful situations that increased HPA axis activity, such as "professional difficulties," were also implicated in the late onset of OCD.[50] Furthermore, in patients with OCD, increased basal activities of HPA were documented.

As OCD and the microbiome is still a largely unexplored area, there has been one direct study in mice treating OCD using the probiotic L. rhamnosus. Kantak and colleagues first RU24969 (5-HT1A/1B receptor agonist) as a way to induce OCD-like symptoms.[51] Then, a probiotic formulation as well as a traditional treatment of OCD fluoxetine as a first-line treatment of 4 weeks. Both treatment groups saw marked improvements in OCD-like behaviors. RU24969 has also been observed to exacerbate OCD symptoms in humans, suggesting the translatability of these findings to humans. Another study by Messaoudi and colleagues also supported the translatability of the findings from Kantak and colleagues In response to daily administrations of probiotic formulations, healthy humans reduced the subscores related to obsessive-compulsive disorders.[52]

While preliminary, much of the data surrounding OCD and the microbiome suggest a direct role of dysbiosis, inflammatory response, and the HPA axis in the development of OCD. Due to the large overlap in the role of the HPA in MDD, anxiety, and OCD, there is a good reason to believe that much of the research in humans for MDD and anxiety can be applied to OCD as well because of the recent view of Anxiety/OCD/Depression being different phenotypes of the same disorder.

PANDAS/PANS AND THE MICROBIOME

Pediatric Acute-Onset Neuropsychiatric Syndrome (PANS) is a pediatric disorder characterized by sudden onset of OCD, severe eating restriction, and at least 2 concomitant neurologic, psychiatric, or cognitive symptoms.[27] Though PANDAS is a rare condition, estimates suggest that up to 1/200 children and/or 25% of children diagnosed with OCD or Tic disorders may be afflicted with PANS/PANDAS. ("Statistics") Theories as to the etiology of PANS are wide-ranging: psychological trauma, postinfectious autoimmune processes, cerebral vasculitis, neuropsychiatric lupus, and others.[27,53] However, up to 80% of patients with PANS have shown evidence of postinfectious autoimmunity or neuroinflammation.[54] When symptoms of PANS are detected in a child who has had a recently confirmed Group A Streptococcus infection. The disorder was classically classified as Pediatric Autoimmune Neuropsychiatric Disorders Associated with Streptococcal Infections (PANDAS). In recent reviews, PANDAS was not found to be a distinctly separate syndrome from PANS, and the proinflammatory state characteristic of PANDAS could be caused by other infectious or inflammatory states.[55] Additionally, Selective Serotonin Reuptake Inhibitors were found to be the most effective treatment of symptoms of PANDAS over antibiotics and nonsteroidal anti-inflammatories (NSAIDs) that had been the traditional mainstay of treatment. Suggesting that the treatment of the streptococcal infection itself may not prevent PANDAS development.[56]

It has been suggested that either the Group A Streptococcus infections or the antibiotic used to treat them alter the gut microbiota, resulting in a bacterial profile that is proinflammatory compared with baseline.[13] Other bacteria (Such as EHEC or EAEC), viral infections, or mixed bacteria viral infections have been shown to have significantly affected the gut microbiome composition.[56] Furthermore, it has long been known that antibiotics significantly affect the composition of the gut microbiome.[57] Interestingly, the pathogenesis of Systemic Lupus erythematosus (SLE, one of the possible etiologic factors contributing to PANS development) was significantly affected by gut microbiome dysbiosis murine models.[58] Thus, the causative autoimmune or proinflammatory state in PANS/PANDAS likely is affected by dysbiosis of the gut microbiome.

The first analysis of the changes in the gut microbiome associated with PANDAS was conducted in 2018 by Quagliariello and colleagues.[15] This study recruited 30 patients with PANS/PANDAS aged 4 to 16 in Rome, Italy, and compared their gut microbiome composition against 70 healthy controls of similar age. The study excluded patients with recent infection, bowel disorder, or recent use of antibiotics to control potential confounding variables. Each patient had 3 samples collected on 3 consecutive days; from these samples, genomic DNA and 16s rRNA were collected from the samples. These sequences were further organized into Operational taxonomical units (OTUs) and compared to the Greengenes database to determine species present and compiled into a phylogenetic tree. Samples were analyzed for *alpha* and *beta* diversity. Finally, the metagenomic functionality was determined using PICRUSt software, using HUMANnV2 v.099. The sample was compared with the KEGG (Kyoto Encyclopedia of Genes and Genomes) to determine functionality.

Overall, patients with PANS/PANDAS were found to have a lower level of alpha-diversity and when analyzing beta diversity, subjects in the 4 to 6 and 7 to 8 years old (grouped together called y-PANS) range were found to have microbiomes that were significantly different from the controls of the same age. In the y-PANS group, patients were found to have a statistically significant increase in the percentage of Bacteroidetes (*Odoribacter*, *Bacteroides*, and *Oscillospira)* OTUs and a statistically significant decrease in Firmicutes and TM7 OTUs. Through further analysis with PICRUSt using the KEGG database, it was found that the PANS/PANDAS strongly expressed pathways associated with glycan biosynthesis and degradation, fatty acid, energy, and vitamin metabolism; however, they showed decreased expression of pathways associated with immune response modulation and neurologic functions.

Though the exploration of the effect of microbiome on PANS/PANDAs is still in its infancy Quagliariello and colleagues propose that streptococcal infections do alter the gut microbiome and lead to altered expression of pathways regulating brain functions such as small chain fatty acids, D-alanine, tyrosine, and dopamine could potentially influence behavior.

SUMMARY

Antidepressants, antipsychotics, and anxiolytics, among other psychotropic medications for psychiatric illnesses have been demonstrated to have antibacterial effects, potentially aggravating microbiome dysbiosis and modifying the medication's intended pharmacologic effects. Although many psychotropics have a specific effect on the gut microbiome, it is yet unknown to what extent these compositional modifications may affect the patient's mental health.

The advent of the transdiagnostic theory of depression, anxiety and OCD has both clinical and broad research utility. Since, it suggests that anxiety, depression, OCD, and by extension PANS/PANDAS are different phenotypes of the same disorder; it is possible to look for general trends within the data for all 4 conditions.

A loss of Alpha Diversity seems to play a key role in the pathogenesis of these diseases. Likely, the increase of proinflammatory genera relative to the decrease in anti-inflammatory genera leads to an overall inflammatory state.[13,25,35,45] This may lead to increases in endogenous hormones, such as cortisol, leading to an increased risk for developing an anxiety disorder. Loss of alpha diversity is reported as the most common finding in studies examining the intestinal microbiome, yet no cause of this loss in diversity has been fully explored.[37] An interesting hypothesis was proposed by Mosca and colleagues, they posited that the "western lifestyle" such as the administration of antibiotics, eating disorders, and irregular sleep–wake cycle could negatively affect the diversity of the gut microbiota.[59] They point to two studies, Yatsunenko and colleagues and Lin and colleagues, that examined the gut microbiome in Americans as compared with Vensulaean and Bangladeshi individuals. Both studies found that Americans had comparatively lower levels of microbiota diversity.[58,60] They suggest that the western lifestyle causes this by removing "predatory bacteria" from the microbiota ecosystem. This allows bacteria that would usually be suppressed, to overtake their ecological niche, leading to the loss of homeostasis and proliferation of proinflammatory strains.

Additionally, increases in anerobic bacteria that produce butyrate and other SCFA were seen in OCD/Anxiety and depression. High levels of butyrate have been shown to stabilize the colonic environment and prevent the colonization of pathogenic bacteria.[61] Furthermore, butyrate has a physiologic effect on the patient. Patients with butyrate-producing genera in their gut have been shown to lower blood pressure during pregnancy and mediate the production of cortisol.[62] However, two butyrate-producing genera (*Odoribacter* and *Oscillospira)* that were elevated in Quagliariello and colleagues, were decreased in Turna and colleagues This effect would paradoxically act to decrease inflammation and dysbiosis in the y-PANS group. Thus, further studies shall be needed to elucidate the causal factors of dysbiosis leading to anxiety disorders.

While preliminary, much of the research on OCD, anxiety, depression, and PANS in relation to the microbiome suggests that dysbiosis, inflammation, and the HPA axis all play a role in their development. A difficulty in applying what is learned in these studies to living patients is how to control the individual composition of the microbiome and parse the multifactorial relationship inflammation has with these conditions. A simple solution to this would be to increase the sample size of the groups and controls being studied to create a statistically significant average microbiome, that dysbiosis could be compared against. To help elucidate causal factors and better control for potential confounding variables, future studies should focus on 3 things. One, the identification of "pathogenic dysbiosis" associated with the severity of multidimensional symptom clusters rather than discrete diagnostic entities. Thus, pathogenic dysbiosis could eventually act as a predictive assay, allowing one to know the possible severity of a condition, and practice evidence-based medicine with this information. Second, examining microbiome associations with brain imaging, neuropsychological and inflammatory assays to mathematically quantify the physiologic changes the "pathologic dysbiosis" causes. Mathematical quantification of data regarding imaging and physiologic changes will allow for more complex mathematical modeling. Finally, proposing and testing interventions capable of changing the gut microbiome and assessing the physiologic and psychological benefits of these treatments. While current studies intending to treat these conditions by altering the microbiome have been mixed, this emerging field of diagnostic medicine may be a promising direction for personalized treatments of mood disorders and pathology.

DISCLOSURE

The authors have nothing to disclose.

REFERENCES

1. Carabotti M, Scirocco A, Maselli MA, et al. The gut-brain axis: interactions between enteric microbiota, central and enteric nervous systems. Ann Gastroenterol 2015;28:203–9.
2. Rubin R. Profile: Institute for Health Metrics and Evaluation, WA, USA. Lancet 2017;389:493.
3. Tomizawa Y, et al. Effects of Psychotropics on the Microbiome in Patients With Depression and Anxiety: Considerations in a Naturalistic Clinical Setting. Int J Neuropsychopharmacol/official scientific J Collegium Internationale Neuropsychopharmacologicum 2021;24:97–107.
4. Macedo D, et al. Antidepressants, antimicrobials or both? Gut microbiota dysbiosis in depression and possible implications of the antimicrobial effects of antidepressant drugs for antidepressant effectiveness. J Affect Disord 2017;208:22–32.
5. Clarke G, et al. The microbiome-gut-brain axis during early life regulates the hippocampal serotonergic system in a sex-dependent manner. Mol Psychiatry 2013;18:666–73.
6. Luczynski P, et al. Growing up in a Bubble: Using Germ-Free Animals to Assess the Influence of the Gut Microbiota on Brain and Behavior. The Int J Neuropsychopharmacol/official scientific J Collegium Internationale Neuropsychopharmacologicum 2016;19.
7. Bercik P, et al. The intestinal microbiota affect central levels of brain-derived neurotropic factor and behavior in mice. Gastroenterology 2011;141:599–609, 609.e591-593.
8. Thabane M, et al. An outbreak of acute bacterial gastroenteritis is associated with an increased incidence of irritable bowel syndrome in children. Am J Gastroenterol 2010;105:933–9.
9. Verdu EF, et al. The role of luminal factors in the recovery of gastric function and behavioral changes after chronic Helicobacter pylori infection. Am J Physiol Gastrointest Liver Physiol 2008;295:G664–70.
10. Collins SM, Surette M, Bercik P. The interplay between the intestinal microbiota and the brain. Nat Rev Microbiol 2012;10:735–42.
11. Yang B, Wei J, Ju P, et al. Effects of regulating intestinal microbiota on anxiety symptoms: A systematic review. Gen Psychiatr 2019;32:e100056.
12. Limbana T, Khan F, Eskander N. Gut Microbiome and Depression: How Microbes Affect the Way We Think. Cureus 2020;12:e9966.

13. Quagliariello A, et al. Gut Microbiota Profiling and Gut-Brain Crosstalk in Children Affected by Pediatric Acute-Onset Neuropsychiatric Syndrome and Pediatric Autoimmune Neuropsychiatric Disorders Associated With Streptococcal Infections. Front Microbiol 2018;9:675.
14. Kennedy SH. Core symptoms of major depressive disorder: relevance to diagnosis and treatment. Dialogues Clin Neurosci 2008;10:271–7.
15. Barden N. Implication of the hypothalamic-pituitary-adrenal axis in the physiopathology of depression. J Psychiatry Neurosci 2004;29:185–93.
16. Bastiaanssen TFS, et al. Gutted! Unraveling the Role of the Microbiome in Major Depressive Disorder. Harv Rev Psychiatry 2020;28:26–39.
17. Sudo N, et al. Postnatal microbial colonization programs the hypothalamic-pituitary-adrenal system for stress response in mice. J Physiol 2004;558:263–75.
18. Miller AH, Raison CL. The role of inflammation in depression: from evolutionary imperative to modern treatment target. Nat Rev Immunol 2016;16:22–34.
19. Collins SM. A role for the gut microbiota in IBS. Nat Rev Gastroenterol Hepatol 2014;11:497–505.
20. Eckburg PB, et al. Diversity of the human intestinal microbial flora. Science 2005; 308:1635–8.
21. Diamant M, Blaak EE, de Vos WM. Do nutrient-gut-microbiota interactions play a role in human obesity, insulin resistance and type 2 diabetes? Obes Rev 2011;12: 272–81.
22. Qin J, et al. A human gut microbial gene catalogue established by metagenomic sequencing. Nature 2010;464:59–65.
23. Madison A, Kiecolt-Glaser JK. Stress, depression, diet, and the gut microbiota: human-bacteria interactions at the core of psychoneuroimmunology and nutrition. Curr Opin Behav Sci 2019;28:105–10.
24. Lurie I, Yang YX, Haynes K, et al. Antibiotic exposure and the risk for depression, anxiety, or psychosis: a nested case-control study. J Clin Psychiat 2015;76. 1522 8.
25. Zheng P, et al. Gut microbiome remodeling induces depressive-like behaviors through a pathway mediated by the host's metabolism. Mol Psychiatry 2016;21: 786–96.
26. Kelly JR, et al. Transferring the blues: Depression-associated gut microbiota induces neurobehavioural changes in the rat. J Psychiatr Res 2016;82:109–18.
27. Chang K, et al. Clinical evaluation of youth with pediatric acute-onset neuropsychiatric syndrome (PANS): recommendations from the 2013 PANS Consensus Conference. J Child Adolesc Psychopharmacol 2015;25:3–13.
28. Abe O, et al. Voxel-based analyses of gray/white matter volume and diffusion tensor data in major depression. Psychiatry Res 2010;181:64–70.
29. Dinan TG, et al. Feeding melancholic microbes: MyNewGut recommendations on diet and mood. Clin Nutr 2019;38:1995–2001.
30. Garcia-Mantrana I, Selma-Royo M, Alcantara C, et al. Shifts on Gut Microbiota Associated to Mediterranean Diet Adherence and Specific Dietary Intakes on General Adult Population. Front Microbiol 2018;9:890.
31. Lassale C, et al. Healthy dietary indices and risk of depressive outcomes: a systematic review and meta-analysis of observational studies. Mol Psychiatry 2019; 24:965–86.
32. Takeda K, Akira S. TLR signaling pathways. Semin Immunol 2004;16:3–9.
33. Zhu C, et al. Loss of Microglia and Impaired Brain-Neurotrophic Factor Signaling Pathway in a Comorbid Model of Chronic Pain and Depression. Front Psychiatry 2018;9:442.

34. Rodes L, et al. Transit time affects the community stability of Lactobacillus and Bifidobacterium species in an in vitro model of human colonic microbiotia. Artif Cells. Blood Substit. Immobil. Biotechnol. 2011;39:351–6.

35. Jiang HY, et al. Altered gut microbiota profile in patients with generalized anxiety disorder. J Psychiatr Res 2018;104:130–6.

36. Morris G, et al. The Role of the Microbial Metabolites Including Tryptophan Catabolites and Short Chain Fatty Acids in the Pathophysiology of Immune-Inflammatory and Neuroimmune Disease. Mol Neurobiol 2017;54:4432–51.

37. Winter G, Hart RA, Charlesworth RPG, et al. Gut microbiome and depression: what we know and what we need to know. Rev Neurosci 2018;29:629–43.

38. Kelly JR, et al. Lost in translation? The potential psychobiotic Lactobacillus rhamnosus (JB-1) fails to modulate stress or cognitive performance in healthy male subjects. Brain Behav Immun 2017;61:50–9.

39. Colica C, et al. Evidences of a New Psychobiotic Formulation on Body Composition and Anxiety. Mediators Inflamm 2017;2017:5650627.

40. Steenbergen L, Sellaro R, van Hemert S, et al. A randomized controlled trial to test the effect of multispecies probiotics on cognitive reactivity to sad mood. Brain Behav Immun 2015;48:258–64.

41. Neufeld KM, Kang N, Bienenstock J, et al. Reduced anxiety-like behavior and central neurochemical change in germ-free mice. Neurogastroenterol Motil 2011;23:255–64, e119.

42. Desbonnet L, Clarke G, Shanahan F, et al. Microbiota is essential for social development in the mouse. Mol Psychiatry 2014;19:146–8.

43. Arentsen T, Raith H, Qian Y, et al. Host microbiota modulates development of social preference in mice. Microb Ecol Health Dis 2015;26:29719.

44. Bloch MH, et al. Long-term outcome in adults with obsessive-compulsive disorder. Depress Anxiety 2013;30:716–22.

45. Turna J, Grosman Kaplan K, Anglin R, et al. What's bugging the gut in OCD?" a review of the gut microbiome in obsessive-compulsive disorder. Depress Anxiety 2016;33:171–8.

46. Rees JC. Obsessive-compulsive disorder and gut microbiota dysregulation. Med Hypotheses 2014;82:163–6.

47. Williams KE, Koran LM. Obsessive-compulsive disorder in pregnancy, the puerperium, and the premenstruum. J Clin Psychiat 1997;58:330–4, quiz 335-336.

48. Forray A, Focseneanu M, Pittman B, et al. Onset and exacerbation of obsessive-compulsive disorder in pregnancy and the postpartum period. J Clin Psychiat 2010;71:1061–8.

49. Neziroglu F, Anemone R, Yaryura-Tobias JA. Onset of obsessive-compulsive disorder in pregnancy. Am J Psychiatry 1992;149:947–50.

50. Millet B, et al. Phenomenological and comorbid features associated in obsessive-compulsive disorder: influence of age of onset. J Affect Disord 2004;79:241–6.

51. Kantak PA, Bobrow DN, Nyby JG. Obsessive-compulsive-like behaviors in house mice are attenuated by a probiotic (Lactobacillus rhamnosus GG). Behav Pharmacol 2014;25:71–9.

52. Messaoudi M, et al. Beneficial psychological effects of a probiotic formulation (Lactobacillus helveticus R0052 and Bifidobacterium longum R0175) in healthy human volunteers. Gut Microbes 2011;2:256–61.

53. Swedo SE, et al. Clinical presentation of pediatric autoimmune neuropsychiatric disorders associated with streptococcal infections in research and community settings. J Child Adolesc Psychopharmacol 2015;25:26–30.

54. Frankovich J, et al. Multidisciplinary clinic dedicated to treating youth with pediatric acute-onset neuropsychiatric syndrome: presenting characteristics of the first 47 consecutive patients. J Child Adolesc Psychopharmacol 2015;25:38–47.
55. Calaprice D, Tona J, Murphy TK. Treatment of Pediatric Acute-Onset Neuropsychiatric Disorder in a Large Survey Population. J Child Adolesc Psychopharmacol 2018;28:92–103.
56. Mathew S, et al. Mixed Viral-Bacterial Infections and Their Effects on Gut Microbiota and Clinical Illnesses in Children. Scientific Rep 2019;9:865.
57. Langdon A, Crook N, Dantas G. The effects of antibiotics on the microbiome throughout development and alternative approaches for therapeutic modulation. Genome Med 2016;8:39.
58. Yatsunenko T, et al. Human gut microbiome viewed across age and geography. Nature 2012;486:222–7.
59. Mosca A, Leclerc M, Hugot JP. Gut Microbiota Diversity and Human Diseases: Should We Reintroduce Key Predators in Our Ecosystem? Front Microbiol 2016;7:455.
60. Lin A, et al. Distinct distal gut microbiome diversity and composition in healthy children from Bangladesh and the United States. PLoS One 2013;8:e53838.
61. Byndloss MX, et al. Microbiota-activated PPAR-γ signaling inhibits dysbiotic Enterobacteriaceae expansion. Science 2017;357:570–5.
62. Gomez-Arango LF, et al. Increased Systolic and Diastolic Blood Pressure Is Associated With Altered Gut Microbiota Composition and Butyrate Production in Early Pregnancy. Hypertension 2016;68:974–81.

Post-traumatic Stress Disorder

Addie N. Merians, PhD[a,b], Tobias Spiller, MD[a,b], Ilan Harpaz-Rotem, PhD[a,b],
John H. Krystal, MD[a,b],*, Robert H. Pietrzak, PhD, MPH[a,b]

KEYWORDS

- Post-traumatic stress disorder • Trauma • Psychiatry • Psychotherapy
- Pharmacotherapy • Assessment

KEY POINTS

- Post-traumatic stress disorder (PTSD) assessment, whether by structured interviews like the CAPS-5 (Clinician-Administered PTSD Scale for DSM-5 [Diagnostic and Statistical Manual of Mental Disorders, 5th edition]) in psychiatric settings or the PCL-5 (PTSD Checklist for DSM-5) in nonpsychiatric settings, is vital for the diagnosis of PTSD to ensure its treatment.
- Evidence-based psychotherapy is the first-line treatment for PTSD.
- Prolonged exposure, cognitive processing therapy, and eye movement desensitization and reprocessing are the forms of psychotherapy with the best evidence for treating PTSD and are recommended by numerous PTSD treatment guidelines.
- Pharmacotherapy is common in clinical practice and often used to reduce overall PTSD severity or target specific symptoms (eg, insomnia).
- The serotonin reuptake inhibiting antidepressants, particularly the US Food and Drug Administration-approved medications sertraline and paroxetine, are the most highly validated pharmacotherapies for PTSD.

POST-TRAUMATIC STRESS DISORDER

Post-traumatic stress disorder (PTSD) is a psychiatric disorder characterized by the development of intrusive symptoms, avoidance of trauma-related cues, negative alterations in cognition and mood, and marked alterations in arousal and reactivity following exposure to a traumatic event (**Table 1**).[1] In a national sample of more than 36,000 US adults, the past-year prevalence of PTSD was 4.7%, and lifetime prevalence was 6.1%.[2] Several sociodemographic characteristics, including younger age, female gender, and lower education and income were associated with higher rates of PTSD.

a Clinical Neurosciences Division, United States Department of Veterans Affairs, National Center for Posttraumatic Stress Disorder, West Haven, CT, USA; b Department of Psychiatry, Yale School of Medicine, 300 George Street #901, New Haven, CT 06511, USA
* Corresponding author. Department of Psychiatry, Yale School of Medicine, 300 George Street #901, New Haven, CT 06511.
E-mail address: john.krystal@yale.edu

Med Clin N Am 107 (2023) 85–99
https://doi.org/10.1016/j.mcna.2022.04.003
0025-7125/23/Published by Elsevier Inc.

Table 1
Criteria of post-traumatic stress disorder

Trauma Exposure	Intrusions	Avoidance	Negative Alterations in Cognitions and Mood	Alterations in Arousal and Reactivity	Other
Actual or threatened death, serious injury, or sexual violence in 1 (or more) of the following ways: 1. Directly experiencing the traumatic event 2. Witnessing, in person, the event(s) as it occurred to others 3. Learning that the traumatic event(s) occurred to a close family member or close friend 4. Experiencing repeated or extreme exposure to aversive details of the traumatic events	1. Recurrently, involuntary, and intrusive distressing memories of the traumatic event(s) 2. Recurrent distressing dreams in which the content and/or affect of the dream are related to the traumatic event(s) 3. Dissociative reactions in which the individual feels or acts as if the traumatic event(s) were reoccurring 4. Intense or prolonged psychological distress at exposure to internal or external cues that symbolize or resemble an aspect of the traumatic event(s) 5. Marked physiologic reactions to internal or external cues that symbolize or resemble an aspect of the traumatic event(s)	Persistent avoidance of stimuli associated with the traumatic event(s), as evidenced by 1. Avoidance of or efforts to avoid distressing memories, thoughts, or feelings about or closely associated with the traumatic event(s) 2. Avoidance of or efforts to avoid external reminders (people, places, conversations, activities, objects, situations) that arouse distressing memories, thoughts, or feelings about or closely associated with the traumatic event(s)	1. Inability to remember an important aspect of the traumatic event(s) 2. Persistent and exaggerated negative beliefs or expectations about oneself, others, or the world 3. Persistent, distorted cognitions about the cause or consequences of the traumatic event(s) that lead the individual to blame themselves or others 4. Persistent negative emotional state 5. Markedly diminished interest or participation I significant activities 6. Feelings of detachment or estrangement from others 7. Persistent inability to experience positive emotions	1. Irritable behavior or angry outbursts typically expressed as verbal or physical aggression toward people or objects 2. Reckless or self-destructive behavior 3. Hypervigilance 4. Exaggerated startle response 5. Problems with concentration 6. Sleep disturbance	1. Duration of symptoms is more than 1 month 2. Disturbance causes clinically significant distress or impairment in social, occupational, or other important areas of functioning 3. Disturbance is not attributable to the physiologic effects of a substance or another medical condition

Data from American Psychiatric Association. *Diagnostic and Statistical Manual of Mental Disorders DSM-5 Fifth Edition.* 5th ed. American Psychiatric Association Publishing; 2013. Accessed May 7, 2020. https://www.appi.org/Products/DSM-Library/Diagnostic-and-Statistical-Manual-of-Mental-Disord?sku=254.

Assessment of Trauma Exposure and Post-traumatic Stress Disorder

There are several measures that can be used to assess exposure to potentially traumatic events and PTSD symptoms in various settings (**Table 2** for the gold-standard measures). The LEC-5 (Life Events Checklist for DSM-5 [Diagnostic and Statistical Manual for Mental Disorders, 5th edition]) is a self-report screening measure for exposure to 16 potentially traumatic events (PTEs) and a different event not listed. It was developed to be administered before the CAPS-5 (Clinician-Administered PTSD Scale for DSM-5) to evaluate exposure to PTEs.[3]

The gold standard of assessing PTSD is the CAPS-5.[4] The CAPS-5 is an in-depth structured diagnostic clinical interview that assesses individual symptoms of PTSD and diagnostic status. Given the scope of assessment, this is a time-intensive instrument, and administration typically takes between 45 and 60 minutes; as such, it is unlikely that it would be administered outside of specialty psychiatric settings.

The PTSD Checklist for DSM-5 (PCL-5) is a 20-item self-report measure that assesses DSM-5 PTSD symptoms.[5] The PCL-5 takes approximately 5 to 10 minutes to complete, making it easier to administer in nonpsychiatric settings where time is limited.

The Primary Care PTSD Screen for DSM-5 (PC-PTSD-5)[6] is a 6-item assessment of exposure to PTEs and PTSD symptoms that is more suitable for time-limited primary care settings. A cut-score of 3 indicates a positive PTSD screen and was determined to maximize quality of sensitivity and specificity.[6,7]

Psychotherapies for Post-Traumatic Stress Disorder

Current treatment guidelines recommend 3 front-line trauma-focused treatments — prolonged exposure (PE), cognitive processing therapy (PE), and eye movement desensitization and reprocessing (EMDR); there is currently insufficient evidence supporting preventive interventions (**Table 3**).[8-10]

Prolonged exposure

PE was developed by Edna Foa, and is a manualized, 8- to 15-session treatment with 90-minute sessions. PE targets avoidance as the symptom that prevents recovery, through helping the client engage in activities they have been avoiding because of trauma and repeated exposure to traumatic memories. PE is one of the most studied treatments for PTSD, with over 20 randomized controlled trials (RCTs).[11] Meta-analytic findings of RCTs and comparing with wait-list control conditions have found that it yields large treatment effect size reductions in PTSD symptoms and loss of diagnosis.[12]

Cognitive processing therapy

CPT was developed by Patricia Resick. and is a manualized, 12-session treatment with 60-miuten sessions. It focuses on addressing cognitive symptoms associated with PTSD that maintain avoidance of negative affect. Like PE, CPT is a rigorously studied treatment, with over 20 RCTs across various traumas, populations, and countries.[11] Meta-analyses assessing RCTs compared with wait-list control conditions and treatment as usual (TAU) have found that CPT yields large effect size reductions in PTSD symptoms and loss of diagnosis.[12,13]

Eye movement desensitization and reprocessing

EMDR[14] was developed by Francine Shapiro., and is typically administered in weekly sessions of up to 90 minutes over the course of 3 months, although length of treatment varies based on the needs of the individual.[15] It focuses on reducing the intensity of traumatic memories through eye movements; however, this mechanism is the ongoing

Table 2
Assessment of potentially traumatic events and post-traumatic stress disorder

Instrument	Type	Usage	Versions	Psychometrics
Life Events Checklist for DSM-5 (LEC-5)[3]	Self-report	To be administered before the CAPS-5 to evaluate exposure to PTEs[3]	Three versions: 1. To determine if an event occurred 2. To determine the worst event for those with multiple exposures to PTEs 3. An interview to establish if a PTE meets the criterion necessary for a diagnosis of PTSD	In various samples, including combat veterans and college students, displayed temporal stability, convergent validity, and predicted distress and PTSD symptoms[3]
CAPS-5[4]	Structured diagnostic interview[4]	Assesses PTSD diagnostic status and symptom severity, including assessment of all PTSD criteria; assessment of the dissociative subtype; and global ratings of distress, impairment, and symptom severity that has been developed for the current diagnostic criteria for PTSD in the DSM-5	One version, which takes approximately 45–60 min, designed to be administered by trained clinicians, clinical researchers, and paraprofessionals	Extensive research in a variety of samples, demonstrating strong internal consistency, interrater reliability, and test-retest reliability, while additionally being strongly correlated with other measures of PTSD[4]
PCL-5[5]	Self-report	Screening individuals for PTSD, provisional diagnosis, and monitoring change during and after treatment	4 versions: 1. Past month 2. Past week 3. With PTE assessment 4. With LEC-5 and PTE assessment	Extensive validation research in a variety of military and civilian samples, displaying high internal consistency, test-retest reliability, and convergent and discriminant reliability[5,62,63]
Primary Care PTSD Screen for DSM-5 (PC-PTSD-5)[6]	Self-report	Screening trauma exposure and PTSD symptoms in time-limited primary care settings	One version with 6 yes/no items	Validation done to create a cut-score of 3 to maximize quality of sensitivity and specificity[6,7]

Table 3
Summary of evidence of psychotherapies for the prevention and treatment of PTSD

Indication	Psychotherapy	Description	VA/DoD Guidelines (2017)[10]	APA Guidelines (2017)[c,64]	NICE Guidelines (2018)[9]	ISTSS Guidelines (2020)[8]
Prevention	Psychological first aid	Early psychosocial intervention applied during or immediately after a trauma that focuses on determining the basic physical and mental needs of an individual[65]	NA	NA	NA	Insufficient evidence
	Critical incident stress debriefing	Individual or group treatment provided hours or days after the trauma that focuses on emotional ventilation, trauma processing, and psychoeducation[66]	Not recommended, harmful	NA	Not recommended, harmful	Insufficient evidence
Treatment	Prolonged exposure	Teaches individuals to gradually approach trauma-related memories, feelings, and situations, leading to reduced avoidance and decreased PTSD symptoms[67]	High quality of evidence	High quality of evidence	High quality of evidence	High quality of evidence
	Cognitive processing therapy	Teaches individuals who to challenge and modify unhelpful beliefs related to the trauma to create new understandings of the trauma, which reduce its impact on daily life[68]	High quality of evidence	High quality of evidence	High quality of evidence	High quality of evidence
	Eye movement desensitization and reprocessing	Processes the memories of traumatic experiences that contain disturbing emotions, thoughts, beliefs, and physical sensations, thus reducing and eliminating symptoms[43,69,70]	High quality of evidence	Moderate rating of evidence	High quality of evidence	High quality of evidence

Abbreviations: DoD, department of defense; ISTSS, international society for traumatic stress studies; NICE, national institute for health and care excellence; PTSD, posttraumatic stress disorder; VA, Veterans Health Administration.

subject of scientific debate.[16] EMDR has been increasingly researched, with over 40 trials assessed in 1 meta-analysis.[16] EMDR has been found to have a strong evidence of effect for treating PTSD.[17,18]

Overall, when it comes to the treatment of PTSD, there is evidence that the treatments with the strongest support are PE and CPT.[17] However, meta-analyses have also found that there is not strong evidence for unequivocal superiority of any particular intervention, indicating that what is important is that affected individuals receive treatment.[19]

Special Group Considerations

When screening and working with individuals with PTSD, there are special group considerations. Women tend to develop PTSD at higher rates compared with men, which is partially accounted for by the high rates of sexual assault that women experience, as sexual assault carries a higher risk of developing PTSD than most other traumas.[20] Veterans are another group with higher rates of PTSD relative to the general population, largely owing to military service-related trauma exposures, with a meta-analysis of PTSD prevalence in the post-9/11 era finding the average prevalence PTSD across 33 studies was 23%.[21]

Minoritized groups, such as refugees, racial/ethnic minorities, and lesbian, gay, bisexual, transgender (LGBT+) people are also at increased risk for PTSD. Refugees are a heterogenous group, with much variation in experiences, such that research has found varying prevalence rates of PTSD within various refugee populations; however, a meta-analysis of 66 articles with 150 prevalence estimates found the prevalence of PTSD in refugees settled in high income countries was 34%.[22] Additionally, refugee populations often experience multiple traumas, including torture, combat, and being close to death.[23] Refugee populations may also have different cultural expressions of psychological distress (eg, increased somatization), which may challenge the assessment and treatment of PTSD.

Certain racial/ethnic minority groups and LGBT + individuals have also been found to have increased risk of PTSD. For example, a study of the general US adult population using the current diagnostic criteria for PTSD, Native Americans had significantly elevated odds of PTSD relative to non-Hispanic whites.[2] In research on specific populations (eg, veterans and 9/11 responders), the prevalence or conditional risk of PTSD was higher among Black/African-American and Latinx/Hispanic individuals.[24–28] Further, among both men and women, those who identify as lesbian/gay or bisexual had higher prevalence of PTSD relative to those who identified as heterosexual.[29] The increased prevalence of PTSD has been found to be associated with different trauma exposures, such that there is greater exposure to types of trauma (eg, interpersonal violence) that carry a greater risk of PTSD,[26,28,29,30,31] and with racial discrimination, which has been found to compromise trauma recovery and be associated with greater severity of PTSD symptoms.[32,33]

Considerations for Pharmacologic Prevention Efforts of Post-Traumatic Stress Disorder

In the first hours and days after a traumatic experience, many individuals report symptoms of acute stress, including increased arousal, insomnia, and agitation.[34] While benzodiazepines (BZDs) are effective in reducing these symptoms, they are ineffective for the prevention of PTSD.[35] Patients newly prescribed with BZDs should be informed about the potential of dependence and carefully monitored. Evidence for other pharmacologic agents, including beta-blockers, opiates, and hydrocortisone, for the prevention of PTSD in the aftermath of a traumatic experience is scarce and of low quality.[36]

Pharmacotherapies for Post-Traumatic Stress Disorder

Treatment guidelines

Most guidelines for the treatment of PTSD, including the VA/DoD,[10] NICE,[9] and Australian guidelines,[37] recommend psychotherapy as first-line treatment and pharmacotherapies only as second-line treatments. This recommendation is based on reviews and meta-analyses showing that pharmacotherapies are less effective than trauma-focused psychotherapeutic interventions in reducing PTSD severity.[18,38,39] However, different groups of patients may be attracted to psychotherapy and pharmacotherapy studies. Also, psychotherapy studies often report higher dropout rates than pharmacotherapy studies. Further, meta-analyses comparing psychotherapy and pharmacotherapy studies often neglect important study design differences between these studies. First, there is no way to hide from therapists and their patients whether the active or placebo psychotherapy is being administered. Second, randomized controlled trials (RCTs) investigating the effectiveness of psychotherapeutic interventions often compare the active treatment against a waitlist condition, in which participants receive no treatment at all. In RCTs testing pharmacologic agents, usually both, the active medication and the placebo group, are often provided with TAU, which can include psychotherapy. Hence, such studies usually report a smaller difference between the 2 investigated conditions.[40] In accordance, 1 landmark study with a head-to-head design found equal efficacy of psychopharmacotherapy, psychotherapy, and the combination of both.[41]

With regard to monotherapy, the highest quality and largest amount of evidence exists for the efficacy of sertraline, paroxetine, fluoxetine (all 3 selective serotonin reuptake inhibitors [SSRIs][a]) and venlafaxine extended release (serotonin norepinephrine reuptake inhibitor [SNRI][b]).[38,30] Based on the mechanism of action of these medications, the whole class of SSRIs can be assumed to be effective.[42] The SSRI and SNRI medications essentially displaced older antidepressants shown to have efficacy for PTSD , the tricyclic antidepressants and monoamine oxidase inhibitors, because of their superior safety and tolerability profiles. However, a tricyclic showed similar efficacy to an SSRI in a head-to-head comparison, suggesting the older medications might be underutilized in patients resistant to the new medications.[43] In addition, the efficacy of quetiapine, an atypical antipsychotic, has been documented also.[44] However, because of its adverse effect profile and lack of additional evidence, its role as a monotherapeutic agent is debated among experts (also see **Table 4**).[8]

Clinical practice

In clinical practice, pharmacotherapy is common for individuals with PTSD.[45,46] For example, in a cohort of more than 700,000 veterans diagnosed with PTSD, the mean number of psychotropic medications prescribed was 3.5 (standard deviation [SD] = 2.7). More than 80% of these veterans received an antidepressant; more than 20% received an atypical antipsychotic agent, and almost 40% were prescribed a sedative hypnotic.[45,47] There are multiple reasons why pharmacotherapy is common among individuals with PTSD. The severity of PTSD symptoms often negatively impacts psychological and daily functioning, requiring pharmacologic stabilization. Importantly, the participation in trauma-focused treatments requires individual to be psychologically stable, which can sometimes only be achieved with pharmacologic treatment. Moreover, even the best currently available psychotherapeutic interventions have limited effectiveness and a relatively high drop-out rate.[48] Thus, psychological treatments alone are often not sufficient to manage symptoms of PTSD, and many individuals therefore receive additional pharmacologic treatment. Such treatment aims to decrease overall severity of PTSD symptoms, or target specific symptoms

Table 4
Summary of evidence for pharmacotherapy for the prevention and treatment of post-traumatic stress disorder

Indication	Drug	FDA Approved	VA/DOD Guidelines (2017)[10]	APA Guidelines (2017)[c,64]	NICE Guidelines (2018)[9]	ISTSS Guidelines (2020)[8]
Prevention	Hydrocortisone	-	Insufficient evidence	NA	-	+ (weak)
	Benzodiazepines[a]	-	Insufficient evidence	NA	-	NA
	Propranolol	-	Insufficient evidence	NA	-	Insufficient evidence
Monotherapy	Sertraline	+	+	+	+	+
	Paroxetine	+	+	+	+	+
	Fluoxetine	-	+	+	+	+
	Venlafaxine	-	+	+	+	+
	Quetiapine	-	-	NA	NA	+ (weak)
	Risperidone	-	-	Insufficient evidence	NA	NA
	Topiramate	-	-	Insufficient evidence	NA	Insufficient evidence
	Other SSRIs[a]	-	Insufficient evidence	NA	+	NA
	Tricyclic antidepressants[a]	-	+ weak[d]	NA	NA	Insufficient evidence
Augmentation	Quetiapine	-	NA	NA	NA	NA
	Risperidone	-	-	NA	NA	+
	Prazosin[b]	-	Insufficient evidence	NA	NA	+

Note. +, recommendation for; -, recommendation against; NA, not addressed.

[a] Class of medications.

[b] For nightmares.

[c] Update ongoing.

[d] Weak recommendation for imipramine and amitriptyline only. Please add the following citation as reference 71: Davidson J, Kudler H, Smith R, Mahorney SL, Lipper S, Hammett E, Saunders WB, Cavenar JO Jr. Treatment of posttraumatic stress disorder with amitriptyline and placebo. Arch Gen Psychiatry. 1990 Mar;47(3):259-66. doi: 10.1001/archpsyc.1990.01810150059010. PMID: 2407208.

(eg, insomnia, agitation) or common comorbidities. Although SSRIs are the first-line treatment for the former, numerous agents can be used for the two latter.

Comorbidity Considerations

PTSD is often comorbid with other conditions,[2] including substance use disorder (SUD), borderline personality disorder (BPD), and insomnia. Given the high levels of comorbidities in individuals with PTSD, treatments that address PTSD and common comorbid conditions have been developed.

SUD is highly comorbid with PTSD, with up to 65% of patients with PTSD have been found to have a comorbid SUD.[49] SUD can be addressed with psychological and pharmacologic treatments. Although there are well-established pharmacologic treatments for PTSD and alcohol use disorder (AUD), evidence regarding treatment for co-occurring PTSD and AUD is limited and generally mixed. This is the case for agents commonly prescribed for either of the 2 conditions (eg, SSRIs or naltrexone) or hypothesized to be beneficial when both conditions co-occur (eg, zonisamide).[50,51] However, the combination of established treatments for PTSD and AUD is mostly well-tolerated and should be considered in clinical practice even in absence of strong evidence.[50] Evidence regarding treatment of PTSD and opioid use disorder (OUD) is even more scarce and mostly limited to retrospective studies.[52] Hence, clinical management often includes the combination of pharmacologic treatments established for PTSD or OUD and should be guided by clinical experience. With regard to psychological treatments, Concurrent Treatment of PTSD and Substance Use Disorder Using Prolonged Exposure (COPE) was developed for treatment of these comorbidities and consists of integrated cognitive-behavioral relapse prevention skills with PE. COPE has been found to significantly reduce PTSD symptom severity compared with TAU and to treat SUD at comparable levels to TAU in an RCT of SUD treatment-seeking participants.[49] Similarly, in an RCT of treatment-seeking veterans, COPE reduced PTSD symptoms and increased PTSD remission compared with an integrated coping skills treatment and decreased substance use equivalently to the coping skills treatment.[53] Overall, COPE has been found to be a feasible, safe, and efficacious treatment for comorbid PTSD and SUD.[49,53]

Dialectical Behavior Therapy-Prolonged Exposure (DBT-PE) was developed to treat those with comorbid PTSD and BPD, as those with PTSD have high odds of also having lifetime (odds ratio [OR] = 2.8) and past-year BPD (OR = 3.3).[2] DBT is a treatment that was developed to treat those with BPD.[54] DBT-PE combined the 2 treatments, integrating individual therapy, group skills training, and phone coaching of DBT with the trauma-focused exposure therapy of PE.[54,55] In both an RCT and an effectiveness study in community mental health settings, DBT-PE was found to be safe and feasible for those with comorbid PTSD and BPD, and resulted in lasting reductions in PTSD, suicidal behaviors, and psychological distress, although the effect sizes were attenuated in the effectiveness study compared with the highly-controlled efficacy study.[54,55]

Among the most debilitating symptoms of PTSD are nightmares, and 70% to 87% of patients with PTSD report comorbid insomnia.[56,57] This is reflected in the class and types of medications that are prescribed to veterans. Many of the most prescribed medications do have hypnotic effects (eg, Trazodone, the most commonly prescribed antidepressant for in veterans with PTSD in Veterans Administration clinics) or atypical antipsychotics.[45] With regard to the latter, adjunctive treatment with risperidone was found to improve sleep quality and nightmares in veterans with chronic, antidepressant-resistant, military-related PTSD.[58] Similarly, there is evidence that prazosin, an α1 adrenergic receptor antagonist approved as an antihypertensive drug, reduces trauma-related nightmares.[59] Yet, the evidence base for this effect is mixed, with a well-powered RCT failing to demonstrate an effect[60] and thus the interpretation of the cumulative evidence is debated among experts (see **Table 4**). Cognitive-behavioral treatments for insomnia, including cognitive-behavioral therapy for insomnia, imagery rehearsal therapy, and exposure, rescripting, and relaxation therapy, were found to reduce both PTSD symptoms and improve insomnia severity and sleep quality in a meta-analysis of 12 RCTs.[61]

CLINICS CARE POINTS

- Nonpsychiatrists can screen for PTSD using the PCL-5, PC-PTSD, and the LEC-5.

- Trauma-focused psychotherapies are first-line treatments for PTSD. Treatments such as PE, CPT, and EMDR are recommended by a variety of treatment guidelines to the quality and depth of empirical evidence.

- SSRIs are first-line pharmacologic treatments for PTSD.

- Comorbidities, including substance use disorder and insomnia, are common among individuals with PTSD and may require additional and specific pharmacologic or psychological treatment

DISCLOSURE

Dr J.H. Krystal is a consultant for Aptinyx, Inc., Atai Life Sciences, AstraZeneca Pharmaceuticals, Biogen, Idec, MA, Biomedisyn Corporation, Bionomics, Limited (Australia), Boehringer Ingelheim International, Cadent Therapeutics, Inc., Clexio Bioscience, Ltd., COMPASS Pathways, Limited, United Kingdom, Concert Pharmaceuticals, Inc., Epiodyne, Inc., EpiVario, Inc., Greenwich Biosciences, Inc., Heptares Therapeutics, Limited (UK), Janssen Research & Development, Jazz Pharmaceuticals, Inc., Otsuk America Pharmaceutical, Inc., Perception Neuroscience Holdings, Inc., Spring Care, Inc., Sunovion Pharmaceuticals, Inc., Takeda Industries, Taisho Pharmaceutical Co., Ltd. J.H. Krystal also reports the following disclosures: Scientific Advisory Board: Biohaven Pharmaceuticals, BioXcel Therapeutics, Inc. (Clinical Advisory Board), Cadent Therapeutics, Inc. (Clinical Advisory Board), Cerevel Therapeutics, LLC, EpiVario, Inc., Eisai, Inc., Lohocla Research Corporation, Novartis Pharmaceuticals Corporation, PsychoGenics, Inc., RBNC Therapeutics, Inc., Tempero Bio, Inc., Terran Biosciences, Inc. Stock: Biohaven Pharmaceuticals, Sage Pharmaceuticals, Spring Care, Inc. Stock Options: Biohaven Pharmaceuticals Medical Sciences, EpiVario, Inc., RBNC Therapeutics, Inc., Terran Biosciences, Inc. Tempero Bio, Inc. Income Greater than $10,000: Editorial Board: Editor - Biological Psychiatry. Patents and Inventions: (1) Seibyl JP, Krystal JH, Charney DS Dopamine and noradrenergic reuptake inhibitors in treatment of schizophrenia. US Patent #:5,447,948.September 5, 1995. (2) Vladimir, Coric, Krystal, John H, Sanacora, Gerard – Glutamate Modulating Agents in the Treatment of Mental Disorders. US Patent No. 8,778,979 B2 Patent Issue Date: July 15, 2014. US Patent Application No. 15/695,164: Filing Date: 09/05/2017. (3) Charney D, Krystal JH, Manji H, Matthew S, Zarate C., - Intranasal Administration of Ketamine to Treat Depression United States Patent Number: 9,592,207, Issue date: 3/14/2017. Licensed to Janssen Research & Development. (4) Zarate, C, Charney, DS, Manji, HK, Mathew, Sanjay J, Krystal, JH, Yale University "Methods for Treating Suicidal Ideation," Patent Application No. 15/379,013 filed on December 14, 2016 by Yale University Office of Cooperative Research. (5) Arias A, Petrakis I, Krystal JH. –

Composition and methods to treat addiction. Provisional Use Patent Application no.61/973/961. April 2, 2014. Filed by Yale University Office of Cooperative Research. (6) Chekroud, A., Gueorguieva, R., & Krystal, JH. "Treatment Selection for Major Depressive Disorder" [filing date 3rd June 2016, USPTO docket number Y0087.70116US00]. Provisional patent submission by Yale University. (7) Gihyun, Yoon, Petrakis I, Krystal JH – Compounds, Compositions and Methods for Treating or Preventing Depression and Other Diseases. U. S. Provisional Patent Application No. 62/444,552, filed on January10, 2017 by Yale University Office of Cooperative Research OCR 7088 US01. (8) Abdallah, C, Krystal, JH, Duman, R, Sanacora, G. Combination Therapy for Treating or Preventing Depression or Other Mood Diseases. U.S. Provisional Patent Application No. 62/719,935 filed on August 20, 2018 by Yale University Office of Cooperative Research OCR 7451 US01. On Non-Federal Research Support: AstraZeneca Pharmaceuticals provides the drug, Saracatinib, for research related to NIAAA grant "Center for Translational Neuroscience of Alcoholism [CTNA-4] Novartis provides the drug, Mavoglurant, for research related to NIAAA grant Center for Translational Neuroscience of Alcoholism [CTNA-4].

REFERENCES

1. American Psychiatric Association. Diagnostic and statistical manual of mental disorders DSM. 5th edition. American Psychiatric Association Publishing; 2013. Available at: https://www.appi.org/Products/DSM-Library/Diagnostic-and-Statistical-Manual-of-Mental-Disord?sku=2554. Accessed May 7, 2020.

2. Goldstein RB, Smith SM, Chou SP, et al. The epidemiology of DSM-5 posttraumatic stress disorder in the United States: results from the national epidemiologic survey on alcohol and related conditions-III. Soc Psychiatry Psychiatr Epidemiol 2016;51(8):1137–48.

3. Gray MJ, Litz BT, Hsu JL, et al. Psychometric properties of the life events checklist. Assessment 2004;11(4).330–41.

4. Weathers FW, Bovin MJ, Lee DJ, et al. The clinician-administered PTSD scale for DSM-5 (CAPS-5): development and initial psychometric evaluation in military veterans. Psychol Assess 2018;30(3):383–95.

5. Blevins CA, Weathers FW, Davis MT, et al. The posttraumatic stress disorder checklist for DSM-5 (PCL-5): development and initial psychometric evaluation. J Trauma Stress 2015;28(6):489–98.

6. Prins A, Bovin MJ, Smolenski DJ, et al. The primary care PTSD screen for DSM-5 (PC-PTSD-5): development and evaluation within a veteran primary care sample. J Gen Intern Med 2016;31(10):1206–11.

7. Bovin MJ, Kimerling R, Weathers FW, et al. Diagnostic accuracy and acceptability of the primary care posttraumatic stress disorder screen for the diagnostic and statistical manual of mental disorders (5th Edition) among US veterans. JAMA Netw Open 2021;4(2):e2036733.

8. Forbes D, Bisson JI, Monson CM, et al. Effective treatments for PTSD: 3rd edition: practice guidelines from the International Society for Traumatic Stress Studies, vol. 3. New York, New York: The Guilford Press; 2020.

9. National Institute for Health and Care Excellence. Post-traumatic stress disorder NICE guideline [NG116]. NICE; 2018. Available at: https://www.nice.org.uk/guidance/ng116. Accessed September 27, 2021.

10. Department of Veterans Affairs, Department of Defense. VA/DOD clinical practice guideline for the management of posttraumatic stress disorder and acute stress

disorder. 2017. Available at: https://www.healthquality.va.gov/guidelines/mh/ptsd/. Accessed December 1, 2021.

11. O'Neil M, McDonagh M, Hsu F, et al. Pharmacologic and nonpharmacologic treatments for posttraumatic stress disorder: groundwork for a publicly available repository of randomized controlled trial data. Rockville, Maryland: Agency for Healthcare Research and Quality (AHRQ); 2019.

12. Cusack K, Jonas DE, Forneris CA, et al. Psychological treatments for adults with posttraumatic stress disorder: a systematic review and meta-analysis. Clin Psychol Rev 2016;128–41. https://doi.org/10.1016/j.cpr.2015.10.003.

13. Bisson JI, Roberts NP, Andrew M, et al. Psychological therapies for chronic posttraumatic stress disorder (PTSD) in adults. Cochrane Database Syst Rev 2013; 12. https://doi.org/10.1002/14651858.CD003388.pub4.

14. Shapiro F. Efficacy of the eye movement desensitization procedure in the treatment of traumatic memories. J Trauma Stress 1989;2(2):199–223.

15. Shapiro F. Eye movement desensitization and reprocessing (EMDR) therapy: basic principles, protocols, and procedures. 3rd Editon. US: The Guilford Press; 2018.

16. Cuijpers P, van Veen SC, Sijbrandij M, et al. Eye movement desensitization and reprocessing for mental health problems: a systematic review and meta-analysis. Cogn Behav Ther 2020;49(3):165–80.

17. Lewis C, Roberts NP, Andrew M, et al. Psychological therapies for post-traumatic stress disorder in adults: systematic review and meta-analysis. [Review]. Eur J Psychotraumatol 2020;11(1):1729633.

18. Mavranezouli I, Megnin-Viggars O, Daly C, et al. Psychological treatments for post-traumatic stress disorder in adults: a network meta-analysis. Psychol Med 2020;50(4):542–55.

19. Kline AC, Cooper AA, Rytwinksi NK, et al. Long-term efficacy of psychotherapy for posttraumatic stress disorder: A meta-analysis of randomized controlled trials. [Review]. Clin Psychol Rev 2018;1:30–40.

20. Tolin DF, Foa EB. Sex differences in trauma and posttraumatic stress disorder: a quantitative review of 25 years of research. Psychol Bull 2006;132(6):959–92.

21. Fulton JJ, Calhoun PS, Wagner HR, et al. The prevalence of posttraumatic stress disorder in Operation Enduring Freedom/Operation Iraqi Freedom (OEF/OIF) veterans: a meta-analysis. J Anxiety Disord 2015;98–107. https://doi.org/10.1016/j.janxdis.2015.02.003.

22. Henkelmann JR, de Best S, Deckers C, et al. Anxiety, depression and post-traumatic stress disorder in refugees resettling in high-income countries: systematic review and meta-analysis. BJPsych Open; 2020. https://doi.org/10.1192/bjo.2020.54.

23. Burnett A, Peel M. Asylum seekers and refugees in Britain: the health of survivors of torture and organised violence. BMJ 2001;322(7286):606–9.

24. Steenkamp MM, Schlenger WE, Corry N, et al. Predictors of PTSD 40 years after combat: findings from the National Vietnam Veterans Longitudinal Study. Depress Anxiety 2017;34(8):711–22.

25. Whealin JM, Ciro D, Dasaro CR, et al. Race/ethnic differences in prevalence and correlates of posttraumatic stress disorder in World Trade Center responders: results from a population-based, health monitoring cohort. Psychol Trauma Published online 2021:No Pagination Specified. doi:10.1037/tra0001081

26. Dohrenwend BP, Turner JB, Turse NA, et al. War-related posttraumatic stress disorder in Black, Hispanic, and majority white Vietnam veterans: the roles of exposure and vulnerability. J Trauma Stress 2008;21(2):133–41.

27. Alcantara C, Casement MD, Lewis-Fernandez R. Conditional risk for PTSD among Latinos: a systematic review of racial/ethnic differences and sociocultural explanations. Clin Psychol Rev 2013;33(1):107–19.
28. Roberts AL, Gilman SE, Breslau J, et al. Race/ethnic differences in exposure to traumatic events, development of post-traumatic stress disorder, and treatment-seeking for post-traumatic stress disorder in the United States. Psychol Med 2011;41(1):71–83.
29. Roberts AL, Austin SB, Corliss HL, et al. Pervasive trauma exposure among US sexual orientation minority adults and risk of posttraumatic stress disorder. Am J Public Health 2010;100(12):2433–41.
30. Beals J, Manson SM, Shore JH, et al. The prevalence of posttraumatic stress disorder among American Indian Vietnam veterans: disparities and context. J Trauma Stress 2002;15(2):89–97.
31. McLaughlin KA, Alvarez K, Fillbrunn M, et al. Racial/ethnic variation in trauma-related psychopathology in the United States: a population-based study. Psychol Med 2019;49(13):2215–26.
32. Brooks Holliday S, Dubowitz T, Haas A, et al. The association between discrimination and PTSD in African Americans: exploring the role of gender. Ethn Health 2020;25(5):717–31.
33. Sibrava NJ, Bjornsson AS, Perez Benitez ACI, et al. Posttraumatic stress disorder in African American and Latinx adults: clinical course and the role of racial and ethnic discrimination. Am Psychol 2019;74(1):101–16.
34. Visser E, Gosens T, Den Oudsten BL, et al. The course, prediction, and treatment of acute and posttraumatic stress in trauma patients: a systematic review. J Trauma Acute Care Surg 2017;82(6):1158–83.
35. Guina J, Rossetter SR, DeRHODES BJ, et al. Benzodiazepines for PTSD: a systematic review and meta-analysis. J Psychiatr Pract 2015;21(4):281–303.
36. Astill Wright L, Sijbrandij M, Sinnerton R, et al. Pharmacological prevention and early treatment of post-traumatic stress disorder and acute stress disorder: a systematic review and meta-analysis. Transl Psychiatry 2019;9(1):334.
37. Australian PTSD guidelines | July 2020. Phoenix Australia. Available at: https://www.phoenixaustralia.org/australian-guidelines-for-ptsd/. Accessed September 27, 2021.
38. Hoskins MD, Bridges J, Sinnerton R, et al. Pharmacological therapy for post-traumatic stress disorder: a systematic review and meta-analysis of monotherapy, augmentation and head-to-head approaches. Eur J Psychotraumatol 2021;12(1): 1802920.
39. de Moraes Costa G, Zanatta FB, Ziegelmann PK, et al. Pharmacological treatments for adults with post-traumatic stress disorder: a network meta-analysis of comparative efficacy and acceptability. J Psychiatr Res 2020;130:412–20.
40. Furukawa TA, Noma H, Caldwell DM, et al. Waiting list may be a nocebo condition in psychotherapy trials: a contribution from network meta-analysis. Acta Psychiatr Scand 2014;130(3):181–92.
41. Rauch SAM, Kim HM, Powell C, et al. Efficacy of prolonged exposure therapy, sertraline hydrochloride, and their combination among combat veterans with posttraumatic stress disorder: a randomized clinical trial. JAMA Psychiatry 2019;76(2):117.
42. Nemeroff CB, Owens MJ. Pharmacologic differences among the SSRIs: focus on monoamine transporters and the HPA axis. CNS Spectr 2004;6(Suppl4):23–31.

43. Petrakis IL, Ralevski E, Desai N, et al. Noradrenergic vs serotonergic antidepressant with or without naltrexone for veterans with PTSD and comorbid alcohol dependence. Neuropsychopharmacology 2012;37(4):996–1004.

44. Villarreal G, Hamner MB, Cañive JM, et al. Efficacy of quetiapine monotherapy in posttraumatic stress disorder: a randomized, placebo-controlled trial. Am J Psychiatry 2016;173(12):1205–12.

45. Krystal JH, Davis LL, Neylan TC, et al. It Is time to address the crisis in the pharmacotherapy of posttraumatic stress disorder: a consensus statement of the PTSD psychopharmacology working group. Biol Psychiatry 2017;82(7):e51–9.

46. Duek O, Pietrzak RH, Petrakis I, et al. Early discontinuation of pharmacotherapy in U.S. Veterans diagnosed with PTSD and the role of psychotherapy. J Psychiatr Res 2021;167–73.

47. Shiner B, Leonard CE, Gui J, et al. Comparing medications for DSM-5 PTSD in routine VA practice. J Clin Psychiatry 2020;81(6). https://doi.org/10.4088/JCP.20m13244.

48. Imel ZE, Laska K, Jakupcak M, et al. Meta-analysis of dropout in treatments for posttraumatic stress disorder. J Consult Clin Psychol 2013;81(3):394–404.

49. Mills KL, Teesson M, Back SE, et al. Integrated exposure-based therapy for co-occurring posttraumatic stress disorder and substance dependence: a randomized controlled trial. JAMA 2012;308(7):690–9.

50. Petrakis IL, Simpson TL. Posttraumatic stress disorder and alcohol use disorder: a critical review of pharmacologic treatments. Alcohol Clin Exp Res 2017;41(2):226–37.

51. Petrakis I, Ralevski E, Arias AJ, et al. Zonisamide as an adjunctive treatment to cognitive processing therapy for veterans with posttraumatic stress disorder and comorbid alcohol use disorder: a pilot study. Am J Addict 2020;29(6):515–24.

52. Meshberg-Cohen S, Ross MacLean R, Schnakenberg Martin AM, et al. Treatment outcomes in individuals diagnosed with comorbid opioid use disorder and Posttraumatic stress disorder: a review. Addict Behav 2021;122:107026.

53. Norman SB, Trim R, Haller M, et al. Efficacy of integrated exposure therapy vs integrated coping skills therapy for comorbid posttraumatic stress disorder and alcohol use disorder: a randomized clinical trial. JAMA Psychiatry 2019;76(8):791–9.

54. Harned MS, Schmidt SC, Korslund KE, et al. Does adding the dialectical behavior therapy prolonged exposure (DBT PE) protocol for PTSD to DBT improve outcomes in public mental health settings? a pilot nonrandomized effectiveness trial with benchmarking. Behav Ther 2021;52(3):639–55.

55. Harned MS, Korslund KE, Linehan MM. A pilot randomized controlled trial of dialectical behavior therapy with and without the dialectical behavior therapy prolonged exposure protocol for suicidal and self-injuring women with borderline personality disorder and PTSD. Behav Res Ther 2014;7–17. https://doi.org/10.1016/j.brat.2014.01.008.

56. Belleville G, Guay S, Marchand A. Impact of sleep disturbances on PTSD symptoms and perceived health. J Nerv Ment Dis 2009;197(2):126–32.

57. Maher MJ, Rego SA, Asnis GM. Sleep disturbances in patients with posttraumatic stress disorder: epidemiology, impact and approaches to management. CNS Drugs 2006;20(7):567–90.

58. Krystal JH, Pietrzak RH, Rosenheck RA, et al. Sleep disturbance in chronic military-related PTSD: clinical impact and response to adjunctive risperidone in the Veterans Affairs cooperative study #504. J Clin Psychiatry 2016;77(4):483–91.

59. Raskind MA, Peskind ER, Hoff DJ, et al. A parallel group placebo controlled study of prazosin for trauma nightmares and sleep disturbance in combat veterans with post-traumatic stress disorder. Biol Psychiatry 2007;61(8):928–34.

60. Reist C, Streja E, Tang CC, et al. Prazosin for treatment of post-traumatic stress disorder: a systematic review and meta-analysis. CNS Spectr 2021;26(4):338–44.

61. Ho FYY, Chan CS, Tang KNS. Cognitive-behavioral therapy for sleep disturbances in treating posttraumatic stress disorder symptoms: a meta-analysis of randomized controlled trials. Clin Psychol Rev 2016;43:90–102.

62. Bovin MJ, Marx BP, Weathers FW, et al. Psychometric properties of the PTSD Checklist for diagnostic and statistical manual of mental disorders-fifth edition (PCL-5) in veterans. Psychol Assess 2016;28(11):1379–91.

63. Morrison K, Su S, Keck M, et al. Psychometric properties of the PCL-5 in a sample of first responders. J Anxiety Disord 2021;1:102339.

64. American Psychological Association. Clinical practice guideline for the treatment of posttraumatic stress disorder (PTSD). :139.

65. Demircioglu M, Seker Z, Aker AT. Psychological first aid: objectives, practicing, vulnerable groups and ethical rules to follow. Psikiyatr Guncel Yaklasimlar 2019;11(3):351–62.

66. North CS, Pfefferbaum B. Mental health response to community disasters: a systematic review. JAMA 2013;310(5):507–18.

67. Prolonged exposure (PE). Available at: https://www.apa.org/ptsd-guideline/treatments/prolonged-exposure. Accessed January 13, 2022.

68. Cognitive processing therapy (CPT). Available at: https://www.apa.org/ptsd-guideline/treatments/cognitive-processing-therapy. Accessed January 13, 2022.

69. Maxfield SL, Solomon RM. Description FTC to T. eye movement desensitization and reprocessing (EMDR) therapy. Available at: https://www.apa.org/ptsd-guideline/treatments/eye-movement-reprocessing. Accessed January 13, 2022.

70. Frank JB, Kosten TR, Giller EL Jr, et al. A randomized clinical trial of phenelzine and imipramine for posttraumatic stress disorder. Am J Psychiatry 1988;145(10):1289–91.

From Mouse to Man: N-Methyl-D-Aspartic Acid Receptor Activation as a Promising Pharmacotherapeutic Strategy for Autism Spectrum Disorders

Stephen I. Deutsch, MD, PhD[a], Jessica A. Burket, PhD[b],*

KEYWORDS

- BALB/c mouse • Autism spectrum disorder • NMDA receptor • mTORC1
- Allosteric modulators

KEY POINTS

- BALB/c mice display hypersensitivity to behavioral effects of MK-801 (dizocilpine), an uncompetitive NMDA receptor "open-channel blocker."
- BALB/c mice show deficits in social preference and social interaction.
- NMDA receptor agonist interventions promote prosocial behavior in the BALB/c mouse model of autism spectrum disorder.
- NMDA receptor hypofunction is a promising translational therapeutic target for some presentations of autism spectrum disorder.

INTRODUCTION

The BALB/c mouse strain differed from comparator strains in terms of heightened sensitivity to behavioral effects of MK-801 (dizocilpine), a noncompetitive NMDA receptor "open-channel" blocker. Moreover, data suggest that MK-801-elicited behavioral readouts in the BALB/c strain index acute pharmacologically induced NMDA receptor hypofunction (NRH), which would facilitate high-throughput screening of promising NMDA receptor agonist therapeutic interventions in an intact behaving mouse.[1–4] Moreover, in the presence of a salient social stimulus mouse, whether

---

[a] Department of Psychiatry and Behavioral Sciences, Eastern Virginia Medical School, 825 Fairfax Avenue, Suite 710, Norfolk, VA 23507, USA; [b] Department of Molecular Biology & Chemistry, Christopher Newport University, 1 Avenue of the Arts, Newport News, VA 23606, USA
* Corresponding author.
E-mail address: jessica.burket@cnu.edu

Med Clin N Am 107 (2023) 101–117
https://doi.org/10.1016/j.mcna.2022.05.002
0025-7125/23/© 2022 Elsevier Inc. All rights reserved.

enclosed or freely behaving, the BALB/c mouse showed reduced locomotor activity and evidence of impaired social preference (ie, showing no preference for an enclosed stimulus mouse over an inanimate object) and impaired social interaction (eg, displaying fewer discrete episodes of social approach).[5,6] Therapeutic targeting of the BALB/c mouse with NMDA receptor agonist strategies showed improvements of both social preference and several measures of social interaction.[6–9] For example, VU0410120, a high-affinity, highly selective inhibitor of the "glycine transporter type 1 (GlyT1)" was shown to improve measures of impaired sociability in the BALB/c mouse.[10,11]

Two complementary mechanisms exist by which NMDA receptor activation dampens the signaling activity of mTORC1, a heteromeric protein complex with serine/threonine kinase activity that integrates a variety of external signals (eg, brain-derived-neurotrophic factor (BDNF) and neurotransmitters, such as L-glutamate and acetylcholine) and internal factors (eg, the nutrient and energy status of the neuron) to determine important outputs, including protein translation in the periphery of neurons.[12–14] Regulatory effects of NMDA receptor activation on mTOR signaling are important because mTOR overactivation is a pathologic point of convergence of several monogenic "syndromal" forms of ASD (eg, Tuberous Sclerosis Complex [TSC]).[12,15–17] In this context, it is interesting that a transcriptomic analysis in frontal cortex of BALB/c mice treated with VU0410120 suggested that *Ddit4*, the gene coding "DNA damage inducible transcript 4" whose functional designation includes "negative regulation of mTOR signaling activity," is upregulated in BALB/c mice that are "low" responders to VU0410120's prosocial effects.[11,18] These data suggest that increased expression of *Ddit4* may be a compensatory mechanism in BALB/c mice responding less well to prosocial effects of VU0410120. The current Review considers preclinical data obtained with the BALB/c mouse model of ASD that support continued translational exploration of NMDA receptor agonist interventional strategies for the treatment of ASD.

N-methyl-D-aspartic Acid Receptors: Structure, Function, and Pharmacotherapeutic Opportunities

The NMDA receptor is a member of a family of tetrameric glutamate-gated cation channel receptors constructed from 4 constituent polypeptide subunits, each of which shares a common motif.[19–23] The subunits are arranged to form an ion-conductive pore with specialized gating properties, especially allowance of ligand-gated Ca^{2+} conductance. The common motif of each subunit includes 3 helical transmembrane segments (M1, M3, and M4) with a short reentry M2 segment between M1 and M3. Increasingly, there is interest in cytoplasmic C-terminal domains of individual NMDA receptor subunits because they show significant evolutionary divergence from each other and contribute to metabotropic functions of the receptor, which can occur independently of receptor-gated ion conductance.[24] The C-terminal domains influence signal transduction cascades and appear to do so as a result of their binding to scaffolding proteins in the complex architecture of the postsynaptic density of the excitatory synapse.[24–27]

NMDA receptors are often referred to as "heterotetrameric" because the subunits are not identical: "conventional" NMDA receptors contain 2 GluN1 subunits that create ligand-binding domains for glycine and D-serine and 2 subunits that are members of the GluN2 family. If the 2 GluN2 family members are identical, the receptors may be referred to as diheterotetrameric, whereas if they are not identical, they may be referred to as triheterotetrameric. The GluN2 subunits create the ligand-binding domain for L-glutamate, the brain's major excitatory neurotransmitter. Expression of the 4 GluN2 subunits (ie, A-D) reflect the transcription of 4 distinct genes, whereas the 8 isoforms of the GluN1 subunit result from the translation of alternative RNA splice variants derived from the transcription of a single gene.[28]

Expression of the 4 types of GluN2 subunits (ie, GluN2A, GluN2B, GluN2C, and GluN2D) is influenced by developmental age, anatomic brain region, and whether the receptor has a synaptic or extrasynaptic location.[27,29,30] For example, expression of the GluN2B subunit predominates in fetal rodent brain, whereas after birth there is a developmental "switch" with the expression of GluN2A increasing; in early postnatal life (eg, postnatal day 14 in the rat), GluN2A expression begins to predominate over GluN2B in cortex, hippocampus, and cerebellum.[27,31,32] Further, in mature brain, expression of GluN2C is enriched in cerebellum and expression of GluN2D is most dense in subcortical regions and brainstem. Also, diheterotetrameric GluN2B receptors are preferentially expressed extrasynaptically, whereby they may promote excitotoxicity, whereas GluN2A-containing receptors have greater relative expression in synaptic locations.

Ligand-gating of ionotropic NMDA receptors is complex and both ion flux and channel opening are often influenced by several factors, including binding of both L-glutamate and either one of the 2 obligatory coagonists glycine or D-serine to distinct extracellular sites, membrane potential, combinatorial diversity of the individual receptor subunits, phosphorylation state of the receptor, presence of endogenous or exogenously administered allosteric modulators, posttranslational modifications of the receptor, such as nitrosylation, pH, oxygen tension and Zn^{2+}.[24,33–35] Combinatorial diversity resulting from the various possible subunit combinations influence biophysical and, ultimately, signaling properties of the diverse variety of NMDA receptors, such as gating characteristics and Ca^{2+}-permeability, kinetics of channel opening, sensitivity to voltage-gated Mg^{2+} blockade, and deactivation kinetics. The specific type of GluN2 subunit in diheterotetrameric receptors has a disproportionate influence on biophysical and signaling properties. Moreover, in the excitatory synapse, phosphorylation of cytoplasmic domains of colocalized NMDA receptors by G-protein-coupled metabotropic glutamate receptors (mGluRs) is a mechanism of "cross-talk" between mGluRs and NMDA receptors.[24,36–40]

In addition to ligand gating, NMDA receptors have the property of voltage gating.[41] Ordinarily, at the membrane's normal negative resting membrane potential, a hydrated Mg^{2+} is bound to a site within the NMDA receptor-associated channel itself. Relief of this Mg^{2+}-blockade, which is necessary to allow NMDA receptor-mediated conductance of Ca^{2+} and other cations to occur, depends on moving the potential in the direction of depolarization. At the excitatory synapse, this depolarization-dependent relief of Mg^{2+}-blockade is accomplished by the activation of a colocalized alpha-amino-3-hydroxy-5-methyl-4-isoxazolepropionic acid (AMPA) receptor and/or an α_7 nicotinic acetylcholine receptor in the neighborhood of the NMDA receptor.[20,42–45] The dependence of NMDA receptor serves as a coincidence detector, responding to both changes in membrane potential and the presence of glutamate and glycine or D-serine in the synaptic cleft.[46] In addition to ligand-gating and voltage-sensing properties, there is additional interest in metabotropic functions of NMDA receptor activation that are not dependent on Ca^{2+} conductance, but rather on the alignment of protein binding partners in the "post-synaptic density (PSD)" of the excitatory synapse.[24,47]

Strategies to Preserve Spatial and Temporal Selectivity of Endogenously Released Glutamate, Glycine, and D-serine

Because electronic configurations of orthosteric binding sites for endogenously released L-glutamate share much in common across a variety of ionotropic and

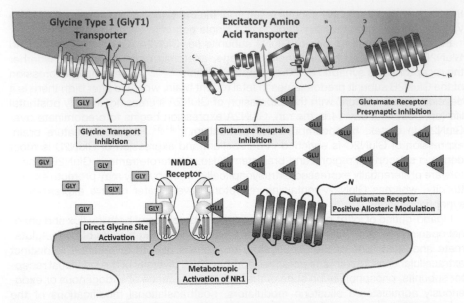

Fig. 1. The figure depicts several promising therapeutic strategies to promote NMDA receptor activation and preserve spatial and temporal selectivity. Mechanisms of NMDA receptor activation include the inhibition of reuptake transporters of both glutamate and glycine (eg, excitatory amino acid transporters and glycine type 1 transporter [GlyT1]), and allosteric modulation of the metabotropic glutamate receptors (mGluR$_S$). See text for details (Data from Deutsch and colleagues, 2015; Deutsch 2022).[22,43]

metabotropic glutamate receptors, selective therapeutic targeting of orthosteric glutamate binding sites is problematic.[22,24] Allosteric modulatory ligands bind to sites distinct from where endogenous glutamate itself binds, lack intrinsic efficacy in the absence of endogenous glutamate, and act to increase (ie, positive allosteric modulators [PAMs]) or decrease (ie, negative allosteric modulators [NAMs]) the likelihood that glutamate and glycine/D-serine will be effective in promoting Ca^{2+} conductance. In addition to PAMs and NAMs developed for ionotropic glutamate receptors, PAMs and NAMs developed for "7 transmembrane domain-GTP binding protein-coupled mGluRs" positively or negatively influence downstream phosphorylation states of relevant substrate proteins, including NMDA receptor subunits.[48–51] Because PAMs and NAMs enjoy greater selectivity for ionotropic and metabotropic glutamate receptor subtypes, they may contribute to the avoidance of off-target effects.[22] Moreover, PAMs and NAMs should be devoid of agonist-induced changes in receptor sensitivity that occur when orthosteric binding sites are targeted.[48] From a therapeutic perspective, it is hoped that PAMs and NAMs will preserve spatial and temporal selectivity of endogenously released glutamate (**Fig. 1**). Other promising strategies for the activation of the NMDA receptor in a spatially and temporally selective manner include increasing concentrations of glycine and D-serine by the inhibition of the glycine transporter type 1 (GlyT1) and inhibition of D-amino acid oxidase, respectively.[11,22,52]

N-methyl-D-aspartic Acid Receptor Activation Improves Sociability in the BALB/c Mouse Model of Autism Spectrum Disorder; Translational Implication for Central Nervous System Medication Development

Because abuse and diversion of phencyclidine (PCP), a noncompetitive "open-channel" blocker of the NMDA receptor, elicited psychosis in susceptible individuals, whose descriptive features resembled idiopathic schizophrenia, interest evolved in "glutamatergic deficiency" and "NMDA receptor hypofunction (NRH)" as a pathogenic mechanism(s) of psychosis.[53–55] The logical translational therapeutic extension of this hypothesis was to explore ways to promote NMDA receptor activation.[43] To facilitate "high-throughput" screening of therapeutically viable NMDA receptor agonist interventions, several laboratories sought to characterize reproducible and reliably rated mouse behaviors elicited in response to noncompetitive NMDA receptor antagonists, such as MK-801 (dizocilpine), and identify mouse strains with heightened sensitivity to these well-defined behavioral effects of MK-801.[1–4,56–58] A promising therapeutic intervention would be one that lessened intensity of MK-801-elicited mouse behaviors, particularly in a test strain with heightened behavioral sensitivity to MK-801.

The genetically inbred BALB/c mouse strain differed from other inbred mouse strains and an outbred comparator strain in terms of increased sensitivity to behavioral effects of MK-801 (dizocilpine).[1,3,4] Moreover, the BALB/c mouse strain was shown to have deficits of both social preference and social interaction in a standard 3-chamber apparatus used to assess social behaviors.[5,59] Social preference compares to time spent by a test mouse (eg, the BALB/c mouse) exploring an enclosed stimulus mouse versus time spent exploring an inanimate object, and social interaction measures operationally defined social interactions between a freely behaving test mouse and stimulus mouse.[5,59]

Early work conducted in an outbred mouse strain genetically related to the Swiss Webster mouse (ie, the NIH Swiss mouse) showed that the acute intraperitoneal administration of MK-801 over a dosage range of 0.32 to 1.00 mg/kg elicited discrete episodes of explosive jumping behavior, referred to as popping.[4,55,60] Moreover, when the intensity of MK-801-elicited popping behavior in the NIH Swiss outbred strain of mouse was compared with MK-801-elicited popping behavior in 4 inbred strains of mice (ie, BALB/c, C57BL/6, AKR, and DBA/2), the BALB/c strain showed a dramatically increased sensitivity to the elicitation of popping that seemed to be dose dependent.[1] Moreover, the intensity of MK-801-elicited popping behavior in C57BL/6, AKR and DBA/2 mice was below that of NIH Swiss mice. These data supported a genetic contribution to the elicitation of popping behavior by MK-801, and focused interest on the BALB/c mouse as a test strain for screening NMDA receptor agonist interventions for neuropsychiatric disorders, whose pathogenesis involves NRH.[61] The data support genetic contributions to strain differences in behavioral sensitivity to MK-801; however, they do not clarify whether differences reflect pharmacodynamic differences in binding and/or NMDA receptor-mediated transduction of L-glutamate and D-serine/glycine or pharmacokinetic differences in distribution, brain uptake and clearance of MK-801 between strains, among other possibilities. In any event, it may be possible to identify and quantify the contributions of discrete chromosomal loci to "sensitivity" and "resistance" to behavioral effects of MK-801 (referred to as quantitative trait loci [QTLs]) by creating recombinant inbred strains through the cross-breeding of sensitive and resistant inbred strains.[62,63] Ideally, QTLs in the mouse would suggest homologous loci in the human genome with relevance to pathogenesis or genetic architecture of disorders with presumptive NRH, such as schizophrenia and autism spectrum disorder (ASD). Of course, the uncertain relevance of behavioral effects of MK-801 in the mouse to complex phenotypes of neuropsychiatric disorders limits meaningful extrapolation.

The BALB/c strain was also more sensitive than C57BL/6, AKR, DBA/2, and NIH Swiss mice to MK-801's ability to raise the threshold voltage required to precipitate tonic hindlimb extension.[3] Specifically, relative to these other strains, a higher percentage of BALB/c mice were maximally protected against electrically precipitated seizures over an MK-801 dosage range of 0.18 to 0.56 mg/kg administered intraperitoneally. These data are consistent with genetic factors influencing anti-seizure effects of MK-801 and increased sensitivity of the BALB/c strain to behavioral effects of MK-801. Moreover, the BALB/c inbred mouse strain was exquisitely sensitive to the elicitation of circling behavior by MK-801 relative to the comparator Swiss Webster outbred strain.[1] Specifically, at intraperitoneally injected doses of 0.32 and 0.56 mg/kg of MK-801, groups of BALB/c mice circled an average of about 100 (0.56 mg/kg) or more times (0.32 mg/kg), whereas the comparator strain circled an average of about 5 times (0.56 mg/kg) or not at all (0.32 mg/kg) in 60 minutes.[1] At MK-801 doses of 1.0 and 1.8 mg/kg, circling behavior in the BALB/c strain decreased to an average of about 40 and less than 10 in a 60 minute observation period, respectively, which reflects the behavioral inhibition of circling due to emergence of ataxia and popping behavior, whereas circling behavior remained close to 0 at these higher doses for the comparator Swiss Webster strain.[1] Thus, the BALB/c strain separates from other mouse strains in terms of providing more intense behavioral readouts of acute pharmacologic induction of NRH.

As noted above, combinatorial diversity is a regulatory mechanism of heterotetra-meric NMDA receptor activation, resulting from the incorporation of different combinations of 8 functional GluN1 splice variants derived from 3 alternatively spliced exons within a single GluN1 gene and 4 different GluN2 subunits derived from 4 separate and distinct genes, designated A through D.[64] Of interest, a study exploring relative protein expression of 6 of the 8 GluN1 splice variant isoforms and GluN2A and GluN2B subunits in mouse hippocampus and cerebral cortex showed no differences between BALB/c mice, a strain with behavioral hypersensitivity to MK-801, and NIH Swiss mice, an outbred comparator strain.[64] Protein subunits were separated and quantified in tissue homogenates using standard gel electrophoresis and Western blotting procedures. However, strain differences in modulatory effects of D-serine, a glycine agonist, and sarcosine, a naturally occurring metabolite that inhibits the glycine transporter, were detected 24-h after the stressful exposure of individual mice to 10 minutes of forced swimming in cold water.[65]

In an early experiment comparing the effects of an enclosed or freely-behaving stimulus mouse on horizontal locomotor activity of individual BALB/c or Swiss Webster mice in the 3-chamber sociability apparatus, the presence of the stimulus mouse significantly reduced horizontal locomotor activity of the BALB/c strain in both conditions.[5] This observation supported an earlier proposal that the BALB/c mouse displayed low sociability, which would be relevant to biological investigations of autism.[66,67] In subsequent work, the BALB/c mouse strain was shown to have deficits of social preference and social interaction in the standard 3-chamber apparatus. As noted, social preference compares the time spent by a test mouse exploring an enclosed stimulus mouse versus time spent exploring an inanimate object. Measures of social interaction include "ratings" of discrete episodes of operationally defined social interactions between a freely behaving test mouse (eg, 4 or 8-week-old male BALB/c mice or age- and gender-matched Swiss Webster comparator mice) and a stimulus mouse (eg, a 4-week-old male ICR mouse), as well as actual time spent engaged in some of these operationally defined behaviors, such as social pursuit.[59] Measures of social interaction were chosen because of descriptive similarities to deficits of social behavior in persons with ASD that could be rated with good reliability. BALB/c and Swiss Webster strains were significantly distinguished from each other on the following measures: social approach, social avoidance, social pursuit (measured in seconds), mounting, anogenital sniffing, and conspecific-provoked immobility.[11,59] Interestingly, the impaired social behavior of the BALB/c strain increased the proportion of discrete episodes of total social approaches made by the ICR stimulus mouse; thus, impaired sociability of a mouse influences social interest shown by other conspecifics. Finally, there was the suggestion that impaired social behaviors could be "dissociated" from stereotypic behaviors in the BALB/c strain. Stereotypic behaviors, such as rearing, were measured during free interaction between test and stimulus mice and were actually significantly less intense in the BALB/c strain than in the Swiss Webster comparator strain.[59]

Heightened sensitivity of the BALB/c mouse to behavioral effects of acute pharmacologic induction of NRH by MK-801 and its impaired sociability stimulated interest in exploring the effects of NMDA receptor agonist interventions on the BALB/c mouse.[43] Thus, an inventory of promising pharmacologic candidates was screened, which included D-serine, a full glycine agonist, D-cycloserine, a partial glycine agonist, and a high-affinity, highly selective glycine transporter type 1 (GlyT1) inhibitor, among other strategies, in a standard paradigm using the BALB/c mouse as the "test" mouse.[6–11,68,69]

D-Cycloserine

Early experiments sought to explore the "therapeutic" effectiveness of D-cycloserine, a partial glycine agonist (320 mg/kg, administered intraperitoneally), to promote prosocial behaviors in 8-week-old male BALB/c mice, and assess possible developmental influences on its effectiveness.[6,9] Thus, in the first study of 8-week-old mice, we tested the effects of D-cycloserine on a variety of operationally defined social behaviors in both the inbred BALB/c strain and the comparator Swiss Webster strain.[6] Importantly, we began our studies of NMDA receptor agonist strategies with D-cycloserine for several reasons: a promising 8-week dose escalation clinical trial reported that D-cycloserine improved ratings on the lethargy/social withdrawal subscale of the Aberrant Behavior Checklist in 10 patients diagnosed with DSM-IV autistic disorder (mean age = 10.0 years; age range 5.1–27.6 years)[70]; a preclinical "resident-intruder social interaction paradigm" reporting that D-cycloserine increased the social investigation of the intruder by resident mice[6]; and the theoretic assumption that a partial agonist, in contrast to a full agonist, would be less likely to cause undesired "excitotoxic" effects and reduced sensitivity of the glycine orthosteric site, especially if studies of chronic administration were to be pursued.[6,7] The 4-week-old male ICR mouse was chosen as a stimulus mouse because its age and gender would be less likely to elicit aggressive or sexual behaviors in test mice. In the vehicle-treated conditions, 8-week-old male BALB/c mice made significantly fewer discrete episodes of social approach during free interaction with a stimulus mouse, and locomotor activity was significantly reduced in the presence of an enclosed and freely behaving stimulus mouse, compared with the Swiss Webster strain; these data replicated earlier findings.[6,9] Importantly, D-cycloserine "normalized" the 8-week-old BALB/c strain such that both discrete episodes of social approach when freely interacting with a stimulus mouse and horizontal locomotor activity in the presence of both an enclosed and freely behaving stimulus mouse were equal to measures obtained in vehicle-treated age and gender-matched Swiss Webster mice. Moreover, there did not seem to be any "neurotoxic" antisocial effects of D-cycloserine on these behaviors in the Swiss Webster strain; in fact, D-cycloserine increased the number of discrete episodes of social approach in the Swiss Webster strain relative to its vehicle-treated condition.[6]

Because ASD is a neurodevelopmental disorder, efforts are directed toward early diagnosis to enable earlier administration of potentially "disease-modifying" psychosocial and psychopharmacological interventions. Thus, we studied possible prosocial effects of D-cycloserine in 4-week old, 1-week postweanling male BALB/c and Swiss Webster mice.[7] D-Cycloserine (320 mg/kg) increased the horizontal locomotor activity of 4-week-old male BALB/c mice, relative to their vehicle-treated condition, when a stimulus mouse was both enclosed in an inverted cup and allowed to behave freely.[7] Moreover, the horizontal locomotor activity of the D-cycloserine-treated 4-week-old male BALB/c mice "normalized" to a level that did not differ significantly from that of vehicle-treated Swiss Webster mice in the presence of enclosed or freely behaving stimulus mice. However, on this measure (ie, horizontal locomotor activity), a possible prosocial effect of D-cycloserine could not be differentiated from a nonspecific effect of D-cycloserine to increase locomotor activity in general, especially as D-cycloserine increased locomotor activity of both strains during their acclimation to the 3-chamber sociability apparatus before exposure to stimulus mice.

Dramatic prosocial effects of D-cycloserine were observed in the 4-week-old male BALB/c mice on social preference and measures of social interaction with 4-week-old male ICR mice serving as the salient social stimulus.[7] Thus, D-cycloserine (320 mg/kg) significantly increased the amount of time immature BALB/c mice spent in the chamber housing enclosed stimulus mice and time they spent sniffing and exploring enclosed stimulus mice within a 2 cm radius of the enclosure; this contrasted with the absence of preference for a social stimulus mouse over an inanimate object in the vehicle-treated condition. Additionally, prosocial effects of D-cycloserine (320 mg) were detected in 4-week-old male BALB/c mice on the following measures of their social interaction with 4-week-old male ICR mice: increased discrete episodes of social approach; decreased discrete episodes of social avoidance; and increased discrete episodes of anogenital sniffing. When a range of D-cycloserine doses was explored (ie, 32, 56, 100, and 180 mg/kg), significantly improved social preference (ie, time spent exploring and sniffing an enclosed stimulus mouse vs an inanimate object) was detected at the 32 mg/kg dose, the lowest dose tested (Deutsch and colleagues, 2012). D-cycloserine did not increase stereotypic behaviors, such as rearing, wall climbing, and grooming in the BALB/c strain, which were emitted infrequently in the vehicle condition, and significantly decreased these stereotypic behaviors in the Swiss Webster strain, which displayed a significantly increased rate of occurrence of these behaviors in the vehicle-treated condition, relative to BALB/c mice. These data suggest that targeting the glycine binding site on the NMDA receptor with D-cycloserine, a partial glycine agonist, has desired prosocial properties at doses that do not increase the intensity of stereotypic behaviors, which may relate to diminished liability for neurologic side effects.[7] Moreover, D-cycloserine improved stereotypic behavior in the Swiss Webster strain, suggesting that targeting the NMDA receptor may also have beneficial therapeutic effects on repetitive stereotypic behaviors.

Experiments conducted with an elevated plus maze (EPM) showed that 8-week-old male BALB/c mice do not spend less time in the open arms than age- and gender-matched Swiss Webster mice, which suggests that BALB/c mice are not more anxious than Swiss Webster mice in the absence of a social stimulus mouse.[9] Decreased time spent in open-arm exploration is thought to be a measure of anxiety. Moreover, vehicle-treated BALB/c mice actually spent significantly more time in the open-arms of the EPM than BALB/c mice treated with D-cycloserine (320 mg/kg), which is the reverse of what was observed with the Swiss Webster strain (ie, D-cycloserine increased the amount of time Swiss Webster mice spent in the open arms). However, although strain differences emerged with respect to D-cycloserine's effect on the total amount of time spent in the open arms, the treatment significantly increased the total number of open-arm entries by both strains, compared with the vehicle-treated controls of these respective strains. Although there were no strain differences in either the amount of time spent in the open-field exploration of an inanimate object or the effect of D-cycloserine on this measure of exploring an inanimate object, the vehicle-treated BALB/c mouse spent significantly less time exploring a 4-week-old male ICR mouse enclosed in an inverted wire cup contained within the open-field than the Swiss Webster comparator mouse. However, treatment with D-cycloserine (320 mg/kg) had a strain-selective effect on the open-field exploration of a 4-week-old male ICR mouse: only D-cycloserine-treated BALB/c mice showed increased time spent exploring the social stimulus mouse compared with its vehicle-treated control.[9] The data suggest that strain differences in exploratory behavior emerge in the presence of a salient social stimulus mouse. The data also suggest that in the absence of a salient stimulus mouse, the BALB/c mouse may not be more anxious than the Swiss Webster comparator strain. The data showing a strain-independent effect of treatment with D-cycloserine (320 mg/kg) on increasing the number of open arm entries may suggest a nonspecific effect of D-cycloserine on locomotor activity. In any event, the data support a strain-selective and somewhat specific prosocial effect of D-cycloserine in the BALB/c strain, which could reflect a functionally relevant impairment of NMDA receptor-mediated neurotransmission in the BALB/c strain.[9]

D-Cycloserine's ability to improve sociability in the BALB/c mouse model of ASD stimulated interest in the generalizability of its prosocial effects in another mouse model of ASD; thus, D-cycloserine (320 mg/kg) was administered to 4-week old, male genetically inbred BTBR T + Itpr 3tf/J (BTBR) mice.[71] D-Cycloserine improved social preference of the BTBR mouse, increasing time spent both in the chamber containing the enclosed stimulus mouse and time spent exploring the enclosed mouse; vehicle-treated BTBR mice showed no social preference.[71] D-Cycloserine improved the following measures of social interaction in the BTBR mouse: increased discrete episodes and time spent in social approach; decreased discrete episodes of social avoidance; and increased discrete episodes of anogenital sniffing. Finally, D-cycloserine decreased both discrete episodes of grooming and time spent by the BTBR mouse engaged in grooming.[71]

In addition to the prosocial effects of D-cycloserine in BALB/c test mice, enclosed D-cycloserine (320 mg/kg)-treated BALB/cJ stimulus mice aroused greater social preference/interest in C57BL/6 test mice than similarly treated and simultaneously enclosed vehicle-treated BALB/cJ stimulus mice.[68] The data suggest the provocative possibility that the treatment of the BALB/c mouse strain with D-cycloserine led to its emission of social cues recognized by the C57BL/6 inbred mouse strain, a strain thought to be "hyper-social."[68]

Exploratory human translational trial of D-cycloserine

Translational "proof of principle/concept" clinical trials exploring NMDA receptor agonist interventions for neuropsychiatric indications are possible with D-cycloserine, which has an approved indication for the treatment of tuberculosis.[70,72–77] The doses used to treat tuberculosis are up to 10 times higher than those used for exploratory studies of this "repurposed" medication for psychiatric indications. Interest in a translational clinical trial of D-cycloserine in ASD was stimulated by our preclinical investigations, suggesting that it might target both impaired sociability and repetitive stereotypic behaviors and a promising 8-week, ascending dose, single-blind pilot study reported by Posey and colleagues (2004).[70] In the study by Posey and colleagues (2004), 10 subjects (8 male; age range = 5.1–27.6 years) with DSM-IV diagnoses of autistic disorder completed all 8 weeks of the study, receiving dose escalations (0.7, 1.4, 2.8 mg/kg/d) at intervals of 2-week after a 2-week placebo lead-in phase.[70] Improvements were noted on severity ratings of the Clinical Global Impressions (CGI) scale and the social withdrawal subscale of the Aberrant Behavior Checklist.[70]

As discussed, because D-cycloserine is a partial glycine agonist, there are theoretic reasons for suggesting it may have lesser liability to cause "agonist-induced desensitization" and side effects related to excitotoxicity. Nonetheless, because of concerns about confounding effects of possible receptor desensitization, the design of our 10-week trial with 8 weeks of active drug was a randomized, double-blind comparison of a pulsed once-weekly dose of 50 mg versus a daily 50 mg dose of D-cycloserine; 20 patients fulfilling DSM-IV Text Revision criteria for an ASD (14 males and 6 females; ages 14–25 years; total IQs ≥70) participated in the trial.[73,74] Statistically and clinically significant improvements were noted on the Social Responsiveness Scale (SRS) and the Aberrant Behavior Checklist (ABC), including the ABC "lethargy/social withdrawal" and "stereotypic behavior" subscales.[73,74] In summary, the NMDA receptor emerged as a promising therapeutic target in ASD.

VU0410120, a high-affinity, highly selective "nonsarcosine" derived GlyT1 inhibitor

Conceivably, "prosocial" effects of released L-glutamate evoked locally by salient social challenges would be potentiated by increasing synaptic concentrations of obligatory coagonists achieved by GlyT1 inhibition.[10] This hypothesis was tested in the BALB/c mouse model by the administration of VU0410120 (2,4-dichloro-N-((4-(cyclopropylmethyl)-1-(ethylsulfonyl)piperidine-4-yl)methyl)benzamide), a high-affinity (IC_{50} for the GlyT1 site = 26 nM), highly selective "nonsarcosine" derived GlyT1 inhibitor. VU0410120 improved social preference in the BALB/c model increasing both time spent in the compartment containing an enclosed stimulus mouse and time spent exploring an enclosed stimulus mouse.[10] VU0410120 dramatically decreased the latency of the BALB/c mouse to approach the enclosed stimulus mouse. Moreover, VU0410120 improved measures of social interaction, including increasing discrete episodes of social approach; decreasing discrete episodes of social avoidance; and increasing time spent in social pursuit. Finally, this GlyT1 inhibitor reduced rearing and grooming in both the BALB/c model and comparator Swiss Webster strain. These data suggest that targeting the GlyT1 site facilitates the activation of NMDA receptors provoked within discrete neural circuits by a salient social stimulus; moreover, in addition to desired prosocial effects, VU0410120 may reduce the intensity of repetitive stereotypic behaviors.[10]

Consistent with its impaired sociability, the immobility of BALB/c mice in the presence of an enclosed or freely behaving stimulus mouse (referred to as "Conspecific-Provoked Immobility [CPI]") was significantly greater than that displayed by the Swiss Webster comparator strain.[11] CPI is used as a behavioral index of social stress. Interestingly, however, although CPI was significantly greater in vehicle-treated BALB/c than vehicle-treated Swiss Webster mice, serum corticosterone levels, a biochemical marker of social stress, did not differ between these groups after exposure to the stimulus mouse.[11] Moreover, treatment with VU0410120, a high-affinity, highly selective GlyT1 inhibitor, significantly decreased CPI in the BALB/c strain; however, serum corticosterone levels did not differ between BALB/c mice showing high or low intensity of CPI in either the vehicle-treated or VU0410120-treated conditions.[11] The serum corticosterone data suggest that disinterest in the socially salient stimulus mouse, in addition to the stressfulness of the social encounter itself, made a significant contribution to the immobility scores of the BALB/c strain. The data also suggest that VU0410120 may act to increase the social salience of the stimulus mouse for the BALB/c strain.[11]

N-methyl-D-aspartic Acid Receptor Activation, a Regulator of Mechanistic Target of Rapamycin Signaling

The mechanistic target of rapamycin (mTOR), a serine/threonine protein kinase, is the defining enzymatic component of mTORC1, a highly regulated multimeric protein. mTORC1 integrates the input of external signals, such as growth factors (eg, brain-derived neurotrophic factor [BDNF]) and neurotransmitters (eg, L-glutamate and acetylcholine), internal nutritional signals (eg, intracellular arginine levels), and the cell's internal energy status (ie, ratio of AMP to ATP) to determine important outputs, including cell cycle kinetics, cellular differentiation, and protein synthesis in the periphery of neurons.[12] Pathological overactivation of mTORC1 has been described as a metabolic point of convergence in several monogenic abnormalities associated with ASD, most notably "Tuberous Sclerosis Complex" (TSC).[13–16,78–83]

The heteromeric TSC protein complex, composed of TSC1 (hamartin), TSC2 (tuberin) and "Tre2-Bub2-Cdc16 1 domain family, member 7 (TBC1D7)," serves as a negative regulator of mTORC1. TSC1 stabilizes the TSC complex and TSC2 is the "GTPase activating protein (GAP)" of the heteromeric TSC protein complex that provides inhibitory input onto mTORC1's activation by the GTP-dependent "Ras homolog enriched in brain (RHEB).'[13–16,78–83] Genetic lesions affecting TSC1 and TSC2 cause impairment or inability of the heteromeric TSC protein complex to hydrolyze the terminal phosphate group on the GTP bound to RHEB, which relieves the inhibitory influence of the heteromeric TSC protein complex on this GTP-dependent Ras protein (ie, RHRB) allowing it to stimulate mTORC1's catalytic serine/threonine kinase activity without regulatory restraint.[12,15,83]

Several prominent psychopathological and phenotypic characteristics of TSC may be more significantly related to metabolic overactivation of mTORC1 and downstream consequences, which include the upregulation of protein translation in the periphery of neurons via phosphorylation of "eukaryotic translation initiation factor 4E-binding protein 1 (eIF-4EBP-1)" and "S6 Kinase (S6K1)," than pathologic hallmarks, such as density of cortical tubers.[15,79,81] Increasingly, there is interest in "proof of principle/proof of concept" translational studies exploring the therapeutic potential of mTORC1 inhibitors (eg, rapamycin and everolimus) in preclinical monogenic mouse models of TSC and hypothesis-testing clinical trials.[13,79,84–88] Moreover, therapeutic strategies for targeting presumptive dysregulation of mTORC1 activity are under investigation in models of "nonsyndromic" ASD and seek to maintain its enzymatic kinase activity and downstream consequences within a "healthy" physiologic range.[83,89]

NMDA receptor activation can inhibit, regulate, and/or fine tune the activity of mTORC1 and its downstream consequences through 2 complementary intracellular signaling mechanisms.[12] NMDA receptor activation causes the internalization of 2 isoforms of the "cationic amino acid transporter (CAT1/3)" that transport arginine into cortical neurons, the latter is detected by internal "nutrient sensors."[13] Detection of lowered intraneuronal concentrations of arginine leads to dampened mTORC1 activity and diminished translational "noise" and dysregulated protein synthesis. NMDA receptor-mediated promotion of transiently increased Ca^{2+} concentrations can lead to downstream activation of "STriatal Enriched protein tyrosine Phosphatase (STEP)," a phosphatase enriched in nodes within circuits critical for sociability and cognition, such as hippocampus and frontal cortex.[90–93] In turn, STEP can dephosphorylate activated "extracellular signal regulated kinase 1/2 (ERK1/2)," inactivating this driver of mTORC1 activity, which serves as an additional mechanism for dampening overactivation of mTORC1.[12] Prosocial effects of rapamycin in the "nonsyndromic" BTBR mouse model of ASD support the exploration of strategies that target mTORC1 to maintain its activity and outputs within an optimal therapeutic range in ASD.[12,94]

SUMMARY

D-Cycloserine has been a useful tool in support of "proof of principle/proof of concept" studies exploring therapeutic targeting of the NMDA receptor in preclinical models of ASD and early translational clinical trials. Increasingly, however, medication development must focus on strategies that are more "physiologic" and better able to preserve and mimic the exquisite spatial and temporal selectivity of endogenously released neurotransmitters within discrete neural circuits while responding to socio-cognitive challenges and performing complex motor behaviors.

Importantly, a variety of genetically unrelated risk alleles associated with clinical presentations of ASD share NMDA receptor hypofunction and/or disruption of a delicate balance between NMDA receptor activation mediated by GluN2B-subtype-containing and GluN2A-subtype-containing NMDA receptors as their common downstream pathophysiological point of convergence.[22] Thus, strategies to selectively increase NMDA receptor activation, via NMDA receptor-subtype-selective PAMs, and/or selectively decrease NMDA receptor activation, via NMDA receptor-subtype-selective NAMs, have great therapeutic appeal, especially for the treatment of at least some distinct monogenic forms of ASD.[22]

CLINICS CARE POINTS

- Current medications for ASD target secondary symptoms, such as irritability and agitation
- Newer medication strategies should address core symptoms, such as deficits in social communication and restricted and narrowed interests and repetitive stereotypic behaviors
- An ideal medication will improve sociability and cognition, while devoid of adverse central nervous system (CNS) side effects
- Several syndromic forms of autism resulting from big effects of single genes are associated with NMDA receptor hypofunction (NRH) or imbalance between neurotransmission mediated by GluR2B and GluR2A-subtype-containing NMDA receptors
- Ideally, correcting NRH or restoring the balance between GluR2B and GluR2A-subtype-containing NMDA receptor activation will facilitate improvements in socialization and cognition
- NMDA receptor-subtype-selective PAMs and NAMs represent potentially viable pharmacotherapeutic strategies for targeting pathogenic disruptions in at least some patients with ASD

DISCLOSURE

The authors (S.I. Deutsch and J.A. Burket) have nothing to disclose.

REFERENCES

1. Burket JA, Cannon WR, Jacome LF, et al. MK-801, a noncompetitive NMDA receptor antagonist, elicits circling behavior in the genetically inbred Balb/c mouse strain. Brain Res Bull 2010;83(6):337–9.
2. Deutsch SI, Mastropaolo J, Riggs RL, et al. The antiseizure efficacies of MK-801, phencyclidine, ketamine, and memantine are altered selectively by stress. Pharmacol Biochem Behav 1997;58(3):709–12.
3. Deutsch SI, Mastropaolo J, Powell DG, et al. Inbred mouse strains differ in their sensitivity to an antiseizure effect of MK-801. Clin Neuropharmacol 1998;21(4):255–7.
4. Deutsch SI, Rosse RB, Paul SM, et al. Inbred mouse strains differ in sensitivity to "popping" behavior elicited by MK-801. Pharmacol Biochem Behav 1997;57(1–2):315–7.

5. Burket JA, Herndon AL, Deutsch SI. Locomotor activity of the genetically inbred Balb/c mouse strain is suppressed by a socially salient stimulus. Brain Res Bull 2010;83(5):255–6.
6. Deutsch SI, Burket JA, Jacome LF, et al. D-Cycloserine improves the impaired sociability of the Balb/c mouse. Brain Res Bull 2011;84(1):8–11.
7. Deutsch SI, Pepe GJ, Burket JA, et al. D-cycloserine improves sociability and spontaneous stereotypic behaviors in 4-week old mice. Brain Res 2012;1439: 96–107.
8. Jacome LF, Burket JA, Herndon AL, et al. D-serine improves dimensions of the sociability deficit of the genetically-inbred Balb/c mouse strain. Brain Res Bull 2011;84(1):12–6.
9. Jacome LF, Burket JA, Herndon AL, et al. D-Cycloserine enhances social exploration in the Balb/c mouse. Brain Res Bull 2011;85(3–4):141–4.
10. Burket JA, Benson AD, Green TL, et al. Effects of VU0410120, a novel GlyT1 inhibitor, on measures of sociability, cognition and stereotypic behaviors in a mouse model of autism. Prog Neuropsychopharmacol Biol Psychiatry 2015;61:10–7.
11. Burket JA, Pickle JC, Rusk AM, et al. Glycine transporter type 1 (GlyT1) inhibition improves conspecific-provoked immobility in BALB/c mice: Analysis of corticosterone response and glucocorticoid gene expression in cortex and hippocampus. Prog Neuropsychopharmacol Biol Psychiatry 2020;99:109869.
12. Burket JA, Benson AD, Tang AH, et al. NMDA receptor activation regulates sociability by its effect on mTOR signaling activity. Prog Neuropsychopharmacol Biol Psychiatry 2015;60C:60–5.
13. Huang Y, Kang BN, Tian J, et al. The cationic amino acid transporters CAT1 and CAT3 mediate NMDA receptor activation-dependent changes in elaboration of neuronal processes via the mammalian target of rapamycin mTOR pathway. J Neurosci 2007;27(3):449–58.
14. Onore C, Yang H, Van de Water J, et al. Dynamic Akt/mTOR signaling in children with autism spectrum disorder. Front Pediatr 2017;5:43.
15. Magdalon J, Sánchez-Sánchez SM, Griesi-Oliveira K, et al. Dysfunctional mTORC1 signaling: a convergent mechanism between syndromic and nonsyndromic forms of autism spectrum disorder? Int J Mol Sci 2017;18(3):E659.
16. Ehninger D. From genes to cognition in tuberous sclerosis: implications for mTOR inhibitor-based treatment approaches. Neuropharmacology 2013;68:97–105.
17. Ehninger D, Silva AJ. Rapamycin for treating tuberous sclerosis and autism spectrum disorders. Trends Mol Med 2011;17(2):78–87.
18. Britto FA, Dumas K, Giorgetti-Peraldi S, et al. Is REDD1 a metabolic double agent? Lessons from physiology and pathology. Am J Physiol Cell Physiol 2020;319(5):C807–24.
19. Hansen KB, Yi F, Perszyk RE, et al. Structure, function, and allosteric modulation of NMDA receptors. J Gen Physiol 2018;150(8):1081–105.
20. Traynelis SF, Wollmuth LP, McBain CJ, et al. Glutamate receptor ion channels: structure, regulation, and function. Pharmacol Rev 2010;62(3):405–96.
21. Nisar S, Bhat AA, Masoodi T, et al. Genetics of glutamate and its receptors in autism spectrum disorder. Mol Psychiatry 2022. https://doi.org/10.1038/s41380-022-01506-w. Published online March 16.
22. Deutsch SI, Luyo ZNM, Burket JA. Targeted NMDA receptor interventions for autism: developmentally determined expression of GluN2B and GluN2A-containing receptors and balanced allosteric modulatory approaches. Biomolecules 2022;12(2):181.

23. Hansen KB, Furukawa H, Traynelis SF. Control of assembly and function of gluta-mate receptors by the amino-terminal domain. Mol Pharmacol 2010;78(4): 535–49.

24. Burket JA, Deutsch SI. Metabotropic functions of the NMDA receptor and an evolving rationale for exploring NR2A-selective positive allosteric modulators for the treatment of autism spectrum disorder. Prog Neuropsychopharmacol Biol Psychiatry 2019;90:142–60.

25. Hardingham GE. NMDA receptor C-terminal signaling in development, plasticity, and disease. F1000Res 2019;8:F1000. Faculty Rev-1547.

26. Liu S, Zhou L, Yuan H, et al. A rare variant identified within the GluN2B C-terminus in a patient with autism affects NMDA receptor surface expression and spine density. J Neurosci 2017;37(15):4093–102.

27. Wyllie DJA, Livesey MR, Hardingham GE. Influence of GluN2 subunit identity on NMDA receptor function. Neuropharmacology 2013;74:4–17.

28. Herbrechter R, Hube N, Buchholz R, et al. Splicing and editing of ionotropic glutamate receptors: a comprehensive analysis based on human RNA-seq data. Cell Mol Life Sci 2021;78(14):5605–30.

29. Vieira M, Yong XLH, Roche KW, et al. Regulation of NMDA glutamate receptor functions by the GluN2 subunits. J Neurochem 2020;154(2):121–43.

30. Vizi ES, Kisfali M, Lőrincz T. Role of nonsynaptic GluN2B-containing NMDA re-ceptors in excitotoxicity: Evidence that fluoxetine selectively inhibits these recep-tors and may have neuroprotective effects. Brain Res Bull 2013;93:32–8.

31. Shipton OA, Paulsen O. GluN2A and GluN2B subunit-containing NMDA recep-tors in hippocampal plasticity. Philos Trans R Soc Lond B Biol Sci 2014; 369(1633):20130163.

32. Monyer H, Burnashev N, Laurie DJ, et al. Developmental and regional expression in the rat brain and functional properties of four NMDA receptors. Neuron 1994; 12(3):529–40.

33. Sapkota K, Dore K, Tang K, et al. The NMDA receptor intracellular C-terminal do-mains reciprocally interact with allosteric modulators. Biochem Pharmacol 2019; 159:140.

34. Choi YB, Tenneti L, Le DA, et al. Molecular basis of NMDA receptor-coupled ion channel modulation by S-nitrosylation. Nat Neurosci 2000;3(1):15–21.

35. Burket JA, Webb JD, Deutsch SI. Perineuronal nets and metal cation concentra-tions in the microenvironments of fast-spiking, parvalbumin-expressing GABAergic interneurons: relevance to neurodevelopment and neurodevelop-mental disorders. Biomolecules 2021;11(8):1235.

36. Awad H, Hubert GW, Smith Y, et al. Activation of metabotropic glutamate receptor 5 has direct excitatory effects and potentiates NMDA receptor currents in neu-rons of the subthalamic nucleus. J Neurosci 2000;20(21):7871–9.

37. Gu L, Luo WY, Xia N, et al. Upregulated mGluR5 induces ER stress and DNA damage by regulating the NMDA receptor subunit NR2B. J Biochem 2022; 171(3):349–59.

38. Takagi N, Besshoh S, Morita H, et al. Metabotropic glutamate mGlu5 receptor-mediated serine phosphorylation of NMDA receptor subunit NR1 in hippocampal CA1 region after transient global ischemia in rats. Eur J Pharmacol 2010; 644(1–3):96–100.

39. Conn PJ, Lindsley CW, Jones CK. Activation of metabotropic glutamate receptors as a novel approach for the treatment of schizophrenia. Trends Pharmacol Sci 2009;30(1):25–31.

40. Choe ES, Shin EH, Wang JQ. Regulation of phosphorylation of NMDA receptor NR1 subunits in the rat neostriatum by group I metabotropic glutamate receptors in vivo. Neurosci Lett 2006;394(3):246–51.
41. Clarke RJ, Johnson JW. Voltage-dependent gating of NR1/2B NMDA receptors. J Physiol 2008;586(23):5727–41.
42. Millan MJ. N-Methyl-D-aspartate receptors as a target for improved antipsychotic agents: novel insights and clinical perspectives. Psychopharmacology (Berl) 2005;179(1):30–53.
43. Deutsch SI, Burket JA, Benson AD, et al. NMDA agonists for autism spectrum disorders: progress and possibilities. Future Neurol 2015;10(5):485–500.
44. Zappettini S, Grilli M, Olivero G, et al. Nicotinic α7 receptor activation selectively potentiates the function of NMDA receptors in glutamatergic terminals of the nucleus accumbens. Front Cell Neurosci 2014;8. Available at: https://www.frontiersin.org/article/10.3389/fncel.2014.00332. Accessed March 27, 2022.
45. Yang Y, Paspalas CD, Jin LE, et al. Nicotinic α7 receptors enhance NMDA cognitive circuits in dorsolateral prefrontal cortex. Proc Natl Acad Sci USA 2013; 110(29):12078–83.
46. Oliet SHR, Mothet JP. Regulation of N-methyl-D-aspartate receptors by astrocytic D-serine. Neuroscience 2009;158(1):275–83.
47. Dore K, Stein IS, Brock JA, et al. Unconventional NMDA receptor signaling. J Neurosci 2017;37(45):10800–7.
48. Conn PJ, Christopoulos A, Lindsley CW. Allosteric modulators of GPCRs: a novel approach for the treatment of CNS disorders. Nat Rev Drug Discov 2009;8(1): 41–54.
49. Geoffroy C, Paoletti P, Mony L. Positive allosteric modulation of NMDA receptors: mechanisms, physiological impact and therapeutic potential. J Physiol 2021. https://doi.org/10.1113/JP280875.
50. Hackos DH, Hanson JE. Diverse modes of NMDA receptor positive allosteric modulation: mechanisms and consequences. Neuropharmacology 2017;112(Pt A):34–45.
51. Silverman JL, Smith DG, Rizzo SJS, et al. Negative allosteric modulation of the mGluR5 receptor reduces repetitive behaviors and rescues social deficits in mouse models of autism. Sci Transl Med 2012;4(131):131ra51.
52. Labrie V, Wang W, Barger SW, et al. Genetic loss of D-amino acid oxidase activity reverses schizophrenia-like phenotypes in mice. Genes Brain Behav 2010;9(1): 11–25.
53. Deutsch SI, Mastropaolo J, Schwartz BL, et al. A "glutamatergic hypothesis" of schizophrenia. Rationale for pharmacotherapy with glycine. Clin Neuropharmacol 1989;12(1):1–13.
54. Halene TB, Ehrlichman RS, Liang Y, et al. Assessment of NMDA receptor NR1 subunit hypofunction in mice as a model for schizophrenia. Genes Brain Behav 2009;8(7):661–75.
55. Deutsch SI, Hitri A. Measurement of an explosive behavior in the mouse, induced by MK-801, a PCP analogue. Clin Neuropharmacol 1993;16(3):251–7.
56. Deutsch SI, Rosse RB, Billingslea EN, et al. Topiramate antagonizes MK-801 in an animal model of schizophrenia. Eur J Pharmacol 2002;449(1–2):121–5.
57. Morales M, Spear LP. The effects of an acute challenge with the NMDA receptor antagonists, MK-801, PEAQX, and ifenprodil, on social inhibition in adolescent and adult male rats. Psychopharmacology (Berl) 2014;231(8):1797–807.
58. Vishnoi S, Raisuddin S, Parvez S. Modulatory effects of an NMDAR partial agonist in MK-801-induced memory impairment. Neuroscience 2015;311:22–33.

59. Jacome LF, Burket JA, Herndon AL, et al. Genetically inbred Balb/c mice differ from outbred Swiss Webster mice on discrete measures of sociability: relevance to a genetic mouse model of autism spectrum disorders. Autism Res 2011;4(6): 393–400.

60. Rosse RB, Mastropaolo J, Sussman DM, et al. Computerized measurement of MK-801-elicited popping and hyperactivity in mice. Clin Neuropharmacol 1995; 18(5):448–57.

61. Deutsch SI, Rosse RB, Mastropaolo J. Behavioral approaches to the functional assessment of NMDA-mediated neural transmission in intact mice. Clin Neuropharmacol 1997;20(5):375–84.

62. Brodkin ES, Goforth SA, Keene AH, et al. Identification of quantitative trait Loci that affect aggressive behavior in mice. J Neurosci 2002;22(3):1165–70.

63. Bhalala OG, Nath AP, Consortium UBE, et al. Identification of expression quantitative trait loci associated with schizophrenia and affective disorders in normal brain tissue. PLOS Genet 2018;14(8):e1007607.

64. Perera PY, Lichy JH, Mastropaolo J, et al. Expression of NR1, NR2A and NR2B NMDA receptor subunits is not altered in the genetically-inbred Balb/c mouse strain with heightened behavioral sensitivity to MK-801, a noncompetitive NMDA receptor antagonist. Eur Neuropsychopharmacol 2008;18(11):814–9.

65. Long KD, Mastropaolo J, Rosse RB, et al. Modulatory effects of d-serine and sarcosine on NMDA receptor-mediated neurotransmission are apparent after stress in the genetically inbred BALB/c mouse strain. Brain Res Bull 2006;69(6):626–30.

66. Brodkin ES. BALB/c mice: low sociability and other phenotypes that may be relevant to autism. Behav Brain Res 2007;176(1):53–65.

67. Sankoorikal GMV, Kaercher KA, Boon CJ, et al. A mouse model system for genetic analysis of sociability: C57BL/6J versus BALB/cJ inbred mouse strains. Biol Psychiatry 2006;59(5):415–23.

68. Benson AD, Burket JA, Deutsch SI. Balb/c mice treated with D-cycloserine arouse increased social interest in conspecifics. Brain Res Bull 2013;99:95–9.

69. Green TL, Burket JA, Deutsch SI. Age-dependent effects on social interaction of NMDA GluN2A receptor subtype-selective antagonism. Brain Res Bull 2016;125: 159–67.

70. Posey DJ, Kem DL, Swiezy NB, et al. A pilot study of D-cycloserine in subjects with autistic disorder. Am J Psychiatry 2004;161(11):2115–7.

71. Burket JA, Benson AD, Tang AH, et al. D-Cycloserine improves sociability in the BTBR T+ Itpr3tf/J mouse model of autism spectrum disorders with altered Ras/Raf/ERK1/2 signaling. Brain Res Bull 2013;96:62–70.

72. Difede J, Cukor J, Wyka K, et al. D-cycloserine augmentation of exposure therapy for post-traumatic stress disorder: a pilot randomized clinical trial. Neuropsychopharmacology 2014;39(5):1052–8.

73. Urbano MR, Okwara L, Manser P, et al. A Trial of D-cycloserine to treat the social deficit in older adolescents and young adults with autism spectrum disorders. J Neuropsychiatry Clin Neurosci 2015;27(2):133–8. Published online April 2015.

74. Urbano M, Okwara L, Manser P, et al. A trial of D-cycloserine to treat stereotypies in older adolescents and young adults with autism spectrum disorder. Clin Neuropharmacol 2014;37(3):69–72.

75. de Kleine RA, Hendriks GJ, Smits JAJ, et al. Prescriptive variables for d-cycloserine augmentation of exposure therapy for posttraumatic stress disorder. J Psychiatr Res 2014;48(1):40–6.

76. Goff DC, Cather C, Gottlieb JD, et al. Once-weekly D-cycloserine effects on negative symptoms and cognition in schizophrenia: an exploratory study. Schizophr Res 2008;106(2–3):320–7.
77. Schade S, Paulus W. D-cycloserine in neuropsychiatric diseases: a systematic review. Int J Neuropsychopharmacol 2016;19(4):pyv102.
78. Crino PB. mTOR: a pathogenic signaling pathway in developmental brain malformations. Trends Mol Med 2011;17(12):734–42.
79. Crino PB. The mTOR signalling cascade: paving new roads to cure neurological disease. Nat Rev Neurol 2016;12(7):379–92.
80. García-Peñas JJ, Carreras-Sááez I. [Autism, epilepsy and tuberous sclerosis complex: a functional model linked to mTOR pathway]. Rev Neurol 2013; 56(Suppl 1):S153–61.
81. Laplante M, Sabatini DM. mTOR signaling in growth control and disease. Cell 2012;149(2):274–93.
82. Lipton JO, Sahin M. The neurology of mTOR. Neuron 2014;84(2):275–91.
83. McCabe MP, Cullen ER, Barrows CM, et al. Genetic inactivation of mTORC1 or mTORC2 in neurons reveals distinct functions in glutamatergic synaptic transmission. In: Monteggia LM, Boudker O, editors. eLife 2020;9:e51440.
84. Fasolo A, Sessa C. Current and future directions in mammalian target of rapamycin inhibitors development. Expert Opin Investig Drugs 2011;20(3):381–94.
85. Albert S, Serova M, Dreyer C, et al. New inhibitors of the mammalian target of rapamycin signaling pathway for cancer. Expert Opin Investig Drugs 2010;19(8): 919–30.
86. Sahin M. Targeted treatment trials for tuberous sclerosis and autism: no longer a dream. Curr Opin Neurobiol 2012;22(5):895–901.
87. Tsai PT, Hull C, Chu Y, et al. Autistic-like behaviour and cerebellar dysfunction in Purkinje cell Tsc1 mutant mice. Nature 2012;488(7413):647–51.
88. Tsai V, Parker WE, Orlova KA, et al. Fetal brain mTOR signaling activation in tuberous sclerosis complex. Cereb Cortex 2014;24(2):315–27.
89. Winden KD, Ebrahimi-Fakhari D, Sahin M. Abnormal mTOR Activation in Autism. Annu Rev Neurosci 2018;41:1–23.
90. Fitzpatrick CJ, Lombroso PJ. The role of striatal-enriched protein tyrosine phosphatase (STEP) in cognition. Front Neuroanat 2011;5:47.
91. Paul S, Connor JA. NR2B-NMDA receptor-mediated increases in intracellular Ca2+ concentration regulate the tyrosine phosphatase, STEP, and ERK MAP kinase signaling. J Neurochem 2010;114(4):1107–18.
92. Paul S, Nairn AC, Wang P, et al. NMDA-mediated activation of the tyrosine phosphatase STEP regulates the duration of ERK signaling. Nat Neurosci 2003;6(1): 34–42.
93. Zhang Y, Venkitaramani DV, Gladding CM, et al. The tyrosine phosphatase STEP mediates AMPA receptor endocytosis after metabotropic glutamate receptor stimulation. J Neurosci 2008;28(42):10561–6.
94. Burket JA, Benson AD, Tang AH, et al. Rapamycin improves sociability in the BTBR T(+)Itpr3(tf)/J mouse model of autism spectrum disorders. Brain Res Bull 2014;100:70–5.

Suicide: An Overview for Clinicians

Leo Sher, MD[a,b,c,]*, Maria A. Oquendo, MD, PhD[d]

KEYWORDS

• Suicide • Psychiatric disorder • Depression • Public health

KEY POINTS

- Suicide is a major public health problem worldwide
- Suicide generally occurs in the context of a psychiatric disorder
- Multiple psychosocial and biological factors contribute to the pathophysiology of suicide
- Careful management of depression and other psychiatric disorders is necessary to reduce suicides
- Certain psychotherapeutic and pharmacologic interventions have specific antisuicidal properties

DEFINITIONS

Suicide attempt is generally defined as a self-destructive act carried out with some degree of intent to end one's life.[1,2] Suicidal behavior refers to suicide death but also includes various types of suicide attempts that range from high lethality attempts to low-lethal attempts that may take place in the setting of a psychosocial crisis and at times encompass a component of a request for help.[3,4] Suicidal ideation is a wide term used to define a variety of thoughts, wishes, and preoccupations with suicide.[5] The severity of suicidal ideation ranges from fleeting, passive thoughts that life is not worth living and not caring if one does not wake up in the morning, to persistent, compelling thoughts of killing oneself with a specific, highly lethal method. Some suicide ideation definitions incorporate suicide planning thoughts, while others regard planning to be a separate stage. Suicidal ideation and suicidal behaviors can be theorized as taking place over a continuum from suicidal ideation, development of a suicide plan, nonfatal suicide attempt(s), or death from suicide, although the progression from one to the other is not necessarily linear.[6]

[a] James J. Peters VA Medical Center, 130 West Kingsbridge Road, Bronx, NY 10468, USA;
[b] Department of Psychiatry, Icahn School of Medicine at Mount Sinai, 1 Gustave L. Levy Place, New York, NY 10029, USA; [c] Department of Psychiatry, Columbia University Vagelos College of Physicians and Surgeons, 1051 Riverside Drive, New York, NY 10032, USA; [d] Department of Psychiatry, Perelman School of Medicine at the University of Pennsylvania, 3535 Market Street, Philadelphia, PA 19104, USA
* Corresponding author. James J. Peters VA Medical Center, 130 West Kingsbridge Road, Bronx, NY 10468.
E-mail address: Leo.Sher@mssm.edu

Med Clin N Am 107 (2023) 119–130
https://doi.org/10.1016/j.mcna.2022.03.008
0025-7125/23/Published by Elsevier Inc.

medical.theclinics.com

EPIDEMIOLOGY

Suicide is a major public health problem worldwide. The World Health Organization estimates that globally more than 800,000 people die by suicide each year.[7] Worldwide, suicide ranks as the 18th leading cause of death across the lifespan and the second leading cause of death among people aged 15 to 29 years.[7] Suicide death occurs at a staggering rate of one person every 40 seconds. Rates of suicide death are very significant in many countries across the world.[7] A report issued in November 2018 by the United States Centers for Disease Control and Prevention (CDC) indicated that from 1999 to 2017, the age-adjusted rate of suicide in the United States increased 33% from 10.5 to 14.0 per 100,000.[8] However, more recently, the CDC reported a decrease in the 2019 suicide rate, from 14.2 per 100,000 individuals in 2018 to 13.9 per 100,000 individuals in 2019.[9] Globally, from 1950 to 1995 in people of all ages, suicide rates increased by about 35% in men and about 10% in women.[3]

It is possible that suicide rates are underestimated. Many suicide deaths may be incorrectly documented as "unnatural" or "undetermined" deaths.[10,11] Actual suicide rates may be 10%–50% higher than reported. The number of nonfatal suicide attempts may be 10 to 20 times higher than the number of suicide death.[12] Suicidal ideation without action is more common than suicidal behavior.[3]

SUICIDAL BEHAVIOR IN PSYCHIATRIC DISORDERS

Suicide generally occurs in the context of a psychiatric disorder.[3] More than 90% of suicide victims have a diagnosable psychiatric illness, and most persons who attempt suicide have a psychiatric disorder.[3,4,13,14] The most common psychiatric conditions associated with suicide or serious suicide attempt are mood disorders.[1,3,4,15,16] 60% of all suicides have a mood disorder at the time of death.[1,16] Personality disorders, alcohol and substance abuse, anxiety disorders, and schizophrenia are also frequently associated with suicidal behavior.[3,16–18]

Estimations of suicidal behavior among psychiatric patients vary broadly. The lifetime mortality because of suicide is estimated at about 20% for patients with bipolar disorder, and 15% for patients with unipolar depression.[1,19,20] However, these suicide rates may pertain to individuals with psychiatric disorders cared for in teaching hospitals who are usually sicker than patients in the community. Cooccurring illnesses that raise the risk for attempted suicide or suicide death in individuals with mood disorders include alcohol and/or substance abuse, and personality disorders.[21,22]

Some suicidologists advocate that suicidal behavior should be a separate diagnosis.[23] It has been suggested that defining suicidal behavior as a separate diagnosis can make approaches to its identification better integrated into clinical practice and that suicidal behavior meets validity and reliability criteria as well as other psychiatric conditions.

SUICIDAL BEHAVIOR IN MEDICAL AND NEUROLOGIC DISORDERS

Disorders of the central nervous system such as epilepsy, Huntington's disease, head injury, and cerebrovascular accidents carry an elevated risk for suicide.[3,24–27] The brain pathology may cause depression and suicidal ideation and may weaken restraint or inhibition of the wish to take action on suicidal thoughts.[3] For example, onset of epilepsy in the first 17 years of life is associated with a significant increase in risk for suicide compared with those whose epilepsy started at an age of more than 29 years.[26]

Medical disorders such as cardiovascular disease or diabetes are also associated with elevated suicide risk.[28–30] For example, a cohort study of the Swedish population demonstrated that individuals with diabetes were 3.36 times more likely to die by suicide than people in the general population.[28]

Many studies have shown that pain is an independent risk factor for suicide.[31–33] For example, a study of factors contributing to cancer-related suicide in US military veterans over the course of 15 years (2002–2017) identified pain as a common suicide risk factor in 47% of the cases.[32] Insufficient management of pain may lead to suicidal behavior in affected persons by causing depression, hopelessness, helplessness and reducing the quality of life.

DEMOGRAPHIC FACTORS

In most countries of the world, men have greater rates of suicide death, while women have greater rates of attempted suicide.[4,7,34–37] The sex differences in suicide rates are especially significant in Eastern European nations.[7,34,37] In the United States, in 2017, the age-adjusted suicide rate for men (22.4 per 100,000) was 3.67 times higher than for women (6.1 per 100,000).[8] Men have a tendency to employ means that are more lethal, may conceive the suicide attempt more carefully, and evade detection.[3,36,38,39] In contrast, women have a tendency to employ less lethal means of suicide, which leads to a greater likelihood of survival.

Regarding age, suicide rates are highest in individuals aged 70 years or over for both men and women in almost all regions of the world.[4] However, increasing rates of suicide among young individuals are an increasing reason for concern. Suicide is the second leading cause of death in people 15 to 29 years.

Most suicides in the US occur in Whites.[39,40] A recent study suggests that suicide rates in 2019 among American Indian or Alaskan Native (22.2 per 100,000 individuals) were higher than among Whites (17.6 per 100,000 individuals).[40] This study also indicates that between 2014 and 2019 the age-adjusted suicide rates increased for African American and Asian or Pacific Islander individuals.

People who are unmarried, divorced, or widowed are at increased risk of suicide death.[39] Highest to lowest rates in the US are found in the following order: widowed, divorced, single or never married, married, and married with children. The protecting influence of marriage against suicide is particularly significant among males and Whites.

PSYCHOSOCIAL FACTORS

Individuals with psychiatric disorders frequently experience psychosocial problems.[41–44] Psychiatric disorders can result in job loss, breakup of marriages or relationships, or the inability to develop close relationships. Furthermore, psychiatric illnesses and psychosocial difficulties can merge to intensify stress on the individual and, thus, possibly elevate the suicide risk. There is heightened risk of suicidal behavior among individuals from disadvantaged backgrounds including people with low socioeconomic status, low income, and limited educational achievement.[41,42,44] Suicide risk is increased among young persons who had dropped out of school or are not enrolled in a college.[41]

Suicide rates may increase during economic crises.[44–46] For example, in the US, suicides increased during the Great Depression.[45] Suicide mortality peaked with unemployment, in the most recessionary years, 1921, 1932, and 1938.

NEUROBIOLOGY

Considerable evidence suggests that dysregulation in stress response systems, especially the hypothalamic–pituitary–adrenal (HPA) axis, is a diathesis for suicide.[3,47,48]

Early life trauma sensitizes the HPA-axis resulting in higher cortisol levels in response to stress later in life. Cortisol modulates the serotonin system, neuronal survival, and inflammatory processes.

Many studies of the neurobiology of suicide focused on the serotonergic system.[1,4,47–49] Altered serotonin transmission was linked to suicide risk. For example, several studies have shown that low CSF levels of 5-hydroxyindoleacetic acid (5-HIAA), an index of serotonin turnover, predict suicide.[4,48,50] Also, investigations using postmortem brain tissues of people who died by suicide have shown decreased levels of 5-HIAA.[4,49] The deficit in serotonin transporter binding has also been implicated in the pathophysiology of suicide.[49]

Changes in glutamatergic function and neuronal plasticity at the cellular and circuitry level have been implicated in the neurobiology of suicide.[48] The role of inflammatory processes in the pathophysiology of suicide has been extensively studied over the past 20 years.[48,51,52] Findings indicate an association between suicidal behavior and inflammation. For example, one study showed that suicide attempters compared with psychiatric controls with only suicidal ideation and nonsuicidal patients with mood and psychotic disorders had higher serum C-reactive protein levels.[51]

Some studies indicate that testosterone may play a role in the pathophysiology of suicidal behavior.[53–57] For example, we observed that higher baseline testosterone levels predicted suicide attempts in men and women with bipolar disorder.[54,57]

There is evidence for elevated suicide risk with diminishing cholesterol levels, whether they take place naturally or whether they are attributable to medications or diet.[3,47,58,59] The rise in suicide risk may be larger when cholesterol is decreased through diet, compared with the use of medications.[58]

THE ROLE OF PRIMARY CARE PHYSICIANS

Primary care physicians are key to prevention efforts as they see 45% of individuals who die by suicide within 30 days of their suicide which offers an opportunity for suicide prevention.[60] Education and training of primary care physicians targeting depression recognition and treatment was found to be one of the most efficient interventions in decreasing suicide rates.[61,62] Over the past 15 years, studies in Sweden, Hungary, and Slovenia have shown that the introduction of such education programs for general practitioners lead to a significant increase in antidepressant use and decreased suicide rates.[62,63]

MANAGEMENT OF SUICIDAL INDIVIDUALS

The management of a suicidal patient comprises 4 major components in no particular order:

- Diagnosis and treatment of existing psychiatric disorders,
- Assessment of suicide risk,
- Restricting access to the means for suicide,
- Specific treatments to reduce the predisposition to attempt suicide.

Diagnosis and Treatment of Existing Disorders

Diagnosis and management of current psychiatric disorders are of utmost importance to prevent suicide.[39,62,63] All psychiatric patients need to be screened for the presence of suicidal ideation. As psychiatric disorders are a major risk factor for suicide their

---

Box 1
Helpful questions that should be included in suicidal risk assessments

How has the patient reacted to stress in the past, and how effective are his or her typical coping strategies?

Has the patient contemplated or attempted suicide in the past? If so, how frequently and under what circumstances?

What are the patient's current social circumstances, and how similar are they to past situations when suicide was attempted?

Is the patient hopeless, helpless, powerless, or angry?

Does the patient have psychotic symptoms such as hallucinations or delusions?

---

pharmacologic and psychological treatment contributes greatly to the prevention of suicidal behavior.

Depression is untreated or undertreated overall and regretfully, this is so even after suicide attempt.[39,64] Treating mood disorders is a critical part of suicide prevention.[39,61,62,64]

Many psychiatric conditions, including depression, are persistent and recurring.[39,64,65] Adherence to medications is frequently limited. Treatments for depression or other psychiatric conditions provided by psychiatrists or primary care physicians are more successful when a case manager follows-up with individuals who skip appointments or necessitate medication renewals.

Assessment of Suicide Risk

Clinicians are expected to gather information about patient's clinical features, to document these features, and to use this information to formulate decisions about patient's dangerousness to self and the treatment plan.[65,66] Suicide assessments consider such factors as previous suicide attempts, mood and anxiety symptoms, coexisting psychiatric disorders including alcohol and drug abuse, the role of any medications (stimulants, antidepressants, other), the lack of family and social support and the accessibility to lethal means.[39,67] The existence of a suicide plan or the possibility of carrying out a suicide plan need also to be assessed. Helpful questions that should be included in any assessment of suicidal risk are shown in **Box 1**.

The best predictor of suicidal behavior is a history of a suicide attempt and current suicidal thoughts.[39,66,68,69] Epidemiologic and clinical research has shown that attempted suicide is associated with a high risk of repetition and with a significantly increased risk of suicide death. Having had one episode of suicidal behavior increases the risk of a subsequent suicidal act.

A study of clinical predictors of suicidal acts in patients with major depressive disorder or bipolar disorder found that the 3 most powerful predictors of future suicidal acts were a history of suicide attempts, subjective rating of the severity of depression, and cigarette smoking, each of which had an additive effect on future risk.[68] The pessimism and aggression/impulsivity factors both predicted suicidal acts, and each factor showed an additive effect.

Clinicians rely primarily on information offered voluntarily by patients regarding past personal suicidal behavior or a family history of suicidal behavior.[65,70] Unfortunately, some of the patients who are most determined to die by suicide may falsely deny suicidal ideation before their suicide because they fear that suicide may be prevented.[70,71]

Many individuals at risk of suicide have either undiagnosed or untreated psychiatric illness.[67] Probably, a family member or loved one may be best placed to notice alarming behaviors. It is important to develop a risk assessment approach that reduces dependence on subjective patient reports and incorporates collateral information.

Many years of suicide research mostly focused on risk factors for suicidal ideation and behavior while neglecting protective factors which are key to the evaluation of individuals with suicidal ideation.[72,73] Protective factors include family responsibilities, having young children, fear of suicide, fear of social disapproval, and life-affirming cultural values.

Restriction of Access to Lethal Means

Means restriction is a major method for reducing suicide rates.[67,74] A significant positive association between the availability of lethal means and suicide events has been observed.[74] Suicide attempts using highly lethal means, such as firearms in US men, or pesticides in rural China, India, and Sri Lanka, result in higher rates of death.

The transient nature of a suicidal crisis means that restricting access to more lethal means could allow the crisis to pass or result in an attempt with a less lethal method.[67] About 90% of those who survive even a nearly lethal suicide attempt do not die by suicide later in life.[75] It means that surviving a suicide crisis indicates a significant chance of long-term survival. Obviously, means restriction is especially important for individuals with suicidal ideation or a history of suicidal behavior.

The absence of guns in homes of psychiatric patients is an effective measure to prevent suicide.[67] To decrease firearm suicide death, firearm owners should be advised to store firearms unloaded, separate from ammunition, and in a secure place like a gun safe. Putting time and space between an individual with a psychiatric disorder and a firearm may reduce impulsive suicides.

Specific Treatments to Reduce the Diathesis to Attempt Suicide

Suicidal ideation can be treated using psychosocial interventions, such as psychotherapy, including cognitive-behavioral therapy (CBT) and somatic methods, including drugs and electroconvulsive therapy (ECT).[39,76–79] Encouraging results in improving treatment adherence and decreasing suicidal behavior exist for CBT, problem-solving therapy, and interpersonal psychotherapy.[76,77,79,80] It has been shown that cognitive therapy halved the suicide reattempt frequency in suicide attempters compared with those getting care as usual.[80] Suicide prevention interventions for individuals with suicidal ideation and/or a history of suicide attempt should include in-person, video or telephone follow-up, and family education and therapy.

When treating patients' psychiatric conditions, clinicians should offer tools and resources to the patients at risk to maximize their chances of working against suicidal urges. For example, suicide planning intervention consists of a written list of coping strategies and sources of support that patients can use to lessen a suicidal crisis. It is developed in close collaboration with the patient and is tool patients may use in the event that suicidal urges do resurface.[81] This plan is made between the clinician and the patient, basically delineating what the patient should/will do if a suicidal crisis is to take place in the future. The safety plan is implemented through 6 steps—please, see **Box 2**. The safety plan is a physical piece of paper that the individual can have with him/her after leaving the clinician.

Clozapine demonstrated efficacy in reducing suicidal behavior in patients with bipolar disorder and schizophrenia.[18,79,82] While extensive observational data support the utility of lithium in suicide prevention in bipolar disorder, the few randomized clinical trials (RCTs) that have studied it have not confirmed this effect.[83–85] All of these

Box 2	
Suicide safety plan	
"Recognition of Warning Signs"	Signs that immediately precede a crisis are outlined
"Internal Coping Strategies"	Patients are asked to list activities they should/can do to distract themselves from suicidal thoughts without contacting another person
"Socialization Strategies for Distraction and Support"	A list of people and social settings that the patient can use to distract themselves from suicidal thoughts and urges
"Social Contacts for Assistance in Resolving Suicidal Crises"	A list of people whom the patient can ask for help; it is mainly composed of family and friends that may provide support if the suicidal urges are too great to combat alone
"Professional and Agency Contacts to Help Resolve Suicidal Crises"	A list of contact information of professionals trained to deal with suicidal crisis
"Means Restriction"	This section addresses how to reduce the availability of means by which the patient would attempt suicide

RCTs have limitations. Nonetheless, it has been observed that lithium discontinuation may elevate suicide risk in bipolar patients[86] so this remains an open question. Clozapine is the only medication approved in the US for lessening suicide risk in psychotic disorders.

Recent clinical research indicates that there is a potential for ketamine or its enantiomer, esketamine, in the treatment of treatment-resistant depression and suicidal ideation.[79] In 2020, esketamine was approved by the US Food and Drug Administration (FDA) for the treatment of depressive symptoms In adults with major depressive disorder with acute suicidal ideation or behavior.[87]

Studies of antidepressants showed that the initiation of pharmacotherapy with antidepressants is not associated with an increased risk of suicide, while the continuation of pharmacotherapy for depression is associated with a reduced risk of suicide.[62,79,88] Antidepressants in combination with psychotherapy can be an effective treatment of depression, for suicidal ideation and for preventing new attempts after a suicide attempt.

Taking into account the immeasurable personal and massive economic impact that suicide has on society, preventing suicide should be a major national and international health priority. However, suicide prevention is a challenging task. Even under the best circumstances, the prediction of a rare behavior such as suicide produces a large number of false-positive and false-negative cases.

CLINICS CARE POINTS

- All psychiatric patients need to be screened for the presence of suicidal ideation.
- Some of the patients who are most determined to die by suicide may falsely deny suicidal ideation before their suicide because they fear that suicide may be prevented. It is important to get collateral information.
- The best predictor of suicidal behavior is a history of a suicide attempt and current suicidal thoughts.
- Treatments for depression or other psychiatric conditions are more successful when a case manager follows-up with patients who skip appointments or need medication renewals.

DISCLOSURE

The authors have nothing to disclose.

REFERENCES

1. Sher L, Oquendo MA, Mann JJ. Risk of suicide in mood disorders. Clin Neurosci Res 2001;1:337–44.
2. Naguy A, Elbadry H, Salem H. Suicide: A Précis. J Fam Med Prim Care 2020;9(8): 4009–15.
3. Mann JJ. A current perspective of suicide and attempted suicide. Ann Intern Med 2002;136(4):302–11.
4. Turecki G, Brent DA, Gunnell D, et al. Suicide and suicide risk. Nat Rev Dis Primers 2019;5(1):74.
5. Harmer B, Lee S, Duong TVH, et al. Suicidal ideation. In: StatPearls [Internet]. Treasure Island (FL: StatPearls Publishing; 2021.
6. Baca-Garcia E, Perez-Rodriguez MM, Oquendo MA, et al. Estimating risk for suicide attempt: are we asking the right questions? Passive suicidal ideation as a marker for suicidal behavior. J Affect Disord 2011;134(1–3):327–32.
7. World Health Organization. Preventing suicide. A global imperative. WHO. 2014. URL Available at: http://www.who.int/mental_health/suicide-prevention/world_report_2014/en/.
8. Hedegaard H, Curtin SC, Warner M. Suicide mortality in the United States, 1999-2017. NCHS Data Brief 2018;(330):1–8.
9. Kochanek KD, Xu JQ, Arias E. Mortality in the United States, 2019. National Center for Health Statistics. 2020. URL Available at: https://www.cdc.gov/nchs/data/databriefs/db395-H.pdf.
10. Tøllefsen IM, Helweg-Larsen K, Thiblin I, et al. Are suicide deaths underreported? Nationwide re-evaluations of 1800 deaths in Scandinavia. BMJ Open 2015;5(11):e009120.
11. Oquendo MA, Volkow ND. Suicide: A silent contributor to opioid-overdose deaths. N Engl J Med 2018;378(17):1567–9.
12. Bilsen J. Suicide and youth: Risk factors. Front Psychiatry 2018;9:540. https://doi.org/10.3389/fpsyt.2018.00540.
13. Beautrais AL, Joyce PR, Mulder RT, et al. Prevalence and comorbidity of mental disorders in persons making serious suicide attempts: a case-control study. Am J Psychiatry 1996;153(8):1009–14.
14. Brådvik L. Suicide risk and mental disorders. Int J Environ Res Public Health 2018;15(9):2028.
15. Rich CL, Fowler RC, Fogarty LA, et al. San Diego Suicide Study. III. Relationships between diagnoses and stressors. Arch Gen Psychiatry 1988;45(6):589–92.
16. Isometsä E, Henriksson M, Marttunen M, et al. Mental disorders in young and middle aged men who commit suicide. BMJ 1995;310(6991):1366–7.
17. Sher L, Kahn RS. Suicide in Schizophrenia: An Educational Overview. Medicina (Kaunas) 2019;55(7):361.
18. Leahy D, Larkin C, Leahy D, et al. The mental and physical health profile of people who died by suicide: findings from the Suicide Support and Information System. Soc Psychiatry Psychiatr Epidemiol 2020;55(11):1525–33.
19. Jamison KR. Suicide and bipolar disorders. Ann NY Acad Sci 1986;487:301–15.
20. Dome P, Rihmer Z, Gonda X. Suicide Risk in Bipolar Disorder: A Brief Review. Medicina (Kaunas) 2019;55(8):403.

21. Cornelius JR, Salloum IM, Mezzich J, et al. Disproportionate suicidality in patients with comorbid major depression and alcoholism. Am J Psychiatry 1995;152: 358–64.
22. Oquendo MA, Malone KM, Mann JJ. Suicide: risk factors and prevention in refractory major depression. Depress Anxiety 1997;5:202–11.
23. Oquendo MA, Baca-Garcia E. Suicidal behavior disorder as a diagnostic entity in the DSM-5 classification system: advantages outweigh limitations. World Psychiatry 2014;13(2):128–30.
24. Schoenfeld M, Myers RH, Cupples LA, et al. Increased rate of suicide among patients with Huntington's disease. J Neurol Neurosurg Psychiatry 1984;47:1283–7.
25. Brent DA. Overrepresentation of epileptics in a consecutive series of suicide attempters seen at a Children's Hospital, 1978-1983. J Am Acad Child Psychiatry 1986;25:242–6.
26. Reeves RR, Panguluri RL. Neuropsychiatric complications of traumatic brain injury. J Psychosoc Nurs Ment Health Serv 2011;49(3):42–50.
27. Coughlin SS, Sher L. Suicidal Behavior and Neurological Illnesses. J Depress Anxiety 2013;Suppl 9(1):12443.
28. Webb RT, Lichtenstein P, Dahlin M, et al. Unnatural deaths in a national cohort of people diagnosed with diabetes. Diabetes Care 2014;37(8):2276–83.
29. Wang B, An X, Shi X, et al. MANAGEMENT OF ENDOCRINE DISEASE: Suicide risk in patients with diabetes: a systematic review and meta-analysis. Eur J Endocrinol 2017;177(4):R169–81.
30. Kwak Y, Kim Y, Kwon SJ, et al. Mental health status of adults with cardiovascular or metabolic diseases by gender. Int J Environ Res Public Health 2021;18(2):514.
31. Calati R, Laglaoui Bakhiyi C, Artero S, et al. The impact of physical pain on suicidal thoughts and behaviors: Meta-analyses. J Psychiatr Res 2015;71:16–32.
32. Aboumrad M, Shiner B, Riblet N, et al. Factors contributing to cancer-related suicide: A study of root-cause analysis reports. Psychooncology 2018;27(9): 2237–44.
33. Petrosky E, Harpaz R, Fowler KA, et al. Chronic pain among suicide decedents, 2003 to 2014: Findings from the National Violent Death Reporting System. Ann Intern Med 2018;169(7):448–55.
34. Rutz W, Rihmer Z. Suicidality in men – practical issues, challenges, solutions. J Men's Health Gend 2007;4(4):393–401.
35. Sullivan EM, Annest JL, Simon TR, et al, Centers for Disease Control and Prevention. Suicide trends among persons aged 10-24 years—United States, 1994-2012. MMWR Morb Mortal Wkly Rep 2015;64(8):201–5.
36. Barrigon ML, Cegla-Schvartzman F. Sex, gender, and suicidal behavior. Curr Top Behav Neurosci 2020;46:89–115. https://doi.org/10.1007/7854_2020_165.
37. Lange S, Rehm J, Tran A, et al. Comparing gender-specific suicide mortality rate trends in the United States and Lithuania, 1990–2019: putting one of the "deaths of despair" into perspective. BMC Psychiatry 2022;22:127. https://doi.org/10.1186/s12888-022-03766-w.
38. Mergl R, Koburger N, Heinrichs K, et al. What are reasons for the large gender differences in the lethality of suicidal acts? An epidemiological analysis in four European countries. PLoS ONE 2015;10(7):e0129062. https://doi.org/10.1371/journal.pone.0129062.
39. Maris RW, Berman AL, Silverman MM. Comprehensive textbook of suicidology. New York: Guilford Press; 2000.

40. Ramchand R, Gordon JA, Pearson JL. Trends in suicide rates by race and ethnicity in the United States. JAMA Netw Open 2021;4(5):e2111563. https://doi.org/10.1001/jamanetworkopen.2021.11563.
41. Gould MS, Fisher P, Parides M, et al. Psychosocial factors for child and adolescent completed suicide. Arch Gen Psychiatry 1996;53:1155–62.
42. Beautrais AL. Risk factors for suicide and attempted suicide among young people. Aust N Z J Psychiatry 2000;34(3):420–36.
43. Mann JJ. Neurobiology of suicidal behaviour. Nat Rev Neurosci 2003;4(10):819–28.
44. Mann JJ, Metts AV. The economy and suicide. Crisis 2017;38(3):141–6.
45. Tapia Granados JA, Diez Roux AV. Life and death during the Great Depression. Proc Natl Acad Sci U S A 2009;106(41):17290–5. Epub 2009 Sep 28.
46. Sher L. The impact of the COVID-19 pandemic on suicide rates. QJM 2020;113(10):707–12.
47. van Heeringen K. The neurobiology of suicide and suicidality. Can J Psychiatry 2003;48(5):292–300.
48. Oquendo MA, Sullivan GM, Sudol K, et al. Toward a biosignature for suicide. Am J Psychiatry 2014;171(12):1259–77.
49. Mann JJ. The serotonergic system in mood disorders and suicidal behaviour. Phil Trans R Soc B Biol Sci 2013;368:20120537.
50. Jokinen J, Nordström AL, Nordström P. CSF 5-HIAA and DST non-suppression: orthogonal biologic risk factors for suicide in male mood disorder inpatients. Psychiatry Res 2009;165:96–102.
51. Gibbs HM, Davis L, Han X, et al. Association between C-reactive protein and suicidal behavior in an adult inpatient population. J Psychiatr Res 2016;79:28–33.
52. Brundin L, Bryleva EY, Thirtamara Rajamani K. Role of inflammation in suicide: From mechanisms to treatment. Neuropsychopharmacology 2017;42(1):271–83.
53. Markianos M, Tripodianakis J, Istikoglou C, et al. Suicide attempt by jumping: a study of gonadal axis hormones in male suicide attempters versus men who fell by accident. Psychiatry Res 2009;170(1):82–5.
54. Sher L, Grunebaum MF, Sullivan GM, et al. Association of testosterone levels and future suicide attempts in females with bipolar disorder. J Affect Disord 2014;166:98–102.
55. Lenz B, Röther M, Bouna-Pyrrou P, et al. The androgen model of suicide completion. Prog Neurobiol 2019;172:84–103.
56. Sher L, Bierer LM, Makotkine I, et al. The effect of oral dexamethasone administration on testosterone levels in combat veterans with or without a history of suicide attempt. J Psychiatr Res 2021;143:499–503.
57. Sher L, Sublette ME, Grunebaum MF, et al. Plasma testosterone levels and subsequent suicide attempts in males with bipolar disorder. Acta Psychiatr Scand 2022;145(2):223–5.
58. Golomb BA. Cholesterol and violence: is there a connection? Ann Intern Med 1998;128(6):478–87.
59. Sudol K, Mann JJ. Biomarkers of Suicide Attempt Behavior: Towards a Biological Model of Risk. Curr Psychiatry Rep 2017;19(6):31.
60. Luoma JB, Martin CE, Pearson JL. Contact with mental health and primary care providers before suicide: a review of the evidence. Am J Psychiatry 2002;159(6):909–16.
61. Mann JJ, Apter A, Bertolote J, et al. Suicide prevention strategies: a systematic review. JAMA 2005;294(16):2064–74.

62. Zalsman G, Hawton K, Wasserman D, et al. Suicide prevention strategies revisited: 10-year systematic review. Lancet Psychiatry 2016;3(7):646–59.
63. Szanto K, Kalmar S, Hendin H, et al. A suicide prevention program in a region with a very high suicide rate. Arch Gen Psychiatry 2007;64:914–20.
64. Oquendo MA, Malone KM, Ellis SP, et al. Inadequacy of antidepressant treatment for patients with major depression who are at risk for suicidal behavior. Am J Psychiatry 1999;156(2):190–4.
65. Goldman HH. Review of general Psychiatry. 5th edn. New York: Lange Medical Books/McGraw-Hill; 2000.
66. Sher L. Preventing suicide. QJM 2004;97(10):677–80.
67. Mann JJ, Michel CA. Prevention of Firearm Suicide in the United States: What Works and What Is Possible. Am J Psychiatry 2016;173(10):969–79.
68. Oquendo MA, Galfalvy H, Russo S, et al. Prospective study of clinical predictors of suicidal acts after a major depressive episode in patients with major depressive disorder or bipolar disorder. Am J Psychiatry 2004;161(8):1433–41.
69. Bostwick JM, Pabbati C, Geske JR, et al. Suicide attempt as a risk factor for completed suicide: even more lethal than we knew. Am J Psychiatry 2016; 173(11):1094–100.
70. Sher L. Teaching medical professionals about suicide prevention: what's missing? QJM 2011;104(11):1005–8.
71. Busch KA, Fawcett J, Jacobs DG. Clinical correlates of inpatient suicide. J Clin Psychiatry 2003;64(1):14–9.
72. McLean J, Maxwell M, Platt S, et al. Risk and protective factors for suicide and suicidal behaviour: a literature review. Scottish Government Social Research; 2008. URL Available at: https://www.webarchive.org.uk/wayback/archive/20180517025526/http://www.gov.scot/Publications/2008/11/28141444/23.
73. Sher L. Resilience as a focus of suicide research and prevention. Acta Psychiatr Scand 2019;140(2):169–80. Epub 2019 Jun 20.
74. Humeau M, Papet N, Jaafari N, et al. Availability of firearms and risk of suicide: A review of the literature. Ann Medico-Psychologiques. 2007;165:269–75.
75. Owens D, Horrocks J, House A. Fatal and non-fatal repetition of self-harm. Systematic review. Br J Psychiatry 2002;181:193–9. https://doi.org/10.1192/bjp.181.3.193.
76. Institute of Medicine (US). In: Goldsmith SK, Pellmar TC, Kleinman AM, et al, editors. Committee on pathophysiology and prevention of Adolescent and adult suicide. Reducing suicide: a national Imperative. Washington (DC): National Academies Press (US); 2002.
77. Brown GK, Ten Have T, Henriques GR, et al. Cognitive therapy for the prevention of suicide attempts: a randomized controlled trial. JAMA 2005;294(5):563–70.
78. Fink M, Kellner CH, McCall WV. The role of ECT in suicide prevention. J ECT 2014; 30(1):5–9.
79. Hawkins EM, Coryell W, Leung S, et al. Effects of somatic treatments on suicidal ideation and completed suicides. Brain Behav 2021;11(11):e2381.
80. Gøtzsche PC, Gøtzsche PK. Cognitive behavioural therapy halves the risk of repeated suicide attempts: systematic review. J R Soc Med 2017;110(10):404–10.
81. Stanley B, Brown G. Safety planning intervention: A brief intervention to mitigate suicide risk. Cogn Behav Pract 2012;19:256–64.
82. D'Anci KE, Uhl S, Giradi G, et al. Treatments for the Prevention and Management of Suicide: A Systematic Review. Ann Intern Med 2019;171(5):334–42.

83. Lauterbach E, Felber W, Müller-Oerlinghausen B, et al. Adjunctive lithium treatment in the prevention of suicidal behaviour in depressive disorders: a randomised, placebo-controlled, 1-year trial. Acta Psychiatr Scand 2008;118(6): 469–79.

84. Oquendo MA, Galfalvy HC, Currier D, et al. Treatment of suicide attempters with bipolar disorder: a randomized clinical trial comparing lithium and valproate in the prevention of suicidal behavior. Am J Psychiatry 2011;168(10):1050–6.

85. Katz IR, Rogers MP, Lew R, et al. Lithium treatment in the prevention of repeat suicide-related outcomes in Veterans with major depression or bipolar disorder: A randomized clinical trial. JAMA Psychiatry 2022;79(1):24–32.

86. Baldessarini RJ, Tondo L, Hennen J. Effects of lithium treatment and its discontinuation on suicidal behavior in bipolar manic-depressive disorders. J Clin Psychiatry 1999;60(Suppl 2):77–84.

87. Mischel NA, Esketamine Balon R. A drug to treat resistant depression that brings more questions than answers. J Clin Psychopharmacol 2021;41(3):233–5.

88. Søndergård L, Lopez AG, Andersen PK, et al. Continued antidepressant treatment and suicide in patients with depressive disorder. Arch Suicide Res 2007; 11(2):163–75.

Psychiatric Issues Among Health Professionals

María Dolores Braquehais, MD, PhD[a,b,*], Sebastián Vargas-Cáceres[c]

KEYWORDS

- Health professionals • Mental symptoms • Mental disorders • Addictions
- COVID-19

KEY POINTS

- During the COVID-19 pandemic, health professionals (HPs) have suffered from high levels of anxiety, insomnia, depressive and trauma-related symptoms.
- Although most of the HPs will be able to recover from these stressful circumstances, the prevalence of mental disorders among them during similar epidemic outbreaks is known to increase in the short and mid-long term.
- HPs usually have difficulties in caring for themselves and if they finally develop mental disorders they are reluctant to seek appropriate help.
- While affective and anxiety disorders are the most common mental disorders among HPs, others, such as addictive disorders, not only worsen their wellbeing but also pose risk to their practice safety.
- This new post–COVID-19 scenario becomes an opportunity to enhance a new culture of professionalism whereby caring for the caregivers becomes a priority both at a personal and institutional level.

INTRODUCTION

A high proportion of health professionals (HPs) neglect their self-care[1,2] a phenomenon that has been popularly reflected in the old saying: "the shoemaker always wears the worst shoes" and, consequently, find it difficult to ask for help when their distress results in a mental disorder. Their sense of duty leads them to maintain a high level of arousal and commitment and may contribute to delay seeking help when suffering from a mental disorder.[3] Although the attitudes of HPs with respect to self-care are slowly changing,[4] they are still consciously or unconsciously trained to care for others

[a] Integral Care Program for Health Care Professionals, Galatea Foundation, Galatea Clinic, Palafolls Street, 15-19, 08017, Barcelona, Spain; [b] Mental Health and Addiction Research Group, Vall d'Hebron Research Institute (VHIR), Vall d'Hebron University Hospital, Vall Hebron Hospital Campus, Passeig Vall d'Hebron, 119-129, 08035, Barcelona, Spain; [c] Adult Mental Health Service, Benito Menni Mental Health Services, Santiago Ramon y Cajal Street, 27-29, 080902, L'Hospitalet de Llobregat, Catalonia, Spain
* Corresponding author. Galatea Clinic, Carrer Palafolls, 15-19, Barcelona 08017, Spain.
E-mail address: mdbraquehais.paimm@comb.cat

Med Clin N Am 107 (2023) 131–142
https://doi.org/10.1016/j.mcna.2022.04.004
0025-7125/23/© 2022 Elsevier Inc. All rights reserved.

and to put their patients' needs before their own. This is even more accentuated in circumstances such as emergencies, disasters, or life-threatening experiences, such as the recent COVID-19 pandemic. HPs also have to deal with non-occupational stressors related to work-home time imbalance and other personal, financial and contextual factors.[5,6] Although most evidence on HPs' wellbeing has focused on physicians and nurses, others (such as psychologists, dentists, social workers, or pharmacists)[2] are also exposed to similar job-related stressors and tend to disregard personal care.

The interest in HPs' wellbeing has increased in the last 2 decades.[4] Preoccupation with HPs' distress has changed into a proactive movement among professional associations and some institutions to raise awareness of the importance for HPs of maintaining healthy habits, achieving a good work-life integration, and promoting resilience despite the adversities found in an increasingly overloaded working environment. It is crucial to underline that not all mental distress turns into mental disorders. However, when this happens, HPs are still reluctant to recognize it and to ask for professional help. Besides the negative implications of this attitude on their wellbeing, in some cases, such as addictions or severe mental disorders, their practice safety can be compromised.

A general perspective on this phenomenon may ignore the role of some idiosyncratic factors associated with the onset of mental disorders and the way they manifest among HPs. Some of them are related to: age (younger HPs are more likely to experience mental distress),[7] gender (women are still confronted by difficulties in balancing work and family, are more likely to develop affective and anxiety disorders compared with men and have less difficulty in seeking help),[8] occupation (physicians, nurses and other HPs have specific work stressors),[2] each country/region's public and private health care system organization, type of mental health resources offered to them,[9,10] and other psychosocial determinants.

In this article, we provide a wide overview of the impact the COVID-19 pandemic on HPs' mental health, analyze the general patterns of their coping strategies when suffering from mental disorders and describe the characteristics of some specialized mental health services designed for them around the world before COVID-19. Despite the serious consequences of this pandemic on HPs' mental health, these unprecedented circumstances can be seen as an opportunity to start promoting a new culture of professionalism that includes self-care as a priority for all HPs and the institutions they work in,[4,11] according to what can be conceptualized as the 2.0 HP wellbeing paradigm.[4]

THE IMPACT OF COVID-19 IN HEALTH PROFESSIONALS

Before the COVID-19 pandemic, HPs were known to have increased rates of occupational distress in the form of burnout. Job-related mental strains increase the risk of developing mental disorders although their etiology is linked to a complex interaction of personal and contextual factors. Among HPs, the most prevalent diagnoses before the pandemic were not different from the general population. Therefore, depressive and anxiety disorders were the most common diagnoses followed by substance use disorders, some of which were related to easy access to medication.[12–14]

In December 2019, a new severe type of pneumonia, later known as COVID-19, was reported in Wuhan, Hubei, China and rapidly extended around the world. By 11 February 2022, the World Health Organization (WHO) reported more than 400 million confirmed cases of COVID-19, including more than 5.5 million deaths while, as of 7 February 2022, 10 million vaccine doses were administered.[15] HPs, especially in countries that had not experienced recent epidemic outbursts, were confronted by unexpected highly stressful experiences during the initial waves of the COVID-19 pandemic and before vaccinations became available to a large number of developed countries. Researchers have widely analyzed the mental health consequences of this epidemic crisis on HPs and their findings have been publicized by traditional and social media around the world.[7,16]

Previous research on other infectious diseases, including the severe acute respiratory syndrome (SARS), the Middle East respiratory syndrome (MERS), and the Ebola virus disease, consistently showed that many HPs reported symptoms of anxiety and depression and were more prone to develop mental disorders, including addictions, both during and after the outbreak, causing a severe impact on their coping abilities, in some cases with long-lasting effects.[17-19]

Many public health care systems in Western societies initially faced this extraordinary situation with significantly reduced material and human resources as a result of the economic cuts that followed the Great Recession (2008). This was in addition to the insecurity inherent in the lack of knowledge about the virus and the absence of effective treatments. The health workforce capacity was even more reduced during the first waves of the COVD-19 pandemic after many HPs became infected and needed to be quarantined.

The health-providing organizations and the socio-economic and political context changed during the pandemic, and the HPs' and general population's responses evolved accordingly. While at the beginning of the COVID-19, the most frequent responses were related to the hyper-activation of arousal and survival mind-body system, several types of loss, fatigue, exhaustion, and skepticism became predominant after the roll out of vaccinations, when the pandemic became apparently less severe despite the emergence of new variants of the virus.

A recent meta-analysis of 40 systematic reviews,[20] including data from 1828 primary studies and 3,245,768 participants estimated that anxiety (16%–41%), depression (14%–37%), and stress/posttraumatic stress disorder (18.6%–56.5%) were the most frequent COVID-19 pandemic-related mental health conditions affecting HPs. Other studies also included high prevalences of insomnia, burnout, fear, obsessive-compulsive disorder, somatization symptoms, phobia, substance abuse, and suicidal thoughts. When comparing countries and regions, the highest anxiety rate was reported in the United Kingdom, the greatest depression rates were in the Middle East and stress-related symptoms were more frequent in the Eastern Mediterranean region. Estimated prevalence figures varied depending on epidemiologic variables such as: number of cases per 100,000 habitants, specific COVID-19 pandemic stage, health service characteristics, and vaccination rates. Regrettably, information regarding maladaptive coping strategies such as alcohol use or sedative self-prescription is less available.[7] Most studies do not specifically screen for potential substance use disorders although experience from previous pandemics points to an increase in the incidence of alcohol use and self-medication among HPs that may result in addictive behavior in the medium-to-long term.[21,22] According to the increased prevalence of mental disorders among HPs in this new scenario, a heightened risk of suicide among is also expected to happen.[20]

Most research evidence was collected at the beginning of the pandemic and later evaluated in several reviews and meta-analyses.[23] During the first stages of the COVID-19, HPs, especially those at the frontline of care, were confronted with unexpected, more intense, and frequent traumatic experiences than the general population. Women, nurses, and frontline HPs have more frequently developed anxiety and depression compared with men, doctors and second-line personnel.[20,24,25] In some studies, younger and less experienced HPs have also been reported to be at higher risk[25] while resilience, perceived intimate and public support, and positive coping styles have been identified as protective factors.[26]

After analyzing the narratives of HPs, their main sources of distress at that point of the pandemic were related to fear of contagion (both in themselves or in relatives), lack of protective measures, social stigma associated with COVID exposure, ethical dilemmas, information and training, and aspects concerning perceived support by families, colleagues, institutions and society.[27,28] The most reported coping strategies included: individual/group psychological support, family/relative support, training/orientation, and securing adequate personal protective equipment.[20]

DIFFICULTIES IN SEEKING APPROPRIATE HELP AND ITS CONSEQUENCES

Certain aspects of the predominant culture of HP professionalism, especially among physicians and other caregivers with highly demanding jobs and responsibilities, have been associated with the resistance to seeking appropriate help when needed. These include: (1) their professional identity construction, with an exaggerated sense of duty combined with an increased sense of invulnerability and perfectionism; (2) their proneness to trying to cope alone; (3) their survival mentality; and (4) their high level of self-doubt, stigma and insecurity with regards to mental distress; and, (5) the fear of licensure problems when there are addictions or other severe mental disorders.[29,30]

Although some coping strategies for working as an HP are initially adaptive, they may become unhealthy defense mechanisms (denial, minimization, and rationalization) when they cannot cope with mental distress[3] Self-medication may also become a maladaptive strategy to cope with distress. In this situation, the evolution and prognosis of the mental disorders are likely to worsen and, if they remain untreated, there is a higher risk of developing addictive behaviors, and, in some cases, of suicide.[31–33]

Stigma and self-stigma associated with mental disorders is even greater among HPs than in the general population. It is known that self-stigma can lead to a delay in asking for help, a tendency to self-medicate, and to a worse prognosis when suffering from a mental disorder.[34,35] However, stigma associated with mental disorders cannot be conceptualized as a dichotomous (yes/no) variable but rather as a spectrum whereby stigma is inversely correlated with social acceptance.

The social recognition that HPs' efforts have received during this pandemic and the mass media diffusion of their testimonies about mental distress may help to lower their internal psychological barriers to seeking help. Therefore, it may become easier for HPs to admit anxiety or depressive symptoms if they are triggered by stressful life events, such as those activated during the COVID-19 pandemic. In contrast, severe disorders, such as bipolar or psychotic disorders, and addictions are experienced with shame and usually hidden. This attitude is not only internalized by HPs but is also present among their peers or in the institutions where they work. The difficulties in asking for help when suffering from severe mental disorders may increase the risk to themselves (suicide risk) and/or to others (practice safety). Prejudices around severe mental disorders and addictions among HPs may be related to the fear of potential disruptive behaviors at some point in their evolution. However, it regretfully persists even when the HP as a patient has consolidated a psychopathological stability and is ready to go back to work safely.

In some individual HPs, psychological barriers to recognizing their own vulnerability may be related to personal characteristics such as high self-criticism, low self-esteem, poor-bonding with relatives, and also to competitive, status-conscious, and humiliating work environments, as well as burn-out symptoms linked to high job demands.[36]

However, vulnerability to developing mental disorders may be linked to other specific personal and family variables together with other psychosocial determinants.

Delaying help seeking is also likely to result in HPs trying to cope on their own and, in some cases, turning to drugs as one of their coping strategies (usually self-prescribed, like sedatives or hypnotics, or socially accepted, such as alcohol). In fact, an estimated 10% to 14% of physicians may become chemically dependent at some point in their careers.[37] However, trends in drug addictions are changing among new HPs and should be appropriately researched in the future. Knowledge and availability of legal drugs may partly explain the higher rates of substance use disorders among some HPs compared with others. Potentially, this combination of factors often leads HPs to experiencing both a substance use and a nonaddictive mental disorder thus complicating their evolution and prognosis.

Suicide risk among HPs is elevated compared with the general population[32,38,39] and suicide incidence data may understate the problem, in part because of difficulties related to reporting reliability.[39] Besides other specific psychosocial factors, delaying help seeking together with easier access and knowledge of potential lethal methods may account for this phenomenon.[40,41] Risk of suicide is higher among nurses, veterinarians, physicians, dentists and pharmacists compared with other HPs and other occupational groups [REF].[40,42]

Denial (conspiracy of silence), minimization, and rationalization are also common defense mechanisms HPs show when a colleague suffers from a mental disorder despite its direct or indirect signs. Some strategies to handle this situation are offered in **Box 1**.

SPECIALIZED MENTAL HEALTH TREATMENT RESOURCES FOR HEALTH PROFESSIONALS

Mental disorders have a negative effect on HPs' practice and may lead both to absenteeism (staying away from work without providing a good reason)[43] and to underperforming presenteeism (attendance at work despite ill health).[44] In any case, evidence shows that sick HPs report more medication errors, patient falls, and give poorer standards of patient care.[45-47] Therefore, providing appropriate treatment help to HPs with mental

---

Box 1
Promoting appropriate voluntary help seeking among health professionals with mental disorders

- A conspiracy of silence does not help the health professional (HP) in trouble.
- Avoid "corridor" consultations.
- Find a quiet, private place to talk without interruptions.
- Try to be empathic and nonjudgmental.
- Show a nonstigmatizing attitude toward mental disorders.
- Underline the benefits of early help seeking as a healthy coping strategy.
- Focus on HP's own strengths and competencies.
- Offer advice on the alternatives for appropriate mental health treatment or help.
- Free, easy access, highly confidential programs may help sick HPs overcome their initial resistance to being appropriately treated.
- Refraining from working should be encouraged if the HP is impaired by their mental disorder.

disorders is critical both to their wellbeing and also reinforces patient safety and society's trust, whereas not doing so increases risk in these areas.[48–50]

The term "impairment" refers to those situations whereby HPs are rendered unable to carry out their professional responsibilities adequately due to a variety of health issues, including a medical disease or mental disorders.[51] Professional impairment due to mental disorders is more frequently related to addictive behaviors. Besides the negative consequences on their practice, other personal and environmental problems can arise when mental disorders impair the HP: (1) sexual, marital, and/or financial difficulties; (2) driving convictions; (3) decreased involvement in family activities and commitments; (4) dependent children behavioral problems; (5) frequent arguments or unexpected mood shifts; (6) social isolation and/or loss of friends: and, (7) cessation of hobbies and other interests.[49,52] In fact, relatives or close friends may be the first to identify addiction or severe mental disorder-related symptoms and may encourage the impaired HP to seek help, although it is not uncommon for the troubled HP to ignore or reject such recommendations.

In addition to the numerous strategies to promote HPs' wellbeing and to the development of numerous counseling services around the world in recent decades, the negative impact of mental disorders when they finally impair HPs was the main reason behind the emergence of specialized mental health programs for them.[53]Physician Health Programs were first developed in the United States in the late 1970s. The purpose was to identify and treat physicians with problems resulting from mental health issues, mainly substance use disorders. Since then, other specialized programs have been developed in Canada, Australia, Spain, the United Kingdom, Argentina, and Uruguay.

The first specialized treatment services for nurses with addictions started even earlier in the US during the 1960s[53] while peer health assistance programs emerged in the 1980s.[54] Since then, treatment resources for nurses with addictions and/or mental disorders have been gradually developed in most of the US states[54] and in other countries such as Australia, Canada or New Zeeland.[55,56] In Catalonia, the program for physicians, the first of its kind in Europe, was progressively offered to other HPs, including nurses, psychologists, dentists, veterinarians, pharmacists, and social workers. This pioneer resource (The Galatea Care Program for Health Professionals) is a free, easy access, highly confidential mental health service, sponsored by both the Catalan Government's Department of Health and the respective HPs' association councils.[53] Although the program design combines promoting voluntary help seeking among HPs with protecting practice safety, the results are similar to other specialized programs around the world.[57]

Across a range of countries and service models, studies from several specialized programs for HPs with addictions that include drug monitoring report long-term follow-up abstinence rates to be around 70% to 80%.[10,57–63] There is a continuum in specialized mental health programs for HPs from the more punitive (mainly those that address practice problems) to the more supportive (merely focused on promoting HPs' wellbeing). Concerns have been raised regarding disciplinary approaches as they may become a controversial and counterproductive solution for those who are willing and potentially able to overcome their mental disorders that pose risks to their practice safety.[55] Therefore, services that are confidential, free, and promote voluntary referrals may reduce barriers to earlier help seeking as has been shown with two such programs for physicians in Europe[3,37] and for nurses in other continents.[55,56]

During the COVID-19 pandemic, Physician Health Programs in the US have adapted their provision of services and protocols both to support physicians and to continue monitoring those with substance use disorders to warrant safe practice.[64] In the

---

Box 2
The COVID-19 crisis as an opportunity to rethink caring for health professionals

- A new culture of professionalism among Health Professionals (HPs) has to include self-care as a priority starting in the undergraduate period and continuing throughout their professional careers.

- Not all mental distress is due to individual factors: the context matters.

- Institutions and policy makers should proactively work in favor of caring for HPs.

- Having sufficient material and human resources to reduce work overload and provide a "good enough" health service should be prioritized.

- The ideal HP leader should be competent, team building, open-minded, fair, transparent, and compassionate.

- Learning healthy coping strategies and compassionate self-care, promoting work-life integration and collaborative teamwork should be fostered throughout the professional career.

- Peer support groups may be helpful to overcome mental distress.

- Destigmatization of mental disorders among HPs needs to be addressed at personal, academic, and institutional levels.

- Help seeking when there are mental disorders should be encouraged and facilitated.

- Offering free, easy access, highly confidential mental health services may help HPs with mental disorders (including addictions) to seek treatment voluntarily even when they are impaired.

UK, the National Health Service (NHS) Practitioner Health Programme, informed that nearly as many patients presented in the 12-month pandemic period (April 2020–March 2021) as in the first 10 years of service (4355 in the last 12 months vs 5000 over the first 10 years).[65] The Integral Care Program for Health Professionals in Catalonia has also experienced a significant increase of HP referrals during the pandemic, especially among physicians.[66] The percentage of HP women at admission and the clinical severity of the first treatment episode remained unchanged before and after COVID-19. The most prevalent main diagnoses after the outbreak were similar as well: adjustment (41.5%), mood (24.9%), anxiety (14.4%), and substance use disorders (11.8%).

SUMMARY

The prevalence of mental disorders, including addictions, has increased during the COVID-19 pandemic and is likely to remain at high rates in its aftermath. Until now, HPs have been consciously or unconsciously trained to prioritize caring for others instead of self-caring. Difficulties in seeking help when needed should be addressed during the undergraduate period and throughout their professional career. Several specialized mental health programs and wellbeing resources have been offered to HPs around the world in recent decades.[4]The impact of the pandemic on HPs mental health has also increased the number of initiatives to support them, although many of them may be temporary.[67–70]

Mental disorders among HPs are only the tip of the iceberg of HPs wellbeing. This issue needs to be approached with a multi-dimensional perspective whereby both the individuals and the context are considered. While offering appropriate treatment programs for those with psychiatric and psychological issues should be a priority, the

COVID-19 pandemic can be seen as an invaluable opportunity to start considering caring for the caregivers not only a moral imperative but also an essential ingredient of professionalism and of health care organizations (**Box 2**). According to Dr Shanafelt proposal for physicians,[4] we were recently moving from the era of distress, when the ideal HP should be perfect, have deity-like qualities, neglect self-care, prioritize autonomous performance and set no work limits, to that of wellbeing 1.0, where resilience, connection with other health care providers and work-life balance was promoted. HPs had hero-like qualities but were frustrated with the institutions they worked in. The COVID-19 pandemic could be a turning point to promote a new wellbeing 2.0 paradigm. HPs' human qualities and self-compassion should now be highly valued, work experienced as meaningful, work-life integration facilitated and team interactions transformed into a collaborative model. Professional organizations, institutions, leaders, HPs and the society, as a whole, need to be involved in the transition to this new paradigm.

CLINICS CARE POINTS

- If you are a health professional (HP), consider self-care as a priority to achieve a good clinical performance.
- If you or one colleague suffers from mental disorders, including addictions, do not delay help seeking.
- HPs should avoid self-medication or alcohol/drug use to cope with mental distress.
- Refraining from working should be encouraged if a HP is impaired by their mental disorder.
- Specialized treatment programs for HPs are a good alternative if you need mental health treatment.

DISCLOSURE

The authors have nothing to disclose.

REFERENCES

1. Bruguera M, Guri J, Arteman A, et al. Care of doctors to their health care. Results of a postal survey. Medicina Clinica 2001;117(13):492–4. https://doi.org/10.1016/s0025-7753(01)72154-9.
2. Available at: https://www.fgalatea.org/ca/recerca-estudis. Accessed February 18, 2022.
3. Gerada C. Clare Gerada: Doctors' mental health and stigma - The tide is turning. BMJ 2019;366. https://doi.org/10.1136/bmj.l4583.
4. Shanafelt TD. Physician Well-being 2.0: Where Are We and Where Are We Going? Mayo Clinic Proc 2021;96(10):2682–93. https://doi.org/10.1016/j.mayocp.2021.06.005.
5. Marshall EJ. Doctors' health and fitness to practise: Treating addicted doctors. Occup Med 2008;58(5):334–40. https://doi.org/10.1093/occmed/kqn081.
6. Carinci AJ, Christo PJ. Physician impairment: Is recovery feasible? Pain Physician 2009;12(3):487–91. https://doi.org/10.36076/ppj.2009/12/487.
7. Braquehais MD, Vargas-Caceres S, Nieva G, et al. Characteristics of resident physicians accessing a specialised mental health service: A retrospective study. BMJ Open 2021;11(12). https://doi.org/10.1136/bmjopen-2021-055184.

8. Braquehais MD, Arrizabalaga P, Lusilla P, et al. Gender Differences in Demographic and Clinical Features of Physicians Admitted to a Program for Medical Professionals with Mental Disorders. Front Psychiatry 2016;7(NOV):181. https://doi.org/10.3389/fpsyt.2016.00181.

9. Braquehais MD, Mozo X, Gausachs E, et al. Nurse admissions at a specialized mental health programme: A pre-Covid-19 retrospective review (2000-2019). J Adv Nurs 2022. https://doi.org/10.1111/jan.15189.

10. Braquehais MD, Tresidder A, DuPont RL. Service provision to physicians with mental health and addiction problems. Curr Opin Psychiatry 2015;28(4):324–9. https://doi.org/10.1097/YCO.0000000000000166.

11. Shapiro J, McDonald TB. Supporting Clinicians during Covid-19 and Beyond — Learning from Past Failures and Envisioning New Strategies. N Engl J Med 2020; 383(27):e142. https://doi.org/10.1056/nejmp2024834.

12. Tay S, Alcock K, Scior K. Mental health problems among clinical psychologists: Stigma and its impact on disclosure and help-seeking. J Clin Psychol 2018; 74(9):1545–55. https://doi.org/10.1002/jclp.22614.

13. Mihailescu M, Neiterman E. A scoping review of the literature on the current mental health status of physicians and physicians-in-training in North America. BMC Public Health 2019;19(1). https://doi.org/10.1186/s12889-019-7661-9.

14. Mark G, Smith AP. Occupational stress, job characteristics, coping, and the mental health of nurses. Br J Health Psychol 2012;17(3):505–21. https://doi.org/10.1111/j.2044-8287.2011.02051.x.

15. WHO Coronavirus (COVID-19) Dashboard. Available at: https://covid19.who.int/. Accessed February 18, 2022.

16. Batra K, Singh TP, Sharma M, et al. Investigating the psychological impact of COVID-19 among healthcare workers: A meta-analysis. Int J Environ Res Public Health 2020;17(23):1–33. https://doi.org/10.3390/ijerph17239096.

17. Gómez-Durán EL, Martin-Fumadó C, Fororo CG. Psychological impact of quarantine on healthcare workers. Occup Environ Med 2020;77(10):666–74. https://doi.org/10.1136/oemed-2020-106587.

18. Bettinsoli ML, di Riso D, Napier JL, et al. Mental Health Conditions of Italian Healthcare Professionals during the COVID-19 Disease Outbreak. Appl Psychol Health Well-Being 2020;12(4):1054–73. https://doi.org/10.1111/aphw.12239.

19. Sirois FM, Owens J. Factors Associated With Psychological Distress in Health-Care Workers During an Infectious Disease Outbreak: A Rapid Systematic Review of the Evidence. Front Psychiatry 2020;11:589545. https://doi.org/10.3389/fpsyt.2020.589545.

20. Chutiyami M, Cheong AMY, Salihu D, et al. COVID-19 Pandemic and Overall Mental Health of Healthcare Professionals Globally: A Meta-Review of Systematic Reviews. Front Psychiatry 2021;12:804525. https://doi.org/10.3389/fpsyt.2021.804525.

21. Madoz-Gúrpide A, Leira-Sanmartín M, Ibañez Á, et al. Self-reported increase in alcohol and drugs intake as a coping strategy in hospital workers during COVID-19 outbreak: A cross-sectional study. Adicciones 2021;0(0):1643. https://doi.org/10.20882/adicciones.1643.

22. McKay D, Asmundson GJG. COVID-19 stress and substance use: Current issues and future preparations. J Anxiety Disord 2020;74. https://doi.org/10.1016/j.janxdis.2020.102274.

23. Fernandez R, Sikhosana N, Green H, et al. Anxiety and depression among healthcare workers during the COVID-19 pandemic: A systematic umbrella review of

the global evidence. BMJ Open 2021;11(9). https://doi.org/10.1136/bmjopen-2021-054528.

24. Cénat JM, Blais-Rochette C, Kokou-Kpolou CK, et al. Prevalence of symptoms of depression, anxiety, insomnia, posttraumatic stress disorder, and psychological distress among populations affected by the COVID-19 pandemic: A systematic review and meta-analysis. Psychiatry Res 2021;295. https://doi.org/10.1016/j.psychres.2020.113599.

25. de Brier N, Stroobants S, Vandekerckhove P, et al. Factors affecting mental health of health care workers during coronavirus disease outbreaks (SARS, MERS & COVID-19): A rapid systematic review. PLoS ONE 2020;15(12 December). https://doi.org/10.1371/journal.pone.0244052.

26. Labrague LJ. Psychological resilience, coping behaviours and social support among health care workers during the COVID-19 pandemic: A systematic review of quantitative studies. J Nurs Manag 2021;29(7):1893–905. https://doi.org/10.1111/jonm.13336.

27. Billings J, Ching BCF, Gkofa V, et al. Experiences of frontline healthcare workers and their views about support during COVID-19 and previous pandemics: a systematic review and qualitative meta-synthesis. BMC Health Serv Res 2021;21(1). https://doi.org/10.1186/s12913-021-06917-z.

28. Koontalay A, Suksatan W, Prabsangob K, et al. Healthcare Workers' Burdens During the COVID-19 Pandemic: A Qualitative Systematic Review. J multidisciplinary Healthc 2021;14:3015–25. https://doi.org/10.2147/JMDH.S330041.

29. Stanton J, Randal P. Doctors accessing mental-health services: an exploratory study. BMJ open 2011;1(1):e000017. https://doi.org/10.1136/bmjopen-2010-000017.

30. Trockel M, Sinsky C, West CP, et al. Self-Valuation Challenges in the Culture and Practice of Medicine and Physician Well-being. Mayo Clinic Proc 2021;96(8):2123–32. https://doi.org/10.1016/j.mayocp.2020.12.032.

31. Merlo LJ, Gold MS. Prescription opioid abuse and dependence among physicians: Hypotheses and treatment. Harv Rev Psychiatry 2008;16(3):181–94. https://doi.org/10.1080/10673220802160316.

32. Center C, Davis M, Detre T, et al. Confronting Depression and Suicide in Physicians: A Consensus Statement. J Am Med Assoc 2003;289(23):3161–6. https://doi.org/10.1001/jama.289.23.3161.

33. Davidson JE, Zisook S, Kirby B, et al. Suicide Prevention: A Healer Education and Referral Program for Nurses. J Nurs Adm 2018;48(2):85–92. https://doi.org/10.1097/NNA.0000000000000582.

34. Rössler W. The stigma of mental disorders: A millennia-long history of social exclusion and prejudices. EMBO Rep 2016;17(9):1250–3. https://doi.org/10.15252/embr.201643041.

35. Ungar T, Knaak S. The hidden medical logic of mental health stigma. Aust N Z J Psychiatry 2013;47(7):611–2. https://doi.org/10.1177/0004867413476758.

36. Firth-Cozens J. Predicting stress in general practitioners: 10 year follow up postal survey. Br Med J 1997;315(7099):34–5. https://doi.org/10.1136/bmj.315.7099.34.

37. Braquehais MD, Lusilla P, Bel MJ, et al. Dual diagnosis among physicians: A clinical perspective. J Dual Diagn 2014;10(3):148–55. https://doi.org/10.1080/15504263.2014.929331.

38. Hem E, Haldorsen T, Aasland OG, et al. Suicide rates according to education with a particular focus on physicians in Norway 1960-2000. Psychol Med 2005;35(6):873–80. https://doi.org/10.1017/S0033291704003344.

39. Davidson JE, Stuck AR, Zisook S, et al. Testing a strategy to identify incidence of nurse suicide in the United States. J Nurs Adm 2018;48(5):259–65. https://doi.org/10.1097/NNA.0000000000000610.
40. Hawton K, Agerbo E, Simkin S, et al. Risk of suicide in medical and related occupational groups: A national study based on Danish case population-based registers. J Affect Disord 2011;134(1–3):320–6. https://doi.org/10.1016/j.jad.2011.05.044.
41. Skegg K, Firth H, Gray A, et al. Suicide by occupation: Does access to means increase the risk? Aust N Z J Psychiatry 2010;44(5):429–34. https://doi.org/10.3109/00048670903487191.
42. Dutheil F, Aubert C, Pereira B, et al. Suicide among physicians and health-care workers: A systematic review and meta-analysis. PloS one 2019;14(12). https://doi.org/10.1371/JOURNAL.PONE.0226361.
43. Dyrbye LN, Shanafelt TD, Johnson PO, et al. A cross-sectional study exploring the relationship between burnout, absenteeism, and job performance among American nurses. BMC Nurs 2019;18(1). https://doi.org/10.1186/S12912-019-0382-7.
44. Letvak SA, Ruhm CJ, Gupta SN. Nurses' presenteeism and its effects on self-reported quality of care and costs. Am J Nurs 2012;112(2).
45. Fahrenkopf AM, Sectish TC, Barger LK, et al. Rates of medication errors among depressed and burnt out residents: Prospective cohort study. BMJ 2008; 336(7642):488–91. https://doi.org/10.1136/bmj.39469.763218.
46. Gärtner FR, Nieuwenhuijsen K, van Dijk FJH, et al. The impact of common mental disorders on the work functioning of nurses and allied health professionals: A systematic review. Int J Nurs Stud 2010;47(8):1047–61. https://doi.org/10.1016/j.ijnurstu.2010.03.013.
47. Emami P, Boozari Pour M, Zahodnezhad H, et al. Investigating the relationship between workplace stressors and caring behaviours of nursing staff in inpatient wards: A cross-sectional study. J Adv Nurs 2021. https://doi.org/10.1111/jan.15080.
48. Edwards D, Burnard P. A systematic review of stress and stress management interventions for mental health nurses. J Adv Nurs 2003;42(2):169–200. https://doi.org/10.1046/j.1365-2648.2003.02600.x.
49. Myers MF. Treatment of the mentally ill physician. Can J Psychiatry Revue canadienne de psychiatrie 1997;42(6). https://doi.org/10.1177/070674379704200625.
50. Melnyk BM, Kelly SA, Stephens J, et al. Interventions to Improve Mental Health, Well-Being, Physical Health, and Lifestyle Behaviors in Physicians and Nurses: A Systematic Review. Am J Health Promot 2020;34(8):929–41. https://doi.org/10.1177/0890117120920451.
51. O'Connor PG, Spickard A. Physician impairment by substance abuse. Med Clin North Am 1997;81(4):1037–52. https://doi.org/10.1016/S0025-7125(05)70562-9.
52. Mayall RM. Substance abuse in anaesthetists. BJA Education 2016;16(7): 236–41. https://doi.org/10.1093/BJAED/MKV054.
53. Poplar JF. Characteristics of nurse addicts. Am J Nurs 1969;69(1):117–9. https://doi.org/10.1097/00000446-196901000-00038.
54. Pace EM, Kesterson C, Garcia K, et al. Experiences and outcomes of nurses referred to a peer health assistance program: Recommendations for nursing management. J Nurs Manag 2020;28(1):35–42. https://doi.org/10.1111/jonm.12874.
55. Monroe T, Kenaga H. Don't ask don't tell: Substance abuse and addiction among nurses. J Clin Nurs 2011;20(3–4):504–9. https://doi.org/10.1111/j.1365-2702.2010.03518.x.

56. Bettinardi-Angres K, Pickett J, Patrick D. Substance Use Disorders and Accessing Alternative-to-Discipline Programs. J Nurs Regul 2012;3(2):16–23. https://doi.org/10.1016/S2155-8256(15)30214-3.

57. Geuijen PM, van den Broek SJM, Dijkstra BAG, et al. Success rates of monitoring for healthcare professionals with a substance use disorder: A meta-analysis. J Clin Med 2021;10(2):1–31. https://doi.org/10.3390/jcm10020264.

58. Boisaubin Ev, Levine RE. Identifying and assisting the impaired physician. Am J Med Sci 2001;322(1):31–6. https://doi.org/10.1097/00000441-200107000-00006.

59. Brewster JM, Kaufmann IM, Hutchison S, et al. Characteristics and outcomes of doctors in a substance dependence monitoring programme in Canada: Prospective descriptive study. BMJ 2008;337(7679):1156–8. https://doi.org/10.1136/bmj.a2098.

60. McLellan AT, Skipper GS, Campbell M, et al. Five year outcomes in a cohort study of physicians treated for substance use disorders in the United States. BMJ 2008; 337(7679):1154–6. https://doi.org/10.1136/bmj.a2038.

61. DuPont RL, McLellan AT, Carr G, et al. How are addicted physicians treated? A national survey of physician health programs. J Subst Abuse Treat 2009;37(1): 1–7. https://doi.org/10.1016/j.jsat.2009.03.010.

62. Bruguera E, Heredia M, Llavayol E, et al. Integral Treatment Programme for Addicted Physicians: Results from the Galatea Care Programme for Sick Physicians. Eur Addict Res 2020;26(3):122–30. https://doi.org/10.1159/000505914.

63. DuPont RL, Skipper GE. Six lessons from state physician health programs to promote long-term recovery. J Psychoactive Drugs 2012;44(1):72–8. https://doi.org/10.1080/02791072.2012.660106.

64. Polles A, Bundy C, Jacobs W, et al. Adaptations to substance use disorder monitoring by physician health programs in response to COVID-19. J Subst Abuse Treat 2021;125. https://doi.org/10.1016/j.jsat.2021.108281.

65. Gerada C. Practitioner Health's COVID Experience. Meeting the mental health needs of doctors during the pandemic. Pract Health Pract Health Programme 2020. Available at: https://www.practitionerhealth.nhs.uk/media/content/files/PHP-covid-report-web version FINAL.pdf.

66. Braquehais MD, Gómez-Duran E, Nieva G, et al. Help seeking of highly specialized mental health treatment before and during the COVID-19 pandemic among health professionals. [Published online 2022]. Int J Environ Res Public Health 2022;19(6): 3665.

67. Kisely S, Warren N, McMahon L, et al. Occurrence, prevention, and management of the psychological effects of emerging virus outbreaks on healthcare workers: rapid review and meta-analysis. BMJ (Clinical research ed) 2020;369:m1642. https://doi.org/10.1136/bmj.m1642.

68. Drissi N, Ouhbi S, Marques G, et al. A Systematic Literature Review on e-Mental Health Solutions to Assist Health Care Workers during COVID-19. Telemed e-Health 2021;27(6):594–602. https://doi.org/10.1089/tmj.2020.0287.

69. Hooper JJ, Saulsman L, Hall T, et al. Addressing the psychological impact of COVID-19 on healthcare workers: Learning from a systematic review of early interventions for frontline responders. BMJ Open 2021;11(5). https://doi.org/10.1136/bmjopen-2020-044134.

70. Cabarkapa S, Nadjidai SE, Murgier J, et al. The psychological impact of COVID-19 and other viral epidemics on frontline healthcare workers and ways to address it: A rapid systematic review. Brain Behav Immun - Health 2020;8:100144. https://doi.org/10.1016/j.bbih.2020.100144.

Overall goal of Cognitive-Behavioral Therapy in Major Psychiatric Disorders and Suicidality: A Narrative Review

Gianluca Serafini, MD, PhD[a,b,]*, Alessandra Costanza, MD[c],
Andrea Aguglia, MD, PhD[a,b], Andrea Amerio, MD, PhD[a,b],
Valeria Placenti, MD[a,b], Luca Magnani, MD[a,b],
Andrea Escelsior, MD[a,b], Leo Sher, MD[d,e], Mario Amore, MD[a,b]

KEYWORDS

- Cognitive-behavioral therapy • Depression • Bipolar disorder • Anxiety
- Obsessive-compulsive disorder • Posttraumatic disorder
- Body dysmorphic disorder • Suicidal behavior

KEY POINTS

- Cognitive-behavioral therapy (CBT) has been shown to be effective for a range of psychiatric conditions, including severe mental illness and suicidality.
- A significant body of research suggests that CBT leads to significant clinical improvements and can be as effective as, or more effective than, other forms of psychological therapy, alone or in combination with psychiatric medications.
- Perspectives for the future include administering CBT online or through mobile phone apps and combining it with other techniques such as mindfulness.

INTRODUCTION

Cognitive-behavioral therapy (CBT) is a form of psychological treatment that is based on the underlying assumption that mental disorders and psychological distress are maintained by cognitive factors, i.e., general beliefs about the world, the self, and

[a] Department of Neuroscience, Rehabilitation, Ophthalmology, Genetics, Maternal and Child Health (DINOGMI), Section of Psychiatry, University of Genoa, Genoa, Italy; [b] IRCCS Ospedale Policlinico San Martino, Largo Rosanna Benzi 10, Genoa 16132, Italy; [c] Department of Psychiatry, Faculty of Medicine, University of Geneva (UNIGE), Geneva, Switzerland; [d] James J. Peters Veterans' Administration Medical Center, Bronx, NY, USA; [e] Icahn School of Medicine at Mount Sinai, New York, NY, USA
* Corresponding author. IRCCS Ospedale Policlinico San Martino, Largo Rosanna Benzi 10, Genoa 16132, Italy.
E-mail address: gianluca.serafini@unige.it

Med Clin N Am 107 (2023) 143–167
https://doi.org/10.1016/j.mcna.2022.05.006
0025-7125/23/© 2022 Elsevier Inc. All rights reserved.

the future contribute to the maintenance of emotional distress and behavioral problems **Tables 1–3**.[1,2] The overall goal of CBT is to replace dysfunctional constructs with more flexible and adaptive cognitions.[3] The most relevant cognitive-behavioral techniques in clinical practice are: *i. Cognitive Restructuring* (also known as the ABCDE method) which is indicated to support patients dealing with negative beliefs or thoughts.[4–6] The different steps in the cognitive restructuring process are summarized by the letters in the ABCDE acronym that describe the different stages of this coaching model: *A*ctivating event or situation associated with the negative thoughts, *B*eliefs and belief structures held by the individual that explain how they perceive the world which can facilitate negative thoughts, *C*onsequences or feelings related to the activating event, *D*isputation of beliefs to allow individuals to challenge their belief system, and *E*ffective new approach or effort to deal with the problem by facilitating individuals to replace unhelpful beliefs with more helpful ones. *ii. Problem-Solving*[7] (also known as SOLVE[8,9]) to raise awareness for specific triggers, and evaluate and choose more effective options. Each letter of the SOLVE acronym identifies different steps of the problem-solving process: *S*elect a problem, generate *O*ptions, rate the *L*ikely outcome of each option, choose the *V*ery best option, and *E*valuate how well each option worked. For example, a suicide attempt is reconceptualized as a failure in problem-solving. This treatment approach attempts to provide patients with a better sense of control over future emerging problems. *iii. Re-attribution* is a technique that enables patients to replace negative self-statements (eg, "it is all my fault") with different statements where responsibility is attributed more appropriately.[10] Furthermore, decatastrophizing may help subjects, especially adolescents decide whether they may be overestimating the catastrophic nature of the precipitating event, and by allowing them to scale the event severity they learn to evaluate situations along a continuum rather than seeing them in black and white.[10] *iv. Affect Regulation* techniques are often used with suicidal adolescents to teach them how to recognize stimuli that provoke negative emotions and how to mitigate the resulting emotional arousal through self-talk and relaxation.[10]

Another useful approach is dialectical behavior therapy (DBT)[11] which can reduce psychological distress and affect dysregulation, particularly in subjects with borderline personality disorder and self-injurious behavior. DBT is a modified CBT. The core goals of DBT are to educate people on how to live in the moment, develop healthy ways to cope with stress, regulate their emotions, and improve their relationships with others.

CBT has been proven to be effective for a range of psychiatric disorders and suicidality (defined as suicidal ideation, SI,[12,13] and suicidal behavior, SB, including the entire spectrum from suicide attempts, SA, and completed suicide). Both research and clinical practice suggested that CBT leads to significant improvement in symptomatology, functioning, and quality of life. Here, we review the main studies exploring the role of CBT in major psychiatric disorders, distinguishing between results obtained for mixed/adult populations and studies focusing on children/adolescents/young adults.

COGNITIVE-BEHAVIORAL THERAPY ON UNIPOLAR/BIPOLAR AFFECTIVE DISORDER

A review of 106 meta-analyses by Hoffman and colleagues examined CBT for a range of psychiatric diseases, including depression and bipolar disorder, in different populations of different ages. The authors concluded that this therapeutic approach delivers a higher response rate compared to other treatment conditions.[14] Furthermore, a meta-analysis of 19 randomized controlled trials for depression

Table 1
Synthesis of the main studies focusing on CBT in unipolar/bipolar affective disorders

Authors	Study Design	Comparisons Investigated	Population Focus	Main Findings
Mixed Populations and Adults				
Hofmann et al,[14] 1999	Meta-analysis	Various	Mixed	Several studies showed CBT to be more effective than controls. CBT was found to be equivalent or superior to some other psychological treatments. CBT had similar effects as pharmacotherapy or the latter was a useful addition. CBT had small to medium overall effect sizes for bipolar disorder that diminished over time.
Von Brachel et al,[17] 2019	475 depressed outpatients	One group only: CBT	Adults	Depression severity declined significantly between pre and posttreatment.
Children/Adolescents/Young Adults				
Lewinsohn and Clarke [25] 1999	Meta-analysis	Various	Children and Adolescents	CBT had an overall effect size of 1.27% and 63% of patients showed clinically significant improvement at the end of treatment.
March et al,[23] 2004	RCT of 439 volunteers with MDD	Four groups: fluoxetine only, CBT only,	Adolescents	Using the Children's Depression Rating Scale-

(continued on next page)

Table 1
(continued)

Authors	Study Design	Comparisons Investigated	Population Focus	Main Findings
		CBT + fluoxetine, or placebo (administered for 12 wk)		Revised, treatment with fluoxetine + CBT was superior to fluoxetine alone which was superior to CBT alone, with respective response rates of 71%, 61%, and 43%.
March et al,[24] 2007	RCT of 327 patients with MDD	Four groups: fluoxetine only, CBT only, CBT + fluoxetine, or placebo (administered for 36 wk)	Adolescents	Response rates were 73% for fluoxetine + CBT, 62% for fluoxetine, and 48% for CBT at week 12; which increased to 86%, 81%, and 81%, respectively, by week 36.
Brent et al,[33] 2008	RCT of a clinical sample of 334 patients with MDD that had not responded to a 2-mo initial treatment with an SSRI	Four groups: switch to a 2nd, different SSRI (paroxetine, citalopram, or fluoxetine), switch to a different SSRI + CBT, switch to venlafaxine, or switch to venlafaxine + CBT.	Adolescents	CBT plus a switch to either medication regimen showed a higher response rate (55%) than a medication switch alone (41%). No difference in response rate between venlafaxine and a second SSRI (48.2% vs 47.0%).
Goodyer et al,[39] 2007	Pragmatic randomized controlled superiority trial in 6 outpatient clinics on 208 patients with moderate to severe MDD or probable MDD	Two groups: SSRI and routine care or SSRI + routine care + CBT, for 12 wk, followed by a 16-wk maintenance phase.	Adolescents	After 28 wk, CBT + SSRI + routine clinical care had not produced any improved outcome compared with SSRI + routine care.

Melvin et al,[35] 2006	RCT of 73 patients with MDD, dysthymic disorder, or unspecified depressive disorder.	Three groups: CBT + sertraline, CBT alone, sertraline alone.	Adolescents	All treatments led to a reduction in depression while CBT alone had a superior acute treatment response (odds ratio: 6.86) compared to sertraline alone. CBT + sertraline had no obvious advantage over CBT alone.
Vázquez et al,[37] 2012	RCT of 133 participants with elevated depression symptoms	Two groups: CBT or relaxation training (RT) administered over 8 wk.	Young adults (university students)	Both interventions led to reduced depression and anxiety scores. Effect size was greatest between pre and immediately postintervention scores for CBT (d = 1.32) and between pre and 6-mo postintervention scores for RT (d = 0.75). In the medium term (3–6 mo), RT produced similar reductions in depressive and anxiety symptoms as CBT.
Weinstein et al,[40] 2018	RCT involving 71 participants diagnosed with pediatric bipolar disorder.	Two groups: Family-focused CBT (CFF-CBT) or psychotherapy treatment as usual.	Children and Adolescents	While SI was prevalent pretreatment (39%), the likelihood and intensity of SI decreased with either treatment without any significant differences between groups.

Abbreviations: CBT, cognitive-behavioral treatment; MDD, major depression disorder; RCT, randomized clinical trial; SSRI, selective serotonin reuptake inhibitors.

Table 2
Synthesis of main studies focusing on anxiety disorders and PTSD

Authors	Study Design	Comparisons Investigated	Population Focus	Main Findings
Adults				
Pigeon et al,[42] 2022	RCT of CBT for insomnia and PTSD in survivors of interpersonal violence	Two groups: CBT for insomnia (CBTi) + cognitive processing therapy (CPT) or attention control + CPT (20 wk).	Adults	CBTi + CPT led to greater improvements in insomnia, depression, and PTSD compared to CPT alone. Effects were larger for insomnia and for depression than for PTSD.
Bryan et al,[43] 2016	RCT of 108 soldiers diagnosed with PTSD	Two groups: cognitive processing therapy-cognitive only version (CBT-C) or present-centered therapy (PCT).	Adults	In both groups, SI significantly improved, particularly in those with pretreatment SI, SI was significantly reduced posttreatment, maintained at 12-mo follow-up. Change in depression symptoms predicted change in suicide risk.
Children/Adolescents/Young Adults				
Wang et al,[48] 2017	Meta-analysis of 115 comparative studies involving 7719 patients.	Randomized and nonrandomized comparative studies on patients with panic disorder, various anxiety disorders, specific phobias who received CBT, pharmacotherapy, or a combination.	Children and Adolescents	CBT significantly improved anxiety symptoms, remission, and response compared to controls. CBT was more effective than fluoxetine for reducing anxiety and improved remission more than sertraline. CBT + sertraline significantly reduced anxiety and response more than

Study	Description	Population	Findings
James et al,[49] 2013	Review of 41 RCTs involving 1806 anxiety patients	Children and Adolescents	RCTs of CBT vs waiting list, active control conditions, TAU, or medication. While CBT is effective for treating anxiety disorder, evidence suggesting that CBT is more effective than active controls or TAU or medication at follow-up is limited and inconclusive. Adverse events were common with medications but not with CBT.
Walkup et al,[50] 2008	RCT of 488 patients diagnosed with separation anxiety disorder, generalized anxiety disorder, or social phobia	Children and Adolescents	Four groups: sertraline only, CBT only, CBT + sertraline, or placebo (administered for 12 wk). For sertraline + CBT 81%, for CBT 60%, for sertraline 55%, and for placebo 24% of participants were rated as very much or much improved on the Clinician Global Impression-Improvement scale.
Kunas et al,[52] 2021	Review of 73 articles and meta-analysis of 23 studies on CBT outcomes for anxiety	Mixed	Higher symptom severity was a predictor of worse CBT outcome. Parental psychopathology was significant and detrimental to CBT outcomes in anxious but not depressed youth. Worse coping skills and more nonsuicidal self-injury were associated with a worse CBT outcome.
McBride et al,[53] 2017	RCT involving 100 participants with anxiety and their parents.	Children	Two groups: CCBT or treatment as usual (TAU). Families were offered the same protocol. CCBT reduced SI/SB from 24% at baseline to 13% during treatment.

Abbreviations: CBT, cognitive-behavioral treatment; CCBT, computer-assisted CBT; PTSD, posttraumatic stress disorder; RCT, randomized clinical trial.

Table 3
Synthesis of main studies focusing on CBT in suicidality

Authors	Study Design	Techniques Used	Population Focus	Main Findings
Adults				
Ecker et al,[81] 2019	Secondary analysis of an RCT in 302 patients with congestive heart failure and/or chronic obstructive pulmonary disease.	Two groups: bCBT or EUC	Adults	bCBT was more effective at reducing the likelihood of high SI compared to EUC posttreatment and at 8-mo follow-up after accounting for baseline suicidal ideation. Participants receiving bCBT were less likely to have high SI at 4, 8, and 12 mo compared to baseline. High suicidal ideation for EUC participants did not differ at 4 or 8 mo but was less likely at 12 mo.
Children/Adolescents/Young Adults				
Donaldson et al,[93] 2005	RCT with 39 patients presented to a pediatric ED or inpatient unit of a child psychiatric hospital after SA.	Two groups: skills-based treatment or supportive relationship treatment. Follow-ups at 3 and 6 mo.	Adolescents	In the 60% of participants completing the entire treatment protocol, they found significant decreases in SI for both treatment approaches without any statistically significant differences between the 2 groups.

Study	Sample	Groups	Population	Findings
Esposito-Smythers et al,[89] 2011	RCT with 40 patients with alcohol and other drug use disorders	Two groups: I-CBT or enhanced TAU	Adolescents	I-CBT was associated with improved substance abuse and SB, and reduced psychiatric hospitalizations and ED visits.
Brent et al,[90] 2009	Partially randomized trial of 124 patients with recent SA and depression	Three groups: specialized CBT for SA, medication, or the combination.	Adolescents	SA was higher in the combination group (24%) compared to either of the monotherapy groups (6.5%). However, patients in the combination group had higher risk at baseline, controlling for this removed any differential effects of treatment type.
Brent et al,[28] 1997	RCT with 107 participants diagnosed with MDD	Three groups: CBT, SBFT or NST.	Adolescents	CBT performed better than SBFT or NST at improving depression diagnoses and reducing remissions and equally well at reducing suicidality and functional impairment.
March et al,[23] 2004, March et al,[24] 2007	RCT of 439 volunteers with MDD	Four groups: fluoxetine only, CBT only, CBT + fluoxetine, or placebo (administered for 12 wk)	Adolescents	Clinically significant SI, present in 29% at baseline, improved significantly in all 4 treatment groups with the combination treatment showing the greatest reduction.

Abbreviations: bCBT, brief CBT; CBT, cognitive-behavioral therapy; EUC, enhanced usual care; MDD, Major Depressive Disorder; NST, nondirective supportive therapy; SB, Suicidal Behavior; SBFT, systemic behavior family therapy; SI, suicidal ideation; TAU, treatment as usual.

prevention found a 14% reduction in depression prevalence.[15] Investigating whether pretreatment SI was a predictor of less beneficial outcomes of CBT for adult depression (also investigated here[16]), von Brachel and colleagues [17] found that depression severity declined significantly between pre- and posttreatment.

Focusing on Children, Adolescents, and Young Adults

Evidence suggests that CBT may be a viable treatment approach for depression in adolescents and young adults where the cognitive approach mainly aims to address maladaptive schemas, automatic thoughts, and cognitive distortions in adolescents.[18] Based on existing guidelines regarding the treatment of depression, evidence-based psychotherapies, and especially CBT represent treatment alternatives to antidepressants for mild depression.[19–22] In adolescent patients with depression, CBT has been shown to have an overall effectivity ranging between 43% and 65%.[23,24] According to existing meta-analyses, the use of CBT is strongly supported among depressed youths with effect sizes ranging from 1.02 to 1.27.[25,26] Based on another meta-analysis that included 11 randomized trials on adolescents with unipolar depression, a mean effect size of .53 was found, presumably as a result of the enhanced severity of the investigated samples or methodological differences.[27] Another interesting report focusing on adolescents with major depressive disorder (MDD) suggested that while CBT performed better than nondirective supportive therapy or systemic behavior family therapy at improving depression diagnoses, resulting in more rapid and complete treatment response, all 3 treatments performed equally well at reducing suicidality.[28]

The effects of attachment-based family therapy (ABFT) were tested by Diamond and collaborators[29] who showed that adolescents randomized to this approach had fewer depression symptoms, family conflict, SI, and lower levels of hopelessness at posttreatment relative to adolescents in the waitlist group. Later studies[30] found that ABFT led to more significant reductions in SI and depressive symptoms than enhanced usual care and similar reductions as family-enhanced nondirective supportive therapy.[31]

Based on the Treatment for Adolescents Depression Study (TADS),[23] the largest multisite treatment study of adolescent depression, the combined treatment of CBT and fluoxetine was more effective (71% response rate after 12 weeks) in reducing depressive symptoms than fluoxetine alone (61%), CBT alone (43%), or placebo (35%). Using fluoxetine (alone or in combination with CBT) also reduced clinically significant SI.[23] In addition, adolescents who were treated with fluoxetine reported a greater prevalence of psychiatric adverse events compared to CBT or placebo.[23] This is in agreement with findings that depressed adolescents who received psychiatric medications (fluoxetine, placebo, or a combination of antidepressants with anxiolytic agents) presented more physical adverse events than those treated with CBT alone.[32] In a later study, similar 12-week response rates were obtained, but 36-week response rates were notably higher: 86% for combination therapy, 81% for fluoxetine therapy, and 81% for CBT.[24]

In the multi-site Treatment of SSRI-Resistant Depression in Adolescents study (TORDIA) involving 334 depressed adolescents who failed to respond to a previous trial of a selective serotonin reuptake inhibitors (SSRI),[33] switching them to medication regimen plus CBT resulted in a higher rate of clinical response (54.8%) than a medication switch alone (40.5%). In a different study, a sample of 46 youths who had responded to 12 weeks of fluoxetine was randomized to receive either 6 months of continued antidepressant medication management or antidepressant medication management plus relapse prevention CBT (MM + CBT). The results showed that the addition of CBT significantly attenuated the risk of relapse compared to medication management alone.[34]

Based on the findings of Melvin and colleagues[35] in a study involving depressed youths, both suicidal ideation and nonsuicidal self-injury were significantly lower in the CBT-plus-fluoxetine group relative to the CBT-only group with this improvement which was maintained at follow-up. CBT has also been investigated in samples of university students at risk for depression.[36,37] While Seligman and colleagues[36] found encouraging short-term reductions in depressive and anxiety symptoms compared to controls, this reduction was only maintained for depression but not anxiety at a 6-month follow-up. In contrast, when comparing CBT to relaxation techniques, Vázquez and colleagues[37] found that both treatment types performed equally well and while the effect sizes were maximal immediately posttreatment, they still observed some long-term benefits at 6-month follow-up for both anxiety and depression. This is supported by Saigo and colleagues[38] who found that group CBT intervention was linked to significant reductions in depression scores compared with baseline and that these improvements were maintained one-year postintervention.

In contrast, Goodyer and colleagues [39] conducted a study on adolescents with moderate to severe MDD or probable MDD and found that the addition of CBT had no benefit over treatment with the SSRI alone.

Child- and family-focused CBT (CFF-CBT) was developed to address child- and family-related issues associated with pediatric bipolar disorder (PBD), a group with a very high suicidality risk. Although not designed to target suicidality, CFF-CBT has been postulated to generalize to the treatment of suicidality.[40] In a randomized clinical trial involving youth with PBD and 39% pretreatment prevalence of suicidal ideation, Weinstein and colleagues[40] found that both CFF-CBT and psychotherapy treatment-as-usual successfully reduced the likelihood and intensity of SI without any significant differences between both treatment groups.

With regard to implications for future developments, a machine learning algorithm that exclusively uses structural connectome data and the baseline depression score may predict with a high accuracy depressive symptom reduction in depressed adolescents with CBT.[41]

COGNITIVE-BEHAVIORAL THERAPY ON ANXIETY DISORDERS AND POSTTRAUMATIC STRESS DISORDER
Focusing on Adults

Pigeon and colleagues[42] conducted a 20-week trial on 110 patients diagnosed with PTSD, depression, and insomnia due to exposure to interpersonal violence. Participants were randomized to sequential treatment with CBT for insomnia (CBTi) followed by cognitive processing therapy (CPT) or attention control followed by CPT. The authors found that CBTi followed by CPT led to more significant improvements in insomnia, depression, and PTSD symptoms than attention control followed by CPT. Group cognitive processing therapy-cognitive only version (CPT-C) was tested on the US Army personnel diagnosed with posttraumatic stress disorder (PTSD) by Bryan and colleagues.[43] They found that soldiers with pretreatment SI exhibited a significantly lower severity SI posttreatment and this improvement persisted for up to 12 months.

Focusing on Children, Adolescents, and Young Adults

Anxiety disorders represent the most frequent mental illness in children and adolescents[44,45] with early onset of anxiety disorders reported to be a significant predictor of anxiety and depression throughout life.[46] Anxiety disorders frequently cooccur with depressive disorders in youths, with prevalence rates ranging between 30% and 44%.[44,47] While CBT has been reported to have a positive effect in the treatment of anxiety disorders in children and adolescents,[48] there is still no conclusive evidence to show that this intervention would be more effective than other existing treatment options.[49]

In a large randomized controlled trial involving 488 children between the ages of 7 and 17 years, diagnosed with anxiety disorders (their primary diagnoses were separation anxiety disorder, generalized anxiety disorder, or social phobia), Walkup and colleagues[50] administered CBT, sertraline, placebo, or a combination of sertraline + CBT treatments and found that although over 0%/0% of children receiving sertraline + CBT/CBT only were very much or much improved on the Clinician Global Impression-Improvement scale, demonstrating that both CBT and sertraline significantly reduced the severity of anxiety disorders with the combination treatment yielding a superior response rate. In patients treated with CBT, there was less insomnia, fatigue, sedation, and restlessness compared to the sertraline group. In addition, there was no significant difference in SI or homicidal ideation between the sertraline and the placebo groups.[50] Independently by CBT, when comparing fluoxetine and placebo for children/adolescents with anxiety disorders, Birmaher and colleagues[51] found no significant difference between both groups in the frequency of suicidal adverse events.

According to a recent systematic review and meta-analysis by Kunas and colleagues,[52] primary symptom severity emerged as a significant negative predictor of CBT outcome for both anxious and depressed youth while the effects of cooccurring anxiety or depression had no significant effect on CBT. However, the effect of parental psychopathology on CBT outcome was significant (negative for anxious youths and nonsignificant for depressed youths).

In youths receiving treatment for anxiety, McBride and colleagues[53] found that computer-assisted CBT (CCBT) led to a reduction in suicidal thoughts and behaviors from 24% at baseline to 13.1% once the treatment had started. Interestingly, over 50% of those harboring suicidal thoughts and behaviors during treatment had not been detected prior to treatment.

Overall, estimates for adult patients' and young adolescents' remission rates of any anxiety or depressive disorder in children and adolescents are approximately 60%.[54]

COGNITIVE-BEHAVIORAL THERAPY FOR BODY DYSMORPHIC DISORDER

Body dysmorphic disorder (BDD), that is, preoccupation with an imagined defect in appearance, is a severe psychiatric condition associated with a significant disability and psychosocial impairment, linked to high rates of depression, hospitalization, and SB.[55–57]

CBT is a well-known psychosocial treatment of BDD[58] with most treatment studies focusing predominantly on short-term CBT, behavior therapy (BT), or cognitive therapy (CT).[59–61] Greenberg and colleagues[58] reported that greater baseline motivation/readiness to change, greater treatment expectancy, and better baseline BDD-related insight all resulted in better CBT response posttreatment, concluding that focusing on these issues at treatment onset can greatly enhance treatment outcomes even for more severe BDD and depression.[58] In these specific patient subgroups, particularly among subjects with impaired insight, motivational interventions and the use of SSRI prior to initiating CBT may ameliorate the general outcome associated with BDD. Overall, patients with a more severe BDD subtype and depressive symptoms may really benefit from CBT which is a safe and efficacious therapy.

Studies on comorbidity supported the strong association between BDD and MDD. For instance, according to Phillips and colleagues,[62] 59% of current and 83% of lifetime prevalence of MDD were reported in a sample of 130 BDD subjects. These results were replicated by Phillips and colleagues[63] who found a 38% current and 74% lifetime prevalence of major depression in a sample of 178 BDD individuals. Subjects with comorbid depression also manifested higher suicidality, poorer functioning, and impaired quality of life.[63] Importantly, most of the SAs in BDD appear to be related to individual appearance concerns stressing the severity of this condition.[64] According to the study by Phillips and Menard[55] who examined 185 subjects with BDD over the course of 4 years, 57.8% of the analyzed individuals reported SI and 2.6% attempted suicide per year. This average annual SI rate is approximately 10 to 25 times higher than the reported national average for the US while the rate of SA (2.6%) is about 3 to 12 times higher.[55] Importantly, cognitive restructuring focusing on depressive beliefs and activity scheduling may be considered useful strategies for attenuating depressive symptoms.[65] In this regard, it is important to consider the role played by inactivity in maintaining depression and preventing the individual from restructuring negative or catastrophic beliefs.

COGNITIVE-BEHAVIORAL THERAPY ON INSOMNIA

Insomnia frequently cooccurs with major psychiatric disorders and represents a risk factor for suicidality. For instance, in depression, both insomnia and depressive symptoms may be considered independent risk factors for SI and SB.[66–69]

Meta-analyses[70,71] reported that cognitive-behavioral treatments, particularly CBT for insomnia (CBTi), were efficacious for alleviating depression and insomnia. Results obtained in a randomized trial by Pigeon and colleagues[72] documented that brief CBTi intervention had large effects on both insomnia severity and sleep diary measures at posttreatment compared to brief sleep hygiene (SH) control condition intervention. However, at a 3-month follow-up, the statistical significance was not maintained except for the number of awakenings.

Effective treatment of insomnia with CBTi may be an important target for reducing suicide risk. For instance, treatment of insomnia among veterans is associated with a reduction in SI, specifically, each 7-point improvement in insomnia severity as a result of CBTi was found to lead to a 65% reduction in the odds ratio of SI, indicating that CBTi may be an important clinical strategy to reduce SI among veterans and patients with insomnia.[73]

In the context of patients with comorbid MDD and insomnia, one study showed that CBTi may be linked to reductions in depression and SI while improving sleep.[74]

Given that the efficacy of brief CBT (bCBT) for reducing SA has been supported by 2 independent randomized clinical trials,[75,76] Roberge and colleagues[77] hypothesized that bCBT could have the same effect on both insomnia and suicidality. The authors reported that bCBT led to clinically significant reductions in insomnia symptoms that persisted for at least 12 months. Furthermore, they found that changes in sleep disturbance predicted changes in suicide risk. Importantly, changes in hopelessness and suicidal beliefs were predictive of changes in insomnia over time.[77]

Based on a two-arm, parallel randomized, controlled clinical study comparing the efficacy of a self-help CBTi smartphone application, proACT-S, with a waitlist control group in subjects with major depression and insomnia, Hui and colleagues[78] proposed that proACT-S was an efficacious brief sleep-focused self-help treatment of subjects with major depression and insomnia.

COGNITIVE-BEHAVIORAL THERAPY FOR SUICIDALITY

Several studies mentioned above already examined the role of CBT on suicidality, typically in the context of major psychiatric disorders. Here, we focus on studies where suicidality was not explicitly related to a major psychiatric disorders (or it was explicitly related to a major psychiatric disorders, such as schizophrenia, but was not included in any of the previous sections), e.g., the occurrence of a suicidal crisis without a specific psychiatric diagnosis.

Focusing on Adults

To test whether CBT was efficacious at reducing SI in patients with schizophrenia, Bateman and colleagues[79] investigated a sample of 90 ambulatory patients with psychotic symptoms resistant to conventional antipsychotic medication. They were randomized to CBT or befriending with CBT providing significant acute reductions in SI which were sustained at follow-up. More recently, Klingberg and colleagues[80] conducted an RCT to explore the frequency and extent of detrimental effects, such as suicides or SA, randomizing 198 patients with schizophrenia to either CBT or cognitive remediation. They found that the severe adverse events remained infrequent and comparable between CBT and cognitive remediation although some patients showed symptom increases with large effect sizes.

In medically ill veterans receiving mental health treatment of depression in primary care, Ecker and colleagues[81] found that patients receiving brief CBT (bCBT) had a reduced likelihood and severity of SI after 4, 8, and 12 months compared to baseline and compared to those receiving enhanced usual care (EUC).

There are also interesting developments planned for the future. For instance, Bozzay and colleagues[82] suggested a protocol that provides a framework for designing multilayered treatment studies for suicide. Overall, 130 veterans with a suicide plan or suicidal behavior in the prior 2 weeks will be recruited from inpatient and outpatient settings. The goal of this study is to test whether combining brief cognitive-behavioral therapy (bCBT) with transcranial magnetic stimulation (TMS) in suicidal veterans reduces rates of suicidal ideation and attempts.

Focusing on Adolescents and Young Adults

SI and SB represent very important public health issues among young adolescents.[83] In this population, particularly, CBT has become an established treatment approach. Maladaptive cognition, behavior, and affective responses to stressors, as well as stress derived from an interpersonal conflict, may trigger a depressive episode and/or suicidal crisis in predisposed adolescents. Importantly, compared to nonsuicidal adolescents with mood disorders, suicidal adolescents have higher cognitive distortion (catastrophizing, personalization, selective abstraction, overgeneralization), reduced assertiveness, more life stressors, and a greater likelihood of history/exposure to familial suicide.[84] Impairments in cognitive processing and problem-solving among depressed adolescents may be related to the occurrence of anger,[85] difficulties in regulating internal states and specific skills compared to nonsymptomatic adolescents.[86] Young adolescents may present maladaptive behaviors such as passive and/or aggressive behaviors and dysfunctional acts predominantly as a result of altered cognitive processing, lack of perceived adaptive solutions, and enhanced affective arousal.[10] Notably, the occurrence of SB may sensitize adolescents to a greater risk of SI and SB in the future.[87]

Stanley and colleagues[88] developed a specific intervention for adolescents at high risk for repeated SAs as the manual-based cognitive behavior psychotherapy for suicide prevention (CBT-SP). In a multisite study, the authors administered CBT-SP to 110 depressed, recent suicide attempters aged 13 to 19 years, and found that 72.4% of participants completed at least 12 sessions.

The study of Esposito-Smythers and colleagues[89] is the only report that found that an integrated CBT (I-CBT) was associated with fewer SA, psychiatric hospitalizations, heavy drinking days, and days of cannabis use over 18 months, relative to treatment as usual. Similar reductions in SI, number of drinking days, and depressive symptoms were observed in CBT and the enhanced treatment as usual treatment groups.

Importantly, based on the treatment of adolescent suicide attempters (TASA), Brent and colleagues,[90] in a study involving youths with past SA and depression, found that suicide reattempts were higher in the group receiving a combination of CBT and medication (24%) compared to either of the monotherapy groups (6.5%). However, patients in the combination group had higher risk of SA at baseline, and once the authors controlled for this, any differential effects of treatment type disappeared.

Klim-Conforti and colleagues[91] conducted a study in Canada on students aged 11 to 14 years who either received a 3-month teacher-delivered Harry-Potter-based CBT embedded in the language arts curriculum (N = 200) or were placed on a wait-list control group (N = 230). They found that composite suicidality scores, life problems, and anxiety/depressive symptoms were significantly improved in the CBT group compared to the control at endpoint, with secondary analyses showing that these improvements were largely driven by significant score changes in female participants.[91]

Rathus and Miller[92] reported that suicidal adolescents treated with DBT had fewer psychiatric hospitalizations and higher rates of treatment completion than the treatment-as-usual (TAU) group at follow-up with no significant differences in terms of SA made during treatment. According to Donaldson and colleagues,[93] adolescents randomized to CBT and the problem-oriented supportive treatment reported important reductions in SI and depression at a 3-month follow-up with no differences between treatment groups. While only 5% of adolescents reattempt after 6 months, both groups retained improvement over baseline.

Overall, existing studies using CBT to treat suicidality in adolescents found improvements in terms of SI and depressed mood which is probably comparable to active comparison treatments.

There have also been findings demonstrating that adolescents with MDD and suicidality may respond differently to CBT. Brent and colleagues[28] conducted a study on 107 adolescents (13–18 years old) diagnosed with MDD and found that participants in the CBT group showed a lower rate of MDD compared with those in the nondirective supportive therapy (NST) group at the end of the study. The CBT group also had significantly higher remission rates (65%) compared to the systemic behavior family therapy (SBFT, 38%) and NST (39%) treatments. The authors also reported a significant decrease in suicidality, across all 3 treatment conditions, with the greatest decrease occurring between intake and 6 weeks.

Similarly, Clarke and colleagues[94] showed that young adolescents manifested comparable reductions in SI, regardless of the randomization to a 16-week group CBT program or care as usual.

Comparable significant improvements in SI after acute treatment that were also maintained at the 6-month follow-up were demonstrated by Melvin and colleagues.[35] No significant differences were found between adolescents receiving serotonergic drugs and clinical care or those receiving CBT along with serotonergic drugs.[39] Riggs and colleagues[95] reported that suicide severity ratings decreased during the first month of treatment, but worsened during weeks 8 and 12 in response to psychosocial stressors, although their sample size was very small (N = 5).

A CBT intervention, namely Adolescent Coping with Depression (CWD-A), was administered to adolescents with comorbid MDD and conduct disorder and was initially more effective (39%) in reducing MDD than the life skills/tutoring control program (19%), although posttreatment, the 6- and 12-month assessments showed no significant difference in the number of SAs.[96]

Finally, while the TADS study[23,24] indicated that there was a slight protective effect of CBT on both SI and SB, the TORDIA study[33] reported that SI decreased from baseline to posttreatment for all participants. Overall, most studies of CBT for depressed adolescents reported a reduction in SI regardless of the CBT format.

INTERNET-BASED APPROACHES
Depression

Martinengo and colleagues[97] systematically evaluated the features, functionality, data security, and congruence with evidence of self-guided CBT apps targeting users affected by depression. Out of 98 included apps, only 28 offered at least 4 evidence-based CBT techniques, particularly apps focusing on depression. Specifically, cognitive restructuring was offered by approximately 80% of the apps while only 30% provided suicide risk management resources.

Anxiety Disorders

The development of internet-based cognitive-behavioral therapy (iCBT) for anxiety disorders provides a promising and innovative therapeutic approach to treating the most relevant anxiety disorders associated with disability and psychosocial impairment.[98,99] iCBT programs for anxiety disorders in children and young people (CYP) have been developed in many countries with evidence emerging that these interventions are effective in reducing anxiety in CYP and are generally acceptable by clinicians and families.[100–103] Hill and colleagues[104] proposed a consensus statement and recommendations from a workshop of international experts in CYP anxiety and iCBT on the development, evaluation, engagement, and dissemination of iCBT for anxiety in CYP. Importantly, a recent randomized clinical trial evaluated the efficacy and cost-effectiveness of therapist-guided iCBT for social anxiety disorder in youths versus internet-delivered supportive therapy (ISUPPORT).[105] The authors found that therapist-guided iCBT was significantly more efficacious than ISUPPORT in reducing social anxiety symptoms, as well as depression, anxiety, and functional impairment. The authors suggested that iCBT was cost-saving, mainly due to lower medication use and higher school productivity. Another recent randomized clinical trial involving anxiety patients[106] reported that group CBT was more effective than a previously validated active control condition (CBT response rate 70.8% compared with 33.0% for the active control condition). The study's main results confirmed CBT as the first-line treatment of anxiety disorders in children.

Rees and colleagues[107] evaluated the effectiveness of self-guided iCBT (the "OCD? Not Me! Program") in youths with obsessive-compulsive disorder (OCD) (see also[108,109]). Study participants showed significant reductions in OCD symptoms and severity between pre- and post-test.

The well-known and validated CBT approach has been integrated with mindfulness meditation resulting in evidence supporting their combined effectiveness with specific psychometric and neurophysiological benefits of online single-arm and randomized controlled trials.[110–116]

According to a recent systematic review of mindfulness-based CBT, similar effects were obtained for both internet-based and in-person approaches.[117] Internet-delivered mindfulness-based CBT programs have been associated with significant changes in adults with anxiety and depression,[118,119] which is supported by the results obtained by the meta-analysis of Karyotaki and colleagues.[120] In addition, to test the feasibility of engaging depressed primary care patients not currently receiving psychotherapy with internet-delivered CBT and supportive coaching, Whiteside and colleagues[121] found that scalable integration of internet-delivered CBT into health care systems is feasible. Specifically, at follow-up recruited patients experienced clinically significant improvements in both the likelihood and intensity of depressive symptoms and suicidal thoughts.

SUMMARY

Cognitive-behavioral therapy (CBT) has been demonstrated to be effective for a range of psychiatric conditions including major psychiatric disorders and suicidality. A significant body of research suggests that CBT leads to significant improvements in clinical symptomatology, functioning, and quality of life and can be as effective as, or more effective than, other forms of psychological therapy, alone or in combination with psychiatric medications. While advances in CBT have been made based on both applied research and clinical practice, there is emerging scientific evidence that CBT actually produces structural changes. For example, from a neurobiological point of view, particularly in the context of neuroinflammation and the etiopathogenesis of suicide,[122,123] recent studies have demonstrated that CBT is capable of suppressing the elevated expression of various inflammatory markers in both somatic illnesses and psychiatric conditions.[124–127] However, further applied studies are needed to confirm the presented findings while additional fundamental research will guide our future expectations.

CLINICS CARE POINTS

- There are various models of cognitive-behavioral therapy (CBT), yet having a globally common goal: to replace dysfunctional constructs with more flexible and adaptative cognitions.
- The use of CBT is recommended in a wide range of mental disorders and suicidality, so across different ages of life.- Clinical practice, supported by numerous scientific evidences, suggested that CBT leads to significant improvements in terms of symptomatology, functioning, and quality of life.

FUNDING

This text did not receive any specific funding from the public, commercial or not-for-profit sectors.

ACKNOWLEDGMENTS

This work was developed within the framework of the Department of Excellence of MIUR (Law 232/2016).

CONFLICTS OF INTEREST

The authors declare no commercial or financial conflicts of interest.

REFERENCES

1. Beck AT. Cognitive therapy: Nature and relation to behavior therapy. Behav Ther 1970;1:184–200.
2. Ellis A. Reason and emotion in psychotherapy. New York: Lyle Stuart; 1962.
3. Rohde P. Cognitive-behavioral treatment for depression in adolescents. J Indian Assoc Child Adolesc Ment Health 2005;1(1):6.
4. Ellis A. The revised ABC's of rational-emotive therapy (RET). J Rational-Emotive Cognitive-Behavior Ther 1991;9(3):139–72.
5. Ellis A. Reason and emotion in psychotherapy, revised and updated. Secaucus (NJ): Carol Publishing Group; 1994.
6. Dryden W. The "ABCs" of REBT I: a preliminary study of errors and confusions in counselling and psychotherapy textbooks. J Rational-Emotive Cognitive-Behavior Ther 2012;30(3):133–72.
7. Haley J. Problem-solving therapy. 2nd edition. San Francisco, USA: Jossey-Bass Publishers; 1987.
8. Donaldson C, Lam D. Rumination, mood and social problem-solving in major depression. Psychol Med 2004;34(7):1309–18.
9. Wolff J, Frazier E, Davis S, et al. Depression and suicidality. In: Flessner CA, Piacentini JC, editors. Clinical handbook of psychological disorders in children and adolescents: a step-by-step treatment manual. New York, USA: Guilford Publications; 2019. p. 578.
10. Spirito A, Esposito-Smythers C, Wolff J, et al. Cognitive-behavioral therapy for adolescent depression and suicidality. Child Adolesc Psychiatr Clin N Am 2011;20(2):191–204.
11. Linehan M. Cognitive-behavioral treatment of borderline personality disorder. New York: Guildford Press; 1993.
12. Costantini L, Pasquarella C, Odone A, et al. Screening for depression in primary care with Patient Health Questionnaire-9 (PHQ-9): A systematic review. J Affect Disord 2021;279:473–83.
13. Baertschi M, Costanza A, Canuto A, et al. The dimensionality of suicidal ideation and its clinical implications. Int J Methods Psychiatr Res 2019;28(1):e1755.
14. Hofmann SG, Asnaani A, Vonk IJJ, et al. The efficacy of cognitive behavioral therapy: a review of meta-analyses. Cognit Ther Res 2012;36(5):427–40.
15. van Zoonen K, Buntrock C, Ebert DD, et al. Preventing the onset of major depressive disorder: a meta-analytic review of psychological interventions. Int J Epidemiol 2014;43(2):318–29.
16. Aguglia A, Solano P, Parisi VM, et al. Predictors of relapse in high lethality suicide attempters: a six-month prospective study. J Affect Disord 2020;271:328–35.
17. von Brachel R, Teismann T, Feider L, et al. Suicide ideation as a predictor of treatment outcomes in cognitive-behavioral therapy for unipolar mood disorders. Int J Clin Health Psychol 2019;19(1):80–4.
18. Kazdin AE, Weisz JR. Identifying and developing empirically supported child and adolescent treatments. J Consult Clin Psychol 1998;66(1):19–36.
19. Iga J-I, Uchiyama M, Ohmori T, et al. The Japanese Society of Mood Disorders Treatment Guideline. Tokyo: The Japanese Society of Mood Disorders Treatment; 2016. Accessed October 14, 2021.
20. Ellis P. Australian and New Zealand clinical practice guidelines for the treatment of depression. Aust N Z J Psychiatry 2004;38(6):389–407.

21. National Collaborating Centre for Mental Health (UK). Depression: the treatment and management of depression in adults. Updated Edition. Leicester (UK): British Psychological Society; 2010.
22. Bauer M, Pfennig A, Severus E, et al. World Federation of Societies of Biological Psychiatry (WFSBP) guidelines for biological treatment of unipolar depressive disorders, part 1: update 2013 on the acute and continuation treatment of unipolar depressive disorders. World J Biol Psychiatry 2013;14(5):334–85.
23. March J, Silva S, Petrycki S, et al. Fluoxetine, cognitive-behavioral therapy, and their combination for adolescents with depression: Treatment for Adolescents With Depression Study (TADS) randomized controlled trial. JAMA 2004;292(7):807–20.
24. March JS, Silva S, Petrycki S, et al. The treatment for adolescents with depression study (TADS): long-term effectiveness and safety outcomes. Arch Gen Psychiatry 2007;64(10):1132–43.
25. Lewinsohn PM, Clarke GN. Psychosocial treatments for adolescent depression. Clin Psychol Rev 1999;19(3):329–42.
26. Reinecke MA, Ryan NE, DuBois DL. Cognitive-behavioral therapy of depression and depressive symptoms during adolescence: a review and meta-analysis. J Am Acad Child Adolesc Psychiatry 1998;37(1):26–34.
27. Klein JB, Jacobs RH, Reinecke MA. Cognitive-behavioral therapy for adolescent depression: a meta-analytic investigation of changes in effect-size estimates. J Am Acad Child Adolesc Psychiatry 2007;46(11):1403–13.
28. Brent DA, Holder D, Kolko D, et al. A clinical psychotherapy trial for adolescent depression comparing cognitive, family, and supportive therapy. Arch Gen Psychiatry 1997;54(9):877–85.
29. Diamond GS, Reis BF, Diamond GM, et al. Attachment-based family therapy for depressed adolescents: a treatment development study. J Am Acad Child Adolesc Psychiatry 2002;41(10):1190–6.
30. Diamond GS, Wintersteen MB, Brown GK, et al. Attachment-based family therapy for adolescents with suicidal ideation: a randomized controlled trial. J Am Acad Child Adolesc Psychiatry 2010;49(2):122–31.
31. Diamond GS, Kobak RR, Krauthamer Ewing ES, et al. A randomized controlled trial: attachment-based family and nondirective supportive treatments for youth who are suicidal. J Am Acad Child Adolesc Psychiatry 2019;58(7):721–31.
32. Emslie G, Kratochvil C, Vitiello B, et al. Treatment for Adolescents with Depression Study (TADS): safety results. J Am Acad Child Adolesc Psychiatry 2006;45(12):1440–55.
33. Brent D, Emslie G, Clarke G, et al. Switching to another SSRI or to venlafaxine with or without cognitive behavioral therapy for adolescents with SSRI-resistant depression: the TORDIA randomized controlled trial. JAMA 2008;299(8):901–13.
34. Kennard BD, Emslie GJ, Mayes TL, et al. Cognitive-behavioral therapy to prevent relapse in pediatric responders to pharmacotherapy for major depressive disorder. J Am Acad Child Adolesc Psychiatry 2008;47(12):1395–404.
35. Melvin GA, Tonge BJ, King NJ, et al. A comparison of cognitive-behavioral therapy, sertraline, and their combination for adolescent depression. J Am Acad Child Adolesc Psychiatry 2006;45(10):1151–61.
36. Seligman ME, Schulman P, Tryon AM. Group prevention of depression and anxiety symptoms. Behav Res Ther 2007;45(6):1111–26.
37. Vazquez FL, Torres A, Blanco V, et al. Comparison of relaxation training with a cognitive-behavioural intervention for indicated prevention of depression in

university students: a randomized controlled trial. J Psychiatr Res 2012;46(11): 1456–63.

38. Saigo T, Hayashida M, Tayama J, et al. Prevention of depression in first-year university students with high harm avoidance: Evaluation of the effects of group cognitive behavioral therapy at 1-year follow-up. Medicine (Baltimore) 2018; 97(44):e13009.

39. Goodyer I, Dubicka B, Wilkinson P, et al. Selective serotonin reuptake inhibitors (SSRIs) and routine specialist care with and without cognitive behaviour therapy in adolescents with major depression: randomised controlled trial. BMJ 2007; 335(7611):142.

40. Weinstein SM, Cruz RA, Isaia AR, et al. Child- and family-focused cognitive behavioral therapy for pediatric bipolar disorder: applications for suicide prevention. Suicide Life Threat Behav 2018;48(6):797–811.

41. Tymofiyeva O, Yuan JP, Huang CY, et al. Application of machine learning to structural connectome to predict symptom reduction in depressed adolescents with cognitive behavioral therapy (CBT). Neuroimage Clin 2019;23:101914.

42. Pigeon WR, Crean HF, Cerulli C, et al. A randomized clinical trial of cognitive-behavioral therapy for insomnia to augment posttraumatic stress disorder treatment in survivors of interpersonal violence. Psychother Psychosom 2022;91(1): 50–62.

43. Bryan CJ, Clemans TA, Hernandez AM, et al. Evaluating potential iatrogenic suicide risk in trauma-focused group cognitive behavioral therapy for the treatment of Ptsd in active duty military personnel. Depress Anxiety 2016;33(6):549–57.

44. Melton TH, Croarkin PE, Strawn JR, et al. Comorbid anxiety and depressive symptoms in children and adolescents: a systematic review and analysis. J Psychiatr Pract 2016;22(2):84–98.

45. Merikangas KR, Nakamura EF, Kessler RC. Epidemiology of mental disorders in children and adolescents. Dialogues Clin Neurosci 2009;11(1):7–20.

46. Beesdo-Baum K, Knappe S. Developmental epidemiology of anxiety disorders. Child Adolesc Psychiatr Clin N Am 2012;21(3):457–78.

47. Manassis K, Menna R. Depression in anxious children: possible factors in comorbidity. Depress Anxiety 1999;10(1):18–24.

48. Wang Z, Whiteside SPH, Sim L, et al. Comparative effectiveness and safety of cognitive behavioral therapy and pharmacotherapy for childhood anxiety disorders: a systematic review and meta-analysis. JAMA Pediatr 2017;171(11): 1049–56.

49. James AC, James G, Cowdrey FA, et al. Cognitive behavioural therapy for anxiety disorders in children and adolescents. Cochrane Database Syst Rev 2015; 2:CD004690.

50. Walkup JT, Albano AM, Piacentini J, et al. Cognitive behavioral therapy, sertraline, or a combination in childhood anxiety. N Engl J Med 2008;359(26): 2753–66.

51. Birmaher B, Axelson DA, Monk K, et al. Fluoxetine for the treatment of childhood anxiety disorders. J Am Acad Child Adolesc Psychiatry 2003;42(4):415–23.

52. Kunas SL, Lautenbacher LM, Lueken PU, et al. Psychological predictors of cognitive-behavioral therapy outcomes for anxiety and depressive disorders in children and adolescents: a systematic review and meta-analysis. J Affect Disord 2021;278:614–26.

53. McBride NM, Johnco C, Salloum A, et al. Prevalence and clinical differences of suicidal thoughts and behaviors in a community sample of youth receiving

cognitive-behavioral therapy for anxiety. Child Psychiatry Hum Dev 2017;48(5): 705–13.

54. Loerinc AG, Meuret AE, Twohig MP, et al. Response rates for CBT for anxiety disorders: Need for standardized criteria. Clin Psychol Rev 2015;42:72–82.

55. Phillips KA, Menard W. Suicidality in body dysmorphic disorder: a prospective study. Am J Psychiatry 2006;163(7):1280–2.

56. Phillips KA, Menard W, Fay C, et al. Psychosocial functioning and quality of life in body dysmorphic disorder. Compr Psychiatry 2005;46(4):254–60.

57. Phillips KA, Quinn G, Stout RL. Functional impairment in body dysmorphic disorder: a prospective, follow-up study. J Psychiatr Res 2008;42(9):701–7.

58. Greenberg JL, Phillips KA, Steketee G, et al. Predictors of response to cognitive-behavioral therapy for body dysmorphic disorder. Behav Ther 2019;50(4): 839–49.

59. Neziroglu F, Khemlani-Patel S. A review of cognitive and behavioral treatment for body dysmorphic disorder. CNS Spectr 2002;7(6):464–71.

60. Neziroglu F, Khemlani-Patel S. Therapeutic approaches to body dysmorphic disorder. Brief Treat Crisis Intervention 2003;3(3):307–22.

61. Williams J, Hadjistavropoulos T, Sharpe D. A meta-analysis of psychological and pharmacological treatments for Body Dysmorphic Disorder. Behav Res Ther 2006;44(1):99–111.

62. Phillips KA, McElroy SL, Hudson JI, et al. Body dysmorphic disorder: an obsessive-compulsive spectrum disorder, a form of affective spectrum disorder, or both? J Clin Psychiatry 1995;56(Suppl 4):41–51 [discussion 52].

63. Phillips KA, Didie ER, Menard W. Clinical features and correlates of major depressive disorder in individuals with body dysmorphic disorder. J Affect Disord 2007;97(1–3):129–35.

64. Phillips KA, McElroy SL, Keck PE Jr, et al. Body dysmorphic disorder: 30 cases of imagined ugliness. Am J Psychiatry 1993;150(2):302–8.

65. Cuijpers P, van Straten A, Warmerdam L. Behavioral activation treatments of depression: a meta-analysis. Clin Psychol Rev 2007;27(3):318–26.

66. Tsuno N, Besset A, Ritchie K. Sleep and depression. J Clin Psychiatry 2005; 66(10):1254–69.

67. Bernert RA, Kim JS, Iwata NG, et al. Sleep disturbances as an evidence-based suicide risk factor. Curr Psychiatry Rep 2015;17(3):554.

68. Bishop TM, Pigeon WR, Possemato K. Sleep disturbance and its association with suicidal ideation in veterans. Mil Behav Health 2013;1(2):81–4.

69. Pigeon WR, Pinquart M, Conner K. Meta-analysis of sleep disturbance and suicidal thoughts and behaviors. J Clin Psychiatry 2012;73(9):e1160–7.

70. Geiger-Brown JM, Rogers VE, Liu W, et al. Cognitive behavioral therapy in persons with comorbid insomnia: a meta-analysis. Sleep Med Rev 2015;23:54–67.

71. Trauer JM, Qian MY, Doyle JS, et al. Cognitive behavioral therapy for chronic insomnia: a systematic review and meta-analysis. Ann Intern Med 2015; 163(3):191–204.

72. Pigeon WR, Funderburk J, Bishop TM, et al. Brief cognitive behavioral therapy for insomnia delivered to depressed veterans receiving primary care services: a pilot study. J Affect Disord 2017;217:105–11.

73. Trockel M, Karlin BE, Taylor CB, et al. Effects of cognitive behavioral therapy for insomnia on suicidal ideation in veterans. Sleep 2015;38(2):259–65.

74. Manber R, Edinger JD, Gress JL, et al. Cognitive behavioral therapy for insomnia enhances depression outcome in patients with comorbid major depressive disorder and insomnia. Sleep 2008;31(4):489–95.

75. Brown GK, Ten Have T, Henriques GR, et al. Cognitive therapy for the prevention of suicide attempts: a randomized controlled trial. JAMA 2005;294(5):563–70.

76. Rudd MD, Bryan CJ, Wertenberger EG, et al. Brief cognitive-behavioral therapy effects on post-treatment suicide attempts in a military sample: results of a randomized clinical trial with 2-year follow-up. Am J Psychiatry 2015;172(5):441–9.

77. Roberge EM, Bryan CJ, Peterson A, et al. Variables associated with reductions in insomnia severity among acutely suicidal patients receiving brief cognitive behavioral therapy for suicide prevention. J Affect Disord 2019;252:230–6.

78. Hui VK, Wong CY, Ma EK, et al. Treating depression with a smartphone-delivered self-help cognitive behavioral therapy for insomnia: study protocol for a parallel group randomized controlled trial. Trials 2020;21(1):843.

79. Bateman K, Hansen L, Turkington D, et al. Cognitive behavioral therapy reduces suicidal ideation in schizophrenia: results from a randomized controlled trial. Suicide Life Threat Behav 2007;37(3):284–90.

80. Klingberg S, Herrlich J, Wiedemann G, et al. Adverse effects of cognitive behavioral therapy and cognitive remediation in schizophrenia: results of the treatment of negative symptoms study. J Nerv Ment Dis 2012;200(7):569–76.

81. Ecker AH, Johnson AL, Sansgiry S, et al. Brief cognitive behavioral therapy reduces suicidal ideation in veterans with chronic illnesses. Gen Hosp Psychiatry 2019;58:27–32.

82. Bozzay ML, Primack JM, Swearingen HR, et al. Combined transcranial magnetic stimulation and brief cognitive behavioral therapy for suicide: study protocol for a randomized controlled trial in veterans. Trials 2020;21(1):924.

83. Lim KS, Wong CH, McIntyre RS, et al. Global lifetime and 12-month prevalence of suicidal behavior, deliberate self-harm and non-suicidal self-injury in children and adolescents between 1989 and 2018: a meta-analysis. Int J Environ Res Public Health 2019;16(22):4581.

84. Brent DA, Kolko DJ, Allan MJ, et al. Suicidality in affectively disordered adolescent inpatients. J Am Acad Child Adolesc Psychiatry 1990;29(4):586–93.

85. Costanza A, Rothen S, Achab S, et al. Impulsivity and impulsivity-related endophenotypes in suicidal patients with substance use disorders: an exploratory study. Int J Ment Health Addict 2021;19(5):1729–44.

86. Fritsch S, Donaldson D, Spirito A, et al. Personality characteristics of adolescent suicide attempters. Child Psychiatry Hum Dev 2000;30(4):219–35.

87. Joiner T. Why people die by suicide. Cambridge, USA: Harvard University Press; 2005.

88. Stanley B, Brown G, Brent DA, et al. Cognitive-behavioral therapy for suicide prevention (CBT-SP): treatment model, feasibility, and acceptability. J Am Acad Child Adolesc Psychiatry 2009;48(10):1005–13.

89. Esposito-Smythers C, Spirito A, Kahler CW, et al. Treatment of co-occurring substance abuse and suicidality among adolescents: a randomized trial. J Consult Clin Psychol 2011;79(6):728–39.

90. Brent DA, Greenhill LL, Compton S, et al. The Treatment of Adolescent Suicide Attempters study (TASA): predictors of suicidal events in an open treatment trial. J Am Acad Child Adolesc Psychiatry 2009;48(10):987–96.

91. Klim-Conforti P, Zaheer R, Levitt AJ, et al. The impact of a harry potter-based cognitive-behavioral therapy skills curriculum on suicidality and well-being in middle schoolers: a randomized controlled trial. J Affect Disord 2021;286:134–41.

92. Rathus JH, Miller AL. Dialectical behavior therapy adapted for suicidal adolescents. Suicide Life Threat Behav 2002;32(2):146–57.

93. Donaldson D, Spirito A, Esposito-Smythers C. Treatment for adolescents following a suicide attempt: results of a pilot trial. J Am Acad Child Adolesc Psychiatry 2005;44(2):113–20.
94. Clarke GN, Hornbrook M, Lynch F, et al. Group cognitive-behavioral treatment for depressed adolescent offspring of depressed parents in a health maintenance organization. J Am Acad Child Adolesc Psychiatry 2002;41(3):305–13.
95. Riggs PD, Mikulich-Gilbertson SK, Davies RD, et al. A randomized controlled trial of fluoxetine and cognitive behavioral therapy in adolescents with major depression, behavior problems, and substance use disorders. Arch Pediatr Adolesc Med 2007;161(11):1026–34.
96. Rohde P, Clarke GN, Mace DE, et al. An efficacy/effectiveness study of cognitive-behavioral treatment for adolescents with comorbid major depression and conduct disorder. J Am Acad Child Adolesc Psychiatry 2004;43(6):660–8.
97. Martinengo L, Stona AC, Griva K, et al. Self-guided Cognitive Behavioral Therapy Apps for Depression: Systematic Assessment of Features, Functionality, and Congruence With Evidence. J Med Internet Res 2021;23(7):e27619.
98. Baxter AJ, Scott KM, Vos T, et al. Global prevalence of anxiety disorders: a systematic review and meta-regression. Psychol Med 2013;43(5):897–910.
99. Kessler RC, Angermeyer M, Anthony JC, et al. Lifetime prevalence and age-of-onset distributions of mental disorders in the World Health Organization's World Mental Health Survey Initiative. World Psychiatry 2007;6(3):168–76.
100. Pennant ME, Loucas CE, Whittington C, et al. Computerised therapies for anxiety and depression in children and young people: a systematic review and meta-analysis. Behav Res Ther 2015;67:1–18.
101. Podina IR, Mogoase C, David D, et al. A meta-analysis on the efficacy of technology mediated CBT for anxious children and adolescents. J Rational-Emotive Cognitive-Behavior Ther 2015;34(1):31–50.
102. Rooksby M, Elouafkaoui P, Humphris G, et al. Internet-assisted delivery of cognitive behavioural therapy (CBT) for childhood anxiety: systematic review and meta-analysis. J Anxiety Disord 2015;29:83–92.
103. Topooco N, Riper H, Araya R, et al. Attitudes towards digital treatment for depression: a European stakeholder survey. Internet Interv 2017;8:1–9.
104. Hill C, Creswell C, Vigerland S, et al. Navigating the development and dissemination of internet cognitive behavioral therapy (iCBT) for anxiety disorders in children and young people: a consensus statement with recommendations from the #iCBTLorentz Workshop Group. Internet Interv 2018;12:1–10.
105. Nordh M, Wahlund T, Jolstedt M, et al. Therapist-guided internet-delivered cognitive behavioral therapy vs internet-delivered supportive therapy for children and adolescents with social anxiety disorder: a randomized clinical trial. JAMA Psychiatry 2021;78(7):705–13.
106. Simon NM, Hofmann SG, Rosenfield D, et al. Efficacy of yoga vs cognitive behavioral therapy vs stress education for the treatment of generalized anxiety disorder: a randomized clinical trial. JAMA Psychiatry 2021;78(1):13–20.
107. Rees CS, Anderson RA, Kane RT, et al. Online obsessive-compulsive disorder treatment: preliminary results of the "OCD? Not Me!" Self-guided internet-based cognitive behavioral therapy program for young people. JMIR Ment Health 2016;3(3):e29.
108. Amerio A, Tonna M, Odone A, et al. Course of illness in comorbid bipolar disorder and obsessive-compulsive disorder patients. Asian J Psychiatry 2016;20:12–4.

109. Tonna M, Amerio A, Ottoni R, et al. The clinical meaning of obsessive-compulsive symptoms in bipolar disorder and schizophrenia. Aust N Z J Psychiatry 2015;49(6):578–9.
110. Azam MA, Mongrain M, Vora K, et al. Mindfulness as an alternative for supporting university student mental health: cognitive-emotional and depressive self-criticism measures. Int J Educ Psychol 2016;5(2):140.
111. Coelho HF, Canter PH, Ernst E. Mindfulness-based cognitive therapy: evaluating current evidence and informing future research. J Consult Clin Psychol 2007; 75(6):1000–5.
112. Guglietti CL, Daskalakis ZJ, Radhu N, et al. Meditation-related increases in GABAB modulated cortical inhibition. Brain Stimul 2013;6(3):397–402.
113. Radhu N, Daskalakis ZJ, Guglietti CL, et al. Cognitive behavioral therapy-related increases in cortical inhibition in problematic perfectionists. Brain Stimul 2012; 5(1):44–54.
114. Radhu N, Daskalakis ZJ, Arpin-Cribbie CA, et al. Evaluating a Web-based cognitive-behavioral therapy for maladaptive perfectionism in university students. J Am Coll Health 2012;60(5):357–66.
115. Ritvo P, Vora K, Irvine J, et al. Reductions in negative automatic thoughts in students attending mindfulness tutorials predicts increased life satisfaction. Int J Educ Psychol 2013;2(3):272–96.
116. Sipe WE, Eisendrath SJ. Mindfulness-based cognitive therapy: theory and practice. Can J Psychiatry 2012;57(2):63–9.
117. Berger T, Hammerli K, Gubser N, et al. Internet-based treatment of depression: a randomized controlled trial comparing guided with unguided self-help. Cogn Behav Ther 2011;40(4):251–66.
118. Boettcher J, Astrom V, Pahlsson D, et al. Internet-based mindfulness treatment for anxiety disorders: a randomized controlled trial. Behav Ther 2014;45(2): 241–53.
119. Carlbring P, Hagglund M, Luthstrom A, et al. Internet-based behavioral activation and acceptance-based treatment for depression: a randomized controlled trial. J Affect Disord 2013;148(2–3):331–7.
120. Karyotaki E, Riper H, Twisk J, et al. Efficacy of Self-guided Internet-Based Cognitive Behavioral Therapy in the Treatment of Depressive Symptoms: A Meta-analysis of Individual Participant Data. JAMA Psychiatry 2017;74(4): 351–9.
121. Whiteside U, Richards J, Steinfeld B, et al. Online cognitive behavioral therapy for depressed primary care patients: a pilot feasibility project. Perm J 2014; 18(2):21–7.
122. Serafini G, Parisi VM, Aguglia A, et al. A specific inflammatory profile underlying suicide risk? Systematic review of the main literature findings. Int J Environ Res Public Health 2020;17(7).
123. Serafini G, Pompili M, Elena Seretti M, et al. The role of inflammatory cytokines in suicidal behavior: a systematic review. Eur Neuropsychopharmacol 2013; 23(12):1672–86.
124. Costanza A, Amerio A, Aguglia A, et al. Hyperinflammation in COVID-19 and suicide etiopathogenesis: hypothesis for a nefarious collision? Neurosci Biobehav Rev 2022;136:104606.
125. Diaz A, Taub CJ, Lippman ME, et al. Effects of brief stress management interventions on distress and leukocyte nuclear factor kappa B expression during primary treatment for breast cancer: a randomized trial. Psychoneuroendocrinology 2021;126:105163.

126. Nemirovsky A, Ilan K, Lerner L, et al. Brain-immune axis regulation is responsive to cognitive behavioral therapy and mindfulness intervention: Observations from a randomized controlled trial in patients with Crohn's disease. Brain Behav Immun Health 2022;19:100407.
127. Sundquist K, Memon AA, Palmer K, et al. Inflammatory proteins and miRNA-144-5p in patients with depression, anxiety, or stress- and adjustment disorders after psychological treatment. Cytokine 2021;146:155646.

Depression and Suicidal Behavior in Adolescents

Aliza Grossberg, MD, MPH, Timothy Rice, MD*

KEYWORDS

- Adolescence • Depression • Suicide • Nonsuicidal self-injury • Development
- Gender • Adverse childhood experiences • Substance abuse

KEY POINTS

- Adolescent depression is a highly prevalent disorder with high lifetime morbidity and mortality.
- While accurate suicide prediction remains difficult even among experts, risk factors for adolescent depression and suicide are increasingly understood and can be surveyed and addressed by clinicians.
- Therapeutic interventions reduce not only risk in adolescence but also lifetime risk as well as lifetime clinical burden and negative developmental progression.

INTRODUCTION

Depression is one of the leading causes of morbidity and mortality globally and in the United States.[1] Depression affects individuals of all ages.[2] Among adolescents aged 13 to 18, the lifetime prevalence of major depressive disorder (MDD) in the United States is 11.0%.[3] The many unique social, psychological, and physical changes and stressors that youth experience at the personal and interpersonal levels impact the mental health of and risk of developing depression among adolescents.[4] Recurrence of depressive episodes is common: After the first episode of depression, approximately 40% to 70% of adolescents have a subsequent depressive episode within 3 to 5 years.[5] Experiencing depression in adolescence often indicates ongoing depression into adulthood.[6] Depression in adolescence has been shown to be associated with several other risk factors such as increased substance use, difficulties with school performance, challenges in interpersonal relationships, and increased suicide rates.[6,7]

Several studies in various settings have demonstrated a link between depressive symptoms, suicidal ideation, and attempted suicide among adolescents.[8] Completed suicide is the second leading cause of death among people between the ages of 10

Department of Psychiatry, Icahn School of Medicine at Mount Sinai, 1111 Amsterdam Avenue, Babcock Building 5 West, New York, NY, USA
* Corresponding author. 1090 Amsterdam Avenue, 13th floor, Suite A, Office 5, New York, NY 10025.
E-mail address: Timothy.Rice@mountsinai.org

Med Clin N Am 107 (2023) 169–182
https://doi.org/10.1016/j.mcna.2022.04.005
0025-7125/23/© 2022 Elsevier Inc. All rights reserved.

and 34.[9] In 2014, 17% of deaths among people ages 10 to 24 in the United States—almost 1 in 5—were due to suicide.[10] Moreover, in a 2019 survey of more than 13,000 US high schoolers, 18.8% reported having seriously considered suicide in the 12 months preceding the survey, 15.7% made a plan about how they would attempt suicide in that same time period, and 8.9% attempted suicide at least once in the year leading up to the survey.[11]

In this article, we introduce the importance of understanding adolescent depression and its developmental and gendered presentations. We elaborate on several important risk factors of adolescent depression, including nonsuicidal self-injury, adverse childhood experiences, and substance abuse. We describe protective factors and contemporary special topics of COVID-19 and adolescent use of social media. This article includes recommendations for assessment and management and conclusions including a commentary on barriers to care.

GENDER AND AGE DIFFERENCES

Several studies document a significant gender difference in the prevalence of adolescent depression. A 2-fold increase in the prevalence of depression among adolescent girls after the age of 15 compared with boys of the same age has been noted.[12] Of note, adolescent girls are more likely to experience suicidal ideation and suicide attempts compared with adolescent boys; however, adolescent boys die by suicide at higher rates than adolescent girls.[12]

Older youth, when compared with younger adolescents, are more likely to die by suicide. For children and early adolescents younger than 14, the global incidence of completed suicide is 0.6 completed suicides per 100,000 individuals.[13] This is significantly lower than the global suicide rate among 15 to 19-year-old adolescents, which is 6.9 completed suicides per 100,000 individuals.[14]

Theoretic underpinnings to adolescent suicide have been proposed.[13,14] Developmental theory can help to understand these differences. The increase in suicide rates from childhood to adolescence relates to the adolescent's attainment of greater capability to effect action through greater independence, physical strength, and planning. In addition to hormonal changes and their impacts on emotion regulation, the awareness of gaining strength and independence can also unsettle adolescents from previous childhood stability and equilibrium. Adolescent young men more commonly choose more lethal methods of suicide which underlay their higher suicide rates despite lower rates of suicide attempts; issues of proving their assertiveness, dedication to an act, and active rather than passive stance intertwined with conceptualizations of masculinity can partly account for this. The meanings of suicidal acts are unique to each adolescent; self-destruction can represent fragile responses to rejection or to a disappointment, alienation from the changing body, counterphobic attitudes against vulnerability, disrupted mourning of old relationships, distorted attempts at self-soothing or bearing painful effects, or a reaction to internalized traumatic objects, among many other meanings.

RISK FACTORS FOR ADOLESCENT DEPRESSION AND SUICIDALITY

There are numerous psychosocial and biological risk factors for adolescents developing depression (**Table 1**).[15] Psychosocial risk factors include childhood neglect or abuse, loss of a loved one, relationship stressors, patterns of cognition, and states of mind such as hopelessness,[16] and socioeconomic stressors. Biological risk factors include a family history of depression, hormonal changes during puberty, chronic medical conditions such as diabetes, female sex, and use of certain medications,

Table 1
Biological, psychological, and social risk factors for adolescent depression

Type of Risk Factor	Biological	Psychological	Social
	Family history of depression or suicide	Feelings of hopelessness	Nonsuicidal self-injurious behavior
	Female sex	Other psychiatric diagnoses *(can also be considered a biological risk factor)*	Being a victim or perpetrator of peer bullying
	Hormonal changes during puberty	Substance Use	Loss of a loved one
	Chronic medical conditions		Relationship Stressors
	Use of certain medications, such as isotretinoin		Socioeconomic stressors
			Other adverse childhood experiences

such as isotretinoin. Additionally, having other psychiatric diagnoses increases the risk of developing depression in adolescents.

Many of these risk factors for depression are also risk factors for adolescent suicidality. For example, substance use is a risk factor for adolescent suicidality.[17] Comorbid psychiatric diagnoses increase the risk for suicidality.[18] Additionally, feelings of hopelessness and sadness are associated with suicidal ideation[19] and suicide attempts.[20] Other risk factors for suicide include being a victim or perpetrator of violence, a prior suicide attempt, and issues at school.[20]

This article will explore in detail 3 risk factors of increasing relevance: nonsuicidal self-injury, substance abuse including cannabis abuse, and adverse childhood experiences.

NONSUICIDAL SELF-INJURY

Nonsuicidal self-injury (NSSI), which includes intentionally harming one's own body tissue without any suicidal intent, is an important factor when assessing for adolescent depression and suicidality.[21,22] The global estimated prevalence of adolescent NSSI in community samples ranges from 14% to 30%.[23,24] In depressed adolescents, the incidence is as high as 40% or greater.[25] The presence of NSSI raises the risk of suicidal ideation and suicidal behavior by a factor of 20.[22] Some of the most common forms of NSSI include cutting, scratching, and hitting or banging.[26] Risk factors for NSSI in depressed adolescents include female gender[27] as well as decreased interpersonal functioning, family cohesion, and adaptability.[25]

The four-factor model can be helpful to understand the reasons that adolescents self-harm.[16] The most common factor is automatic negative reinforcement whereby NSSI helps alleviate negative feelings such as tension. Another factor is the automatic positive reinforcement, which involves positive feelings, such as relief, while engaging in self-harm. The third factor is social positive reinforcement, such as receiving attention for the self-harm behavior. The final factor is social negative reinforcement, which allows adolescents to remove themselves from unwanted social interactions.[28] The interpersonal theory of suicide proposes that engaging in NSSI increases the acquired capability of suicide, which includes a heightened fearlessness toward death and pain tolerance, and which, in combination with suicidal desire, is associated with suicide attempts.[29,30]

In addition to the risk factors noted above, histories of childhood emotional abuse and neglect are independent risk factors for NSSI in depressed adolescents,[25] signaling the need to consider adverse childhood experience (ACE) as a fundamental factor in understanding adolescent depression and suicidality.

ADVERSE CHILDHOOD EXPERIENCES AND SUICIDALITY

Adverse childhood experiences, which include but are not limited to parental interpersonal violence, sexual abuse, parental incarceration, physical abuse, emotional abuse, and neglect, are assayed in the 10-item self-administered ACE questionnaire[31] and further explored in the broader Pediatric ACEs and Related Life-Event Screener.[32]

Adverse experiences in childhood are extremely common, and adolescents with a history of ACEs are at an increased risk of depression.[33] In a study of more than 21,000 youth ages 12 to 17 that explored the impact of ACEs on anxiety and depression, 48% of the study sample had experienced at least one ACE.[34] In a cross sectional-survey of nearly 40,000 children and adolescents between the ages of 8 and 17 being exposed to 2 or more ACEs increased the odds of current depression (adjusted OR = 2.6) compared with those with fewer than 2 ACEs.[35]

Several studies have shown the association between ACEs and suicidal ideation and attempts. Adults with ACEs have a higher prevalence of suicidal ideation and attempts.[36] Having just one ACE, while controlling for depression, drug use, problem alcohol use, gender, race, age, urbanicity, can increase the risk of suicidal ideation and suicide attempts in adulthood by 1.4 to 2.7 times.[37] It is also important to note that having more than one ACE increases the incidence of suicidal ideation and attempts and that for those with 3 or more ACEs, while controlling for the same factors, the odds of attempting suicide or seriously considering suicide was 3 times that of those with no ACEs.[37]

ACEs and attendant risk need not occur within the home. As an example, peer bullying is a risk factor for depression, suicidal ideation, and suicide attempts prevalent among adolescents.[38] Being bullied can contribute to one's sense of belonging, and those who feel less of a sense of belonging are more likely to develop depression. Effects can be longstanding, as both cross-sectional and prospective studies demonstrate that bullying in adolescence predicts depression in early adulthood.[39,40]

SUBSTANCE USE AND DEPRESSION AND SUICIDALITY IN ADOLESCENCE

Alcohol, nicotine, and cannabis are the 3 most commonly abused substances in adolescence. Prepandemic data from 2019 reveal a 29.3% 30-day prevalence among American high school seniors of alcohol, 22.3% of cannabis, and 25.5% of nicotine vaping.[41] Substance use rates declined as the pandemic progressed. Societal reopening will require new vigilance on adolescent substance use trends.

Large amount of nicotine vaping in adolescents is a relatively new phenomenon with significant data supporting mental health correlates.[42] These include depression: As of 2021, of 7 identified quantitative or mixed-methods studies exploring the association between adolescent nicotine vaping and depression,[43–48] 6 found positive associations.[43–49] One of the studies was of longitudinal design and demonstrated escalating depressive symptoms over time with sustained nicotine vaping and a bidirectional association in which depression increased nicotine vaping onset across mid-adolescence as well.[49]

Three studies demonstrate that nicotine vaping commonly precedes cannabis use.[50–52] While the association between youth cannabis use and the risk of schizophrenia[53] is widely known, perhaps just as important is its association with an increased risk of depression and suicidality.[54] In a review of 4 different Australian cohort studies, the adjusted difference between mean depression scores for those at age 15 who used cannabis weekly compared with 15 year olds who did not use cannabis had an effect size of 0.31.[55] At 15, the highest effect size was noted and the association between cannabis use and depression scores decreased at later ages. This risk is also longitudinal: In a recent meta-analysis of 11 longitudinal and prospective studies and more than 23,000 individuals, the estimated population attributable risk of developing depression between the ages of 18 and 32 from cannabis use before the age of 18 was 7.2%.[54] This suggests that more than 400,000 young adult cases of depression are potentially attributable to cannabis use.[54] Risk seems dose-dependent: one older cohort study[56] showed a 2-fold versus a 5-fold increase in the risk of depression and anxiety in young adulthood with weekly versus daily cannabis use in adolescence, respectively. While the recent meta-analysis[54] did not find an increased risk of anxiety in young adulthood at a level of statistical significance, the increased risk of suicidal ideation (OR: 1.50) and suicide attempt (OR: 3.46) were significant. In the first population-based cohort study exploring predictors of adolescent suicide attempts with suicidal ideation or NSSI, cannabis use was identified as a strong predictor.[57]

Adolescence presents a vulnerability window for development. Up until the age of 25, brain development is ongoing. A recent longitudinal imaging study of 799 cannabis-naïve youth in middle adolescence[58] demonstrated that cannabis exposure altered normal neurodevelopmental processes and cortical architecture, replicating findings from earlier animal studies.

A 2020 meta-analysis found that nicotine vaping was associated with a 6-fold risk of alcohol use and binge drinking in adolescence.[59] Male adolescents and young adults were more likely to engage in both social solitary drinking at the start of the COVID-19 pandemic.[60] This is concerning when male adolescents more commonly complete suicide and solitary drinking among late adolescents and young adults is known to be directly associated with depression and suicidal ideation.[61] In a cross-sectional study of more than 6000 Norwegian adolescents between the ages of 16 and 18, high levels of depressive symptoms were associated with frequent alcohol consumption.[62] The highest quartile of youth in the study showed increased frequent alcohol consumption (OR = 1.6 for boys and OR = 1.9 for girls), increased frequent alcohol intoxication (OR = 1.6 for boys and OR = 2.1 for girls), and an earlier onset of alcohol consumption (OR = 1.4 for boys and OR = 1.9 for girls). This study also demonstrates that as depressive symptoms worsen, so too do the alcohol-related outcomes above.

PROTECTIVE FACTORS AND RESILIENCE IN ADOLESCENT DEPRESSION AND SUICIDALITY

Protective factors can mediate the impact of stress on adolescent depression and suicidality. Among many, community, peer, and family support warrant emphasis. All provide a protective mechanism against mental health issues faced by adolescents.

Higher social cohesion is associated with less depression and anxiety among adolescents.[63] Strong peer relationships not only protect against these mental health issues but also build resilience.[64] Strong peer relationships can aid youth in feeling as though they are a part of a group and having a sense of group membership is also protective for youth in mediating depression and the risk of suicide. Mentorship moderates the relationship between stress and depression.[65]

In addition to peer support and a sense of group membership, family support provides a similar function. Adolescents who experienced early life stress, but who had strong family support, showed a reduction in developing depressive symptoms.[66]

ASSESSMENT FOR ADOLESCENT DEPRESSION AND SUICIDALITY

There are several pieces of the assessment that together help inform one's risk of depression or suicidality. Some of these pieces include the clinical interview with the adolescent, observations of the adolescent's behavior, surveying risk and protective factors, both acute and chronic, assessing for suicidal ideation, plan, or intent, and collecting collateral information. Guidelines for the primary care provider in the identification, assessment, and initial management of adolescent depression exist.[67]

There are unique aspects of the adolescent patient encounter to keep in mind in contrast to working with adults. For example, it is important to interview the adolescent alone and to assess for biological factors that may be contributing to the adolescent's presentation, as well as psychosocial aspects, such as work, school, and peer, family, and romantic relationships.[7] These diverse pieces of one's life may be considered risk factors or may be protective in nature.

In addition to symptoms of depression, it is important to ask about suicidality and to distinguish between the types of suicidality to best work with and treat the patient. For example, patients with passive suicidal ideation may have thoughts of wishing they were not alive or that their life would end. This is in contrast with active suicidal ideation, which is defined by the desire, intent, or plan to end one's own life.

There are significant discrepancies between self-reports from adolescents and reports from parents and teachers with regard to adolescent depression and suicidality. For example, in a study of more than 1200 Canadian youth, 13.3% of the adolescents themselves reported suicidal ideation or behavior compared with 2.0% of parents and 1.8% of teachers reporting such ideation or behavior among these adolescents.[68] Despite such discrepancies, it is helpful to retrieve collateral information from parents, teachers, coaches, or other significant figures in the adolescent's life. Completing a comprehensive assessment will help to ensure the safety of at-risk youth.

ADOLESCENT DEPRESSION AND THE COVID-19 PANDEMIC

It is unclear how the many changes brought about by the COVID-19 pandemic have impacted the mental health of adolescents. The pandemic has been associated with a risk of depressive symptoms.[69] For example, in a study of more than 8000 adolescents in China, 43% of youth from the ages of 13 to 18 reported moderate to severe symptoms of depression in March 2020.[70] The long-term effects of the COVID-19 pandemic on adolescent mental health are still being studied and will help inform care for youth moving forward.

There are several possible reasons for adolescents experiencing depressive symptoms related to COVID-19. Social distancing protocols, which were put in place to limit the spread of the virus, but which also inevitably limit in-person social interaction, can significantly affect the mental health of adolescents.[71,72] However, the effects of adolescents spending an increased amount of time at home have varying effects depending on one's home environment. Adolescents with healthy and positive relationships with those who live at home, such as parents or siblings, may be less negatively affected by these protocols. However, for many, home is not a safe place and may be whereby an adolescent endures physical, sexual, verbal, or emotional abuse. Overall, due to COVID-19, many adolescents have fewer options for in-person interactions with peers, which can lead to a detrimental effect on their socialization.

During the COVID-19 pandemic, in-person schooling shifted to virtual schooling for children and adolescents. For some, this transition means protection from the social exclusion and bullying they experienced with in-person schooling. However, for others, school is whereby they feel safest, and this safe space was eliminated from their lives for a period of time. This dichotomy demonstrates the varied experiences and the possible protections and challenges that come with suddenly spending less time at school and more time at home.

SOCIAL MEDIA'S INFLUENCE ON ADOLESCENT MENTAL HEALTH

Social media use, which consists of interactive digital participation, has become extremely prevalent among adolescents. Among those aged 13 to 17, 97% are active on at least one social networking site.[73] There seem to be both advantages and detriments to social media use among youth. Some of the negative aspects include no in-person interactions, there can be increased peer pressure from comparisons made with other peers, cyberbullying, and it can be addictive in nature.[74] Positive aspects include feeling more connected to peers, having the ability to connect with diverse peers who can be a source of support, having a platform to explore their identities, and greater access to information.[74,75] Feedback on social media, depending on whether the feedback is positive or negative, can impact the self-esteem of adolescents, both positively and negatively.[76] In a study of more than 400 students aged 11 to 15, increased social media use and emotional investment in social media were both associated with increased depression.[77]

Given the ever-changing landscape of social media content and participation from adolescents, continued research on this topic will help guide practitioners working with youth.

RECOMMENDATIONS

Whereas 64% and 53% of primary care providers report routinely screening for adolescent depression and suicidal thoughts, only 16% and 7% of their patients reported receiving these services at their last visit, respectively.[78] As noted above, some youth are more susceptible to developing depression and/or suicidality, and a thorough assessment of adolescents can help to mitigate risk factors and to ensure the appropriate level of care. **Box 1** includes topics to discuss for the evaluation and screening of adolescent depression and suicidality.

Using the above recommendations will aid in establishing a risk assessment and will help to navigate most adolescent mental health encounters to ensure patient safety.

TREATMENT OPTIONS

A comprehensive assessment will help determine whether a patient would be most safely treated in the outpatient, partial hospitalization, inpatient, or residential setting. With any treatment of depression and suicidality, it is important to include patient and family education and support. The 2 mainstays of treatment of adolescent depression and thus adolescent suicidality include psychosocial interventions such as therapy and medication management.[5]

Box 1
Evaluation and screening recommendations to assess for adolescent depression and suicidality

Adolescent Depression and Suicidality Screening Recommendations:
  Assess peer relationships, including bullying
  Assess family relationships
  Ask about romantic relationships
  Screen for nicotine, cannabis, and alcohol use
  Ask about social media use
  Inquire about the presence of isolation
  Inquire about the effects of COVID-19 on mood
  Ask family psychiatric history
  Evaluate for prior suicide attempts
  Screen for nonsuicidal self-injury

The greatest evidence base in psychosocial interventions for adolescent depression exists within cognitive-behavioral therapy and interpersonal therapy.[79] CBT has a wide evidence basis in child and adolescent poopulations.[80] CBT, with a focus on healthy coping skills, can help adolescents address and change maladaptive behaviors, to identify their feelings and to better understand themselves, and to interact more effectively with others. Moreover, CBT helps patients identify and confront the cognitive distortions they maintain regarding how they view themselves and the world around them with guidance on how these cognitive distortions may be contributing to their feelings of depression. CBT which involves parents or which combines behavioral activation with thought challenge is associated with better outcomes.[80] CBT may also be helpful in not only treating, but also preventing, adolescent depression; however, more research is needed on prevention interventions.[81]

Interpersonal therapy (IPT) with skills training can also be helpful to treat depressive symptoms among adolescents.[82] The focus of IPT is on interpersonal roles, personal challenges, and other problems adolescents deal with such as grief, conflict, and transitions. For adolescents with depression, IPT can be particularly helpful in acute treatment. Once remission of depressive symptoms occurs, patients should continue with therapeutic treatment for at least 6 to 12 months to prevent recurrence of depressive symptoms.

Dialectical behavioral therapy (DBT), commonly used in adult populations for individuals with borderline personality disorder, is increasingly studied in adolescent populations at risk for suicide. One recent study demonstrated efficacy in reducing NSSI and suicide attempts in a high-risk population.[83] Further study of this modality may support its inclusion into practice parameters as a first-line treatment approach for depressed adolescents.

In addition to psychotherapy, some adolescents may require pharmacologic interventions to treat their depression. First-line pharmacotherapy treatment of patients with depression not due to bipolar disorder or psychosis includes selective serotonin reuptake inhibitors (SSRIs).[5] SSRIs are dosed once a day, which can help with easing administration. SSRIs may lead to the improvement of depressive symptoms in the 4 to 6 weeks after initiation, so it is important to talk with patients and their parents or guardians about overall expectations, including expectations in efficacy time course. If there is no improvement by this time period, increasing the dose or changing the medication may be necessary. If the patient is a minor, the patient's parent or legal guardian must provide informed consent to initiate any medication for the patient. Thus, it is important to share the risks and benefits of any medication with the parent or guardian.

In 2004, the Food and Drug Administration's (FDA) review of antidepressants found that among those taking antidepressants, there was a 2% increase in suicidal thoughts or behaviors compared with those taking placebo.[84] This prompted the "black box" warning for pediatric patients regarding the increased risk of suicidality with antidepressant use. In addition to discussing the risks of antidepressant initiation, including the black box warning, with parents, it is important to examine the potential benefits of starting an antidepressant for their child so that the parent can make an informed decision on how to best keep their child safe, healthy, and well.

After a suicide attempt, an adolescent often requires a tremendous amount of care and attention to understand the meaning of the event in the service of preventing a future recurrence. Prior suicidal behavior is the strongest predictor of a future suicidal behavior.[85] Adolescents who have completed first-line psychosocial and pharmacologic interventions and who remain at elevated risk will often require expert longitudinal psychotherapy with medication management for years after immediate stabilization and step-down. Relapse is common, and morbidity and mortality remain high.[5]

BARRIERS TO CARE

There are several variables that can influence whether one receives treatment of depression. In a sample of more than 1600 nationally representative adolescents, approximately 53% of those with elevated depressive symptoms accessed treatment of any kind, whether in the outpatient, inpatient, or school setting.[86] However, adolescents of low socioeconomic status are less likely to access specialty inpatient or outpatient mental health services.[87] In addition to socioeconomic status, some of the barriers to accessing or using the treatment of adolescent depression include insurance status, parent challenges in identifying symptoms of depression, the severity of symptoms, mental health stigma, limited communication between the parent and child, and structural limitations such as geographic access, transportation, and financial means.[88,89] To achieve equity in access to care, health care systems must focus on minority inclusion and on proactively countering mental health stigma.

SUMMARY

Adolescent depression and suicidality are prevalent throughout society. A comprehensive biopsychosocial assessment, in collaboration with the adolescent and his/her parent, can help distinguish a patient's risk level and what level of care from which the patient will benefit. Identifying risk factors, as well as protective factors, is a significant part of the evaluation. If an adolescent suffers from depression and/or suicidality, treatment options, which include psychotherapy and medication, exist; however, many adolescents face significant barriers to accessing care.

CLINICS CARE POINTS

- When assessing for suicidality in adolescents, it is important to identify and address relevant biological, psychological, and social risk factors.
- When identifying treatment options for adolescent depression, consider therapeutic interventions which can reduce adolescent and lifetime risk of worsening depression.
- Adolescents who remain at elevated risk of suicide after completing first-line psychosocial and pharmacologic interventions will often require expert longitudinal psychotherapy with medication management for years after immediate stabilization.

DISCLOSURE

The authors have nothing to disclose.

REFERENCES

1. Liu Q, He H, Yang J, et al. Changes in the global burden of depression from 1990 to 2017: Findings from the Global Burden of Disease study. J Psychiatr Res 2020; 126:134–40.
2. Hammen C, Garber J, Ingram R. Vulnerability to depression accross the lifespan. In: Vulnerability to Psychopathology: risk across the Lifespan. ; 2001:258-267.
3. Avenevoli S, Swendsen J, He J-P, et al. Major Depression in the National Comorbidity Survey–adolescent supplement: prevalence, correlates, and treatment. J Am Acad Child Adolesc Psychiatry 2015;54(1):37–44.e2.
4. Cicchetti D, Toth SL. The development of depression in children and adolescents. Am Psychol 1998;53(2):221–41.
5. Birmaher B, Brent D. Practice Parameter for the Assessment and Treatment of Children and Adolescents With Depressive Disorders. J Am Acad Child Adolesc Psychiatry 2007;46(11):1503–26.
6. Zisook S, Lesser I, Stewart JW, et al. Effect of Age at Onset on the Course of Major Depressive Disorder. Am J Psychiatry 2007;164(10):1539–46.
7. Choe CJ, Emslie GJ, Mayes TL. Depression. Child Adolesc Psychiatr Clin N Am 2012;21(4):807–29.
8. Labelle R, Breton J-J, Pouliot L, et al. Cognitive correlates of serious suicidal ideation in a community sample of adolescents. J Affect Disord 2013;145(3):370–7.
9. Centers for Disease Control and Prevention. Web-based Injury Statistics Query and Reporting System (WISQARS). 2020. Available at: https://webappa.cdc.gov/sasweb/ncipc/mortrate.html. Accessed June 24, 2020.
10. Kann L, McManus T, Harris WA, et al. Youth Risk Behavior Surveillance - United States, 2015. MMWR Surveill Summ 2016;65(6):1–174.
11. Underwood JM, Brener N, Thornton J, et al. Overview and Methods for the Youth Risk Behavior Surveillance System — United States, 2019. MMWR Suppl 2020; 69(1):1–10.
12. Roh B-R, Jung EH, Hong HJ. A Comparative Study of Suicide Rates among 10–19-Year-Olds in 29 OECD Countries. Psychiatry Investig 2018;15(4):376–83.
13. Anderson R. A psychoanalytical approach to suicide in adolescents. In: Relating to self-harm and suicide: psychoanalytic perspectives on practice, theory and prevention. New York, NY: Routledge; 2008. p. 61–71.
14. King RA, Apter A. Psychoanalytic Perspectives on Adolescent Suicide. Psychoanal Study Child 1996;51(1):491–511.
15. Clark MS, Jansen KL, Cloy JA. Treatment of childhood and adolescent depression. Am Fam Physician 2012;86(5):442–8. Available at: http://www.ncbi.nlm.nih.gov/pubmed/22963063.
16. Joiner TE, Rudd MD. Disentangling the interrelations between hopelessness, loneliness, and suicidal ideation. Suicide Life Threat Behav 1996;26(1):19–26. Available at: http://www.ncbi.nlm.nih.gov/pubmed/9173606.
17. Hallfors D, Waller M, Ford C, et al. Adolescent depression and suicide riskAssociation with sex and drug behavior. Am J Prev Med 2004;27(3):224–31.
18. Lewinsohn PM, Rohde P, Seeley JR. Adolescent Psychopathology: III. The Clinical Consequences of Comorbidity. J Am Acad Child Adolesc Psychiatry 1995; 34(4):510–9.

19. Peltzer K, Pengpid S. Suicidal Ideation and Associated Factors among School-Going Adolescents in Thailand. Int J Environ Res Public Health 2012;9(2):462–73.
20. Borowsky IW, Ireland M, Resnick MD. Adolescent Suicide Attempts: Risks and Protectors. Pediatrics 2001;107(3):485–93.
21. Nock MK. Self-Injury. Annu Rev Clin Psychol 2010;6(1):339–63.
22. Whitlock J, Muehlenkamp J, Eckenrode J, et al. Nonsuicidal Self-Injury as a Gateway to Suicide in Young Adults. J Adolesc Heal 2013;52(4):486–92.
23. Guan K, Fox KR, Prinstein MJ. Nonsuicidal self-injury as a time-invariant predictor of adolescent suicide ideation and attempts in a diverse community sample. J Consult Clin Psychol 2012;80(5):842–9.
24. Muehlenkamp JJ, Claes L, Havertape L, et al. International prevalence of adolescent non-suicidal self-injury and deliberate self-harm. Child Adolesc Psychiatry Ment Health 2012;6(1):10.
25. Shao C, Wang X, Ma Q, et al. Analysis of risk factors of non-suicidal self-harm behavior in adolescents with depression. Ann Palliat Med 2021;10(9):9607–13.
26. Zetterqvist M. The DSM-5 diagnosis of nonsuicidal self-injury disorder: a review of the empirical literature. Child Adolesc Psychiatry Ment Health 2015;9(1):31.
27. Bresin K, Schoenleber M. Gender differences in the prevalence of nonsuicidal self-injury: A meta-analysis. Clin Psychol Rev 2015;38:55–64.
28. Brown RC, Plener PL. Non-suicidal Self-Injury in Adolescence. Curr Psychiatry Rep 2017;19(3):20.
29. Heffer T, Willoughby T. The role of emotion dysregulation: A longitudinal investigation of the interpersonal theory of suicide. Psychiatry Res 2018;260:379–83.
30. Van Orden KA, Witte TK, Cukrowicz KC, et al. The interpersonal theory of suicide. Psychol Rev 2010;117(2):575–600.
31. Felitti VJ, Anda RF, Nordenberg D, et al. Relationship of childhood abuse and household dysfunction to many of the leading causes of death in adults. The Adverse Childhood Experiences (ACE) Study. Am J Prev Med 1998;14(4):245–58.
32. Koita K, Long D, Hessler D, et al. Development and implementation of a pediatric adverse childhood experiences (ACEs) and other determinants of health questionnaire in the pediatric medical home: A pilot study. Tu W-J, ed. PLoS One. 2018;13(12):e0208088. doi:10.1371/journal.pone.0208088.
33. Lee HY, Kim I, Nam S, et al. Adverse childhood experiences and the associations with depression and anxiety in adolescents. Child Youth Serv Rev 2020;111:104850.
34. Kim I, Galván A, Kim N. Independent and cumulative impacts of adverse childhood experiences on adolescent subgroups of anxiety and depression. Child Youth Serv Rev 2021;122:105885.
35. Elmore AL, Crouch E. The Association of Adverse Childhood Experiences With Anxiety and Depression for Children and Youth, 8 to 17 Years of Age. Acad Pediatr 2020;20(5):600–8.
36. Fuller-Thomson E, Baird SL, Dhrodia R, et al. The association between adverse childhood experiences (ACEs) and suicide attempts in a population-based study. Child Care Health Dev 2016;42(5):725–34.
37. Thompson MP, Kingree JB, Lamis D. Associations of adverse childhood experiences and suicidal behaviors in adulthood in a U.S. nationally representative sample. Child Care Health Dev 2019;45(1):121–8.
38. Brunstein Klomek A, Marrocco F, Kleinman M, et al. Bullying, depression, and suicidality in adolescents. J Am Acad Child Adolesc Psychiatry 2007;46(1):40–9.

39. Bowes L, Joinson C, Wolke D, et al. Peer victimisation during adolescence and its impact on depression in early adulthood: prospective cohort study in the United Kingdom. BMJ 2015;350(jun02 2):h2469.

40. Ttofi MM, Farrington DP, Lösel F, et al. Do the victims of school bullies tend to become depressed later in life? A systematic review and meta-analysis of longitudinal studies. Ttofi MM, ed. J Aggress Confl Peace Res. 2011;3(2):63-73.

41. National Institute on Drug Abuse. Monitoring the Future.

42. Becker TD, Rice TR. Youth vaping: a review and update on global epidemiology, physical and behavioral health risks, and clinical considerations. Eur J Pediatr 2022;181(2):453–62.

43. Chadi N, Li G, Cerda N, et al. Depressive Symptoms and Suicidality in Adolescents Using e-Cigarettes and Marijuana: A Secondary Data Analysis From the Youth Risk Behavior Survey. J Addict Med 2019;13(5):362–5.

44. Chen Y-L, Wu S-C, Chen Y-T, et al. E-Cigarette Use in a Country With Prevalent Tobacco Smoking: A Population-Based Study in Taiwan. J Epidemiol 2019; 29(4):155–63.

45. Jee Y-J. Comparison of emotional and psychological indicators according to the presence or absence of the use of electronic cigarettes among Korea youth smokers. Information 2016;19(10):4325–532.

46. Lee Y, Lee KS. Association of Depression and Suicidality with Electronic and Conventional Cigarette Use in South Korean Adolescents. Subst Use Misuse 2019; 54(6):934–43.

47. Leventhal AM, Strong DR, Sussman S, et al. Psychiatric comorbidity in adolescent electronic and conventional cigarette use. J Psychiatr Res 2016. https://doi.org/10.1016/j.jpsychires.2015.11.008.

48. Goldenson NI, Khoddam R, Stone MD, et al. Associations of ADHD Symptoms With Smoking and Alternative Tobacco Product Use Initiation During Adolescence. J Pediatr Psychol 2018;43(6):613–24.

49. Lechner WV, Janssen T, Kahler CW, et al. Bi-directional associations of electronic and combustible cigarette use onset patterns with depressive symptoms in adolescents. Prev Med (Baltim) 2017;96:73–8.

50. Unger JB, Soto DW, Leventhal A. E-cigarette use and subsequent cigarette and marijuana use among Hispanic young adults. Drug Alcohol Depend 2016;163: 261–4.

51. Dai H, Catley D, Richter KP, et al. Electronic cigarettes and future marijuana use: A longitudinal study. Pediatrics 2018;141(5):e20173787.

52. Audrain-Mcgovern J, Stone MD, Barrington-Trimis J, et al. Adolescent e-cigarette, hookah, and conventional cigarette use and subsequent marijuana use. Pediatrics 2018;142(3):e20173616.

53. Casadio P, Fernandes C, Murray RM, et al. Cannabis use in young people: The risk for schizophrenia. Neurosci Biobehav Rev 2011;35(8):1779–87.

54. Gobbi G, Atkin T, Zytynski T, et al. Association of Cannabis Use in Adolescence and Risk of Depression, Anxiety, and Suicidality in Young Adulthood. JAMA Psychiatry 2019;76(4):426.

55. Horwood LJ, Fergusson DM, Coffey C, et al. Cannabis and depression: An integrative data analysis of four Australasian cohorts. Drug Alcohol Depend 2012; 126(3):369–78.

56. Patton GC. Cannabis use and mental health in young people: cohort study. BMJ 2002;325(7374):1195–8.

57. Mars B, Heron J, Klonsky ED, et al. Predictors of future suicide attempt among adolescents with suicidal thoughts or non-suicidal self-harm: a population-based birth cohort study. Lancet Psychiatry 2019;6(4):327–37.

58. Albaugh MD, Ottino-Gonzalez J, Sidwell A, et al. Association of Cannabis Use During Adolescence With Neurodevelopment. JAMA Psychiatry 2021;78(9):1031.

59. Rothrock AN, Andris H, Swetland SB, et al. Association of E-cigarettes with adolescent alcohol use and binge drinking-drunkenness: A systematic review and meta-analysis. Am J Drug Alcohol Abuse 2020;46(6):684–98.

60. Dumas TM, Ellis W, Litt DM. What Does Adolescent Substance Use Look Like During the COVID-19 Pandemic? Examining Changes in Frequency, Social Contexts, and Pandemic-Related Predictors. J Adolesc Heal 2020;67(3):354–61.

61. Ju YJ, Kim W, Oh SS, et al. Solitary drinking and the risk of depressive symptoms and suicidal ideation in college students: Findings from a nationwide survey in Korea. J Affect Disord 2019;257:710–5. https://doi.org/10.1016/j.jad.2019.07.080.

62. Johannessen EL, Andersson HW, Bjørngaard JH, et al. Anxiety and depression symptoms and alcohol use among adolescents - a cross sectional study of Norwegian secondary school students. BMC Public Health 2017;17(1):494.

63. Kingsbury M, Clayborne Z, Colman I, et al. The protective effect of neighbourhood social cohesion on adolescent mental health following stressful life events. Psychol Med 2020;50(8):1292–9.

64. van Harmelen A-L, Kievit RA, Ioannidis K, et al. Adolescent friendships predict later resilient functioning across psychosocial domains in a healthy community cohort. Psychol Med 2017;47(13):2312–22.

65. Hurd N, Zimmerman M. Natural Mentors, Mental Health, and Risk Behaviors: A Longitudinal Analysis of African American Adolescents Transitioning into Adulthood. Am J Community Psychol 2010;46(1–2):36–48.

66. van Harmelen A-L, Gibson JL, St Clair MC, et al. Friendships and Family Support Reduce Subsequent Depressive Symptoms in At-risk adolescents. In: Alway SE, editor. PLoS One 2016;11(5):e0153715. https://doi.org/10.1371/journal.pone.0153715.

67. Zuckerbrot RA, Cheung AH, Jensen PS, et al. Guidelines for Adolescent Depression in Primary Care (GLAD-PC): I. Identification, Assessment, and Initial Management. Pediatrics 2007;120(5):e1299–312.

68. Joffe BI, Van Lieshout RJ, Duncan L, et al. Suicidal Ideation and Behavior in Adolescents Aged 12-16 Years: A 17-Year Follow-Up. Suicide Life-threatening Behav 2014;44(5):497–509.

69. Guessoum SB, Lachal J, Radjack R, et al. Adolescent psychiatric disorders during the COVID-19 pandemic and lockdown. Psychiatry Res 2020;291:113264. https://doi.org/10.1016/j.psychres.2020.113264.

70. Zhou S-J, Zhang L-G, Wang L-L, et al. Prevalence and socio-demographic correlates of psychological health problems in Chinese adolescents during the outbreak of COVID-19. Eur Child Adolesc Psychiatry 2020;29(6):749–58.

71. Clemens V, Deschamps P, Fegert JM, et al. Potential effects of "social" distancing measures and school lockdown on child and adolescent mental health. Eur Child Adolesc Psychiatry 2020;29(6):739–42.

72. Orben A, Tomova L, Blakemore S-J. The effects of social deprivation on adolescent development and mental health. Lancet Child Adolesc Heal 2020;4(8):634–40.

73. Anderson M, Jiang J. Teens, Social Media and Technology 2018; 2018.

74. Vidal C, Lhaksampa T, Miller L, et al. Social media use and depression in adolescents: a scoping review. Int Rev Psychiatry 2020;32(3):235–53.
75. Bell J. Harmful or helpful? The role of the internet in self-harming and suicidal behaviour in young people. Ment Heal Rev J 2014;19(1):61–71.
76. Valkenburg PM, Peter J, Schouten AP. Friend Networking Sites and Their Relationship to Adolescents' Well-Being and Social Self-Esteem. Cyberpsychology Behav 2006;9(5):584–90.
77. Woods HC, Scott H. #Sleepyteens: Social media use in adolescence is associated with poor sleep quality, anxiety, depression and low self-esteem. J Adolesc 2016;51:41–9.
78. Klein JD, Allan MJ, Elster AB, et al. Improving adolescent preventive care in community health centers. Pediatrics 2001;107(2):318–27. Availble at: http://www.ncbi.nlm.nih.gov/pubmed/11158465. Accessed August 14, 2014.
79. Weersing VR, Jeffreys M, Do M-CT, et al. Evidence Base Update of Psychosocial Treatments for Child and Adolescent Depression. J Clin Child Adolesc Psychol 2017;46(1):11–43.
80. Oud M, de Winter L, Vermeulen-Smit E, et al. Effectiveness of CBT for children and adolescents with depression: A systematic review and meta-regression analysis. Eur Psychiatry 2019;57:33–45.
81. Carnevale TD. Universal Adolescent Depression Prevention Programs. J Sch Nurs 2013;29(3):181–95.
82. Young JF, Mufson L, Davies M. Efficacy of Interpersonal Psychotherapy-Adolescent Skills Training: an indicated preventive intervention for depression. J Child Psychol Psychiatry 2006. https://doi.org/10.1111/j.1469-7610.2006.01667.x. 061006030313006-.
83. McCauley E, Berk MS, Asarnow JR, et al. Efficacy of Dialectical Behavior Therapy for Adolescents at High Risk for Suicide. JAMA Psychiatry 2018;75(8):777.
84. Wagner KD, Asarnow JR, Vitiello B, et al. Out of the Black Box: Treatment of Resistant Depression in Adolescents and the Antidepressant Controversy. J Child Adolesc Psychopharmacol 2012;22(1):5–10.
85. Horwitz AG, Czyz EK, King CA. Predicting Future Suicide Attempts Among Adolescent and Emerging Adult Psychiatric Emergency Patients. J Clin Child Adolesc Psychol 2015;44(5):751–61.
86. Dobias ML, Sugarman MB, Mullarkey MC, et al. Predicting Mental Health Treatment Access Among Adolescents With Elevated Depressive Symptoms: Machine Learning Approaches. Adm Policy Ment Heal Ment Heal Serv Res 2022;49(1):88–103.
87. Amone-P'Olak K, Ormel J, Oldehinkel AJ, et al. Socioeconomic Position Predicts Specialty Mental Health Service Use Independent of Clinical Severity. J Am Acad Child Adolesc Psychiatry 2010;49(7):647–55.
88. Upadhyay N, Aparasu R, Rowan PJ, et al. The association between geographic access to providers and the treatment quality of pediatric depression. J Affect Disord 2019;253:162–70.
89. Radovic A, Reynolds K, McCauley HL, et al. Parents' Role in Adolescent Depression Care: Primary Care Provider Perspectives. J Pediatr 2015;167(4):911–8.

Frailty
A Multidimensional Biopsychosocial Syndrome

Carl I. Cohen, MD*, Rivka Benyaminov, BA,
Manumar Rahman, MD, Dilys Ngu, MD, Michael Reinhardt, MD

KEYWORDS

• Frailty • Cognitive frailty • Social frailty • Psychological frailty

KEY POINTS

- The original conceptual landscape of frailty has evolved into a complex, multidimensional biopsychosocial syndrome including physical, cognitive, social, and psychological domains.
- Many new tools are available to assess the frailty domains.
- Frailty is a dynamic, potentially reversible state, and numerous biological, lifestyle, environmental, and clinical risk and protective factors have been identified.
- Research and care of persons with frailty have been hampered by a lack of consensus in defining the frailty domains and a limited understanding of the mechanisms of how the domains affect each other.

INTRODUCTION

Frailty is thought to be one of the most serious public health challenges of the twenty-first century.[1] All older adults are at risk for developing frailty, and it is associated with many adverse outcomes including diminished quality of life and increased rates of mortality, hospitalizations, falls, depression, and dementia.[2] Recognition of frailty and its risk factors can inform treatment decisions and prognosis. In recent years, several features of frailty have become well-established: (1) Although the physical dimension has been privileged, it is increasingly recognized that frailty is multidimensional and complex, and includes physical, cognitive, psychological, and social domains; that is, it is a "biopsychosocial" syndrome; (2) Frailty is a dynamic process

Partial support was provided by funding from HRSA Award No. U1QHP33077 and the SUNY Health Network of Excellence.
SUNY Downstate Health Sciences University, 450 Clarkson Avenue, Brooklyn, NY 11203, USA
* Corresponding author. SUNY Downstate Health Sciences University, MSC 1203, 450 Clarkson Avenue, Brooklyn, NY 11203.
E-mail address: carl.cohen@downstate.edu

Med Clin N Am 107 (2023) 183–197
https://doi.org/10.1016/j.mcna.2022.04.006

that can fluctuate between various states of frailty; and (3) Frailty is potentially preventable, reversible, or can be slowed, until a point of "no return."[1,3] The conceptual change of frailty as a biopsychosocial syndrome has broadened the field to include social and behavioral scientists and clinicians from a wide range of specialties.

Among the issues that have dominated discussions of frailty have been efforts to more precisely define these domains and attain consensus regarding these definitions; whether these conceptual domains can be best viewed as a single phenotype, separate phenotypes, or overlapping of physical, cognitive, and social conditions; and whether prevention and treatment strategies will have to target each type of frailty or are there strategies that might act across these conditions? In this article, we will address these issues by reviewing the concepts and definitions of each domain, their epidemiology, the measures used for assessment, their risk factors, pathogenesis, and suggestions for treatment and prevention. We conclude with a discussion of controversies in the frailty literature and future directions for research.

DEFINITIONS
Physical Frailty

When first classified in 1986, frailty was associated with older individuals having multiple comorbidities that restricted their activities of daily living and were dependent on assistance from others.[4] Later definitions became more inclusive toward persons that would be considered in a precursor state of disability. This perspective shifted the focus toward early intervention in high-risk individuals. frailty can be dichotomized into 2 broad conceptual systems that should be considered complementary but not substitutable[4,5]: (1) Risk accumulation model.[6] As people grow older, they will accumulate diseases and impairments that will cause them to obtain a predisposition for adverse outcomes. This model proposes that interventions be aimed at modifying these risk factors. (2) Frailty as a syndrome.[3] Frailty is seen as a set of signs and symptoms that define a health condition.

Although the accumulation model considers frailty solely as a "preclinical" entity (ie, a risk), the syndrome model regards it primarily as a health condition or phenotype that can be viewed as a progressive process to be staged across a range of severity states, with lower and higher risk for adverse outcomes considered "prefrail" and "frail," respectively. Fried's[7] conceptualization operationalized frailty on the presence of weak muscle strength, slow gait speed, unintentional weight loss, exhaustion, and low physical activity. It did not include disabilities in its operationalization. However, the deficit accumulation model includes health deficits such as signs, symptoms, disabilities, and abnormal medical tests. Both models have been found to predict adverse outcomes such as a higher risk for mortality and hospitalizations.

Many popular conceptualizations of physical frailty are hybrids of these 2 models that focus on the risks for future adverse events. However, hybridization risks conflating a syndrome (ie, phenotype) that should have specific symptoms and signs with an accretion of deficits across multiple systems. For example, Panza and colleagues[8] proposed a hybrid framework in which frailty would be considered "primary" or "preclinical" when the state is not associated directly with a specific disease or has no substantial disability. This definition is more akin to the physical phenotype of frailty. Frailty is considered "secondary" or "clinical" when associated with known comorbidities such as dementia or overt cardiovascular disease or disability. Secondary frailty is more congruent with the accumulation of deficits model. Kelaiditi and colleagues[9] ruefully observed that despite several decades of research, there is a lack of consensus about a unique operational definition of frailty.

Cognitive Frailty

Cognitive frailty results from preexisting physical frailty and cognitive impairment, generally considered mild or subjective. In 2013, the International Academy on Nutrition and Aging and the International Association of Gerontology and Geriatrics (IANA-IAGG)[9] defined cognitive frailty as the presence of both physical frailty and mild cognitive impairment (MCI), operationalized as a Clinical Dementia Rating score of 0.5, and the exclusion of concurrent dementias such as Alzheimer disease (AD). The definition suggests reduced cognitive reserve which is differentiated from normal aging. Moreover, there is a potential for reversibility in the cognitive and physical components. The authors allow for the possibility that various neurocognitive disorders may ultimately arise, although they should not be present when diagnosing cognitive frailty.

Recently, several investigators have proposed a modification of the framework for the definition of cognitive frailty by identifying 2 subtypes: "potentially reversible" cognitive frailty and "reversible" cognitive frailty; the aim being to make the potential reversibility of physical frailty consistent with the potential reversibility of cognitive deficits.[10] Thus, the physical frailty components for both cognitive frailty subtypes include physical "prefrailty" and "frailty." The cognitive impairment components of "potentially reversible cognitive frailty" should be MCI (ie, mild objective cognitive deficits without declines in daily functioning), whereas "reversible cognitive frailty" is defined as pre-MCI "subjective" cognitive deficits. Subjective cognitive disorders are characterized by self-reported memory complaints but no objective cognitive deficits or deficits in daily living. Subjects with reversible cognitive frailty and no biomarker evidence of AD pathologic condition may include individuals with normal cognitive aging or undetectable preclinical AD.

Social Frailty

This syndrome has not received the attention given to physical and cognitive frailty. There has been no consensus in the literature regarding the concept and methods for assessment. Bunt and colleagues'[11] review found that social frailty is most typically defined on a continuum of being at risk of losing, or having lost, resources that are important for fulfilling one or more basic social needs during the life span. They also found that social frailty includes the threat or absence of self-management abilities necessary to fulfill these social needs. Other items sometimes included within social frailty are low income and housing insecurity. For the most part, social frailty has not been operationalized to require the co-occurrence of physical frailty.

Psychological Frailty

This syndrome has been largely neglected or incorporated into other frailty dimensions. A review by McKelvie and coauthors[12] found that only 8% of articles on social or psychological frailty were specifically devoted to psychological frailty. Psychological frailty has been operationalized to include the co-occurrence of physical frailty with low mood, apathy, depression, loneliness, and cognitive deficits.[8,12] The latter 2 variables may sometimes be classified under social frailty and cognitive frailty, respectively. Most studies have focused on depression, and Brown and colleagues[13] proposed a "depressed frail" phenotype.

Table 1 describes the frailty domains.

EPIDEMIOLOGY

Siriwardhana and colleagues'[31] meta-analysis of persons aged 50 years and older in 15 countries found that the pooled prevalence of physical frailty was 17.4% (range

Table 1
Frailty domains: Description and assessment scales

Frailty Domain	Physical Frailty	Cognitive Frailty	Psychological Frailty	Social Frailty
Description	Two popular models: Model 1: Risk accumulation model—with increased age, a person will accumulate diseases and impairments that will cause them to obtain a predisposition for adverse outcomes and hospitalization. This model proposes that interventions be aimed at modifying these risk factors Model 2: Frailty as a syndrome—frailty is seen as a set of signs and symptoms that define a health condition usually divided into risk levels of "prefrail" and frail	The co-occurrence of physical frailty and cognitive impairment, usually defined as mild. A modified framework for the definition of cognitive frailty was developed based on identifying 2 subtypes: (1) Potentially reversible—simultaneous presence of physical prefrailty or physical frailty and mild cognitive impairment (MCI) (2) Reversible—the simultaneous presence of physical prefrailty or physical frailty and pre-MCI subjective cognitive deficits	Often operationalized to include low mood, apathy, and depression with the co-occurrence of physical frailty	Typically defined on a continuum of being at risk of losing, or having lost, resources that are important for fulfilling one or more basic social needs. Sometimes includes sociodemographical risk factors. Co-occurrence of physical frailty not usually required.
Selected Assessment Tools	Fried Frailty Scale,[7] FRAIL questionnaire,[14] Deficit Accumulation Index (Frailty Index),[15] Clinical Frailty Scale,[36] Edmonton Frailty Scale,[16] Tilburg Frailty Scale[17]	Brief screens: Mini-Cog,[18] the MMSE,[19] 3-MS,[20] SLUMs,[38] and the MoCA[21] Comprehensive cognitive tests: Mattis DRS,[22] Alzheimer's Disease Assessment Scale,[23] and the CERAD neuropsychological battery[24] Subjective Cognitive Decline Questionnaire[25] ADL assessment scales[26]	Geriatric Depression Scale[27]; CES-D[28]	SOCIAL[29]; Social Frailty Scale[30]

3.9% to 51.4%) and prefrailty was 49.3% (range: 13.4% to 71.6%). The study found that the prevalence of frailty seems higher among community-dwelling older adults in upper-middle-income countries than in high-income countries; there were insufficient data on low-income countries.

Since the 2013 IANA-IAGG consensus on cognitive frailty,[9] various studies have emerged studying the epidemiology of cognitive frailty using its newly proposed definition. There has been a wide variability in prevalence rates that has been attributed to differences in models of cognitive frailty, age, gender, and setting.[8] Once stratified, it was found that studies of participants in a clinical setting had a higher prevalence (10.7%–22.0%) of cognitive frailty when compared with population-based studies (1.0%–4.4%).[32] A recent meta-analysis by Qui and colleagues[33] of 24 studies involving 73,643 participants aged 60 years or older living in the community found an estimated pooled prevalence of cognitive frailty of 9%. Because of the diverse definitions of cognitive frailty, the prevalence varied from 1% to 50% across the studies. Of note, there have been changes in prevalence over time, with rates of 6% from 2012 to 2017 and 11% from 2018 to 2020. The estimated pooled prevalence of cognitive frailty was 11% in men and 15% in women.

There have been no meta-analyses or systematic reviews of the prevalence of social frailty. Studies by Tsutsumimoto and colleagues[30] and Yamada and Arai[34] in Japan found a prevalence rate of 26.8% and 18%, respectively. The latter study found rates of social prefrailty of 32%. Rates of social frailty increased from 16% in the 65 to 69 age group to 41% in those aged 90 years and older.

Vaughan and coauthors'[35] literature review found that the prevalence rates of the co-occurrence of depressive symptomatology and physical frailty in older adults aged 55 years and older varied widely (range: 16.4%–53.8%). A large study in Japan found that among older adults with any form of frailty status, the incidence of depressive symptoms increased significantly in the presence of physical, cognitive, or social frailty.[30]

DIAGNOSIS AND ASSESSMENT

Ruan and colleagues[10] pointed out that many well-validated physical frailty models have operationalized screening measures incorporating the various conceptual models. The Fried phenotype of the Cardiovascular Health Study[7] is the most common frailty-screening tool used worldwide. It is fast and easy to administer. Patients are rated based on the presence of the following 5 signs/symptoms: unintentional weight loss, self-reported exhaustion, poor grip strength, slow walking speed, or low physical activity (scoring: 0 = robust, 1–2 = prefrail, 3–5 = frail). The validated simple FRAIL questionnaire[14] screening tool is a good alternative physical frailty screening instrument without objective measures, and it can rapidly identify individuals with physical frailty or physical prefrailty in large clinical cohort studies. It contains 5 items—fatigue, resistance, aerobic, illness accumulation, and loss of weight (0 = robust, 1–2 = prefrail, 3–5 = frail). A variety of more comprehensive batteries exist. The deficit accumulation index (or frailty index) includes scales that assess diseases, signs, symptoms, laboratory abnormalities, cognitive impairments, mood, and disabilities in activities of daily living; most scales contain between 30 and 70 items. [15] Scores are calculated by summing the number of positive items divided by the total number of items; scores range from 0 to 1.0. The use of cutoffs is controversial, although 0.25 or greater has been proposed to indicate frailty. Rockwood also developed the Clinical Frailty Scale[36] which appraises medical disease burden and functionality based on 7 components ranging from 1 (robust health) to 7 (complete functional dependence on others). An intermediate-length instrument within this framework is the Edmonton Frail Scale,[16] which consists of 10 items examining cognition, functional performance, general health, functional independence, social support, medication use, nutrition, mood, and continence. The Tilburg Frailty Index[17] conceptualizes frailty as a multidimensional concept (physical, psychological, social) and includes 10 determinants and 15 components of frailty that classify patients into frail or not. Other instruments include the Program of Research on Integration of Services for the Maintenance of Autonomy (PRISMA-7) questionnaire, Timed Get-Up and Go Test, and the Gerontopole Frailty Screening Tool (see Sukkriang[37]).

Diagnosing cognitive frailty requires the clinician to diagnose physical prefrailty and frailty, MCI, subjective cognitive impairment (SCI), and to rule out dementia. Cognitive deficits can be assessed with a variety of instruments. Brief measures that can be administered quickly in an office setting include the Mini-Cog,[18] the Mini-Mental State Examination (MMSE),[19] the Modified Mini-Mental State Examination (3-MS),[2] the St. Louis Mental Status Examination (SLUMs),[38] and the Montreal Cognitive Assessment (MoCA).[21] More comprehensive cognitive tests that include a detailed assessment of cognitive dimensions include the Dementia Rating Scale (DRS),[22] Alzheimer's Disease Assessment Scale,[23] and the Consortium to Establish a Registry for Alzheimer's Disease (CERAD) neuropsychological battery.[24]

Many researchers classify SCI based on a positive response to a single question about perceived difficulty, change, or worry/concern about one's memory or cognition, whereas others use cut scores/median split approaches on a questionnaire or other methods.[39] There are several batteries to test SCI; one of the most cited is the Subjective Cognitive Decline Questionnaire.[25] Rabin and colleagues[39] argue that it is critical to distinguish between those people whose concerns about cognition reach a threshold for significance that may be attributed to underlying neurodegenerative changes consistent with prodromal AD (or other dementia subtypes) from those whose concerns are generally mild and attributed to benign conditions associated with normal aging. This is problematic because both the distinction between SCI and cognitively normal aging are made based on subjective cognitive reports. Both groups are considered unimpaired on standardized neurocognitive tests. Methods to discriminate more benign conditions from those that may progress to AD have incorporated the use of biomarkers, for example, cerebrospinal fluid aβ42, tau, and phosphorylated tau concentrations; amyloid deposition and glucose metabolism in positron emission tomography; and hippocampal atrophy on magnetic resonance imaging. Finally, to distinguish between dementia and MCI/SCI, an assessment of daily functioning must be done. There are a variety of simple measures to assess Instrumental Activities of Daily Living (ADL) and Basic Activities of Daily Living.[26]

There are several questionnaires to assess social frailty. These instruments assay a broader spectrum of psychosocial risk factors for creating frailty, some focus on psychological as well as social factors. Most are brief questionnaires such as the SOCIAL (sadness, outside activities, cognition, income adequacy, attachment to neighborhood, lethargy) with scores of 4 to 6 indicating social frailty and 2 to 3 indicating presocial frailty.[29] A questionnaire developed by Tsutsumimoto and coauthors[30] focuses only on social network factors (going out less frequently, visiting friends, living alone, feeling helpful, talking with someone daily) with scores of 2 to 5 indicating social frailty and a score of 1 indicating presocial frailty.

There are no specific scales for psychological frailty. The 15-item Geriatric Depression Scale[27] and the Center for Epidemiologic Studies-Depression (CES-D) questionnaire[28] have been used in several studies.[35,40]

The scales are listed in **Table 1**.

PREDICTORS, PATHOGENESIS, AND COURSE

Frailty is a dynamic potentially reversible state, and identifying the risk factors of frailty will facilitate prevention and management.[41] Recent studies have identified many risks and protective factors including biological, lifestyle, environmental, and clinical elements (**Table 2**).

In addition to the risk factors and biomarkers summarized in **Table 2**, there are important interactions between the various frailty domains. Physical frailty is associated with late-life cognitive impairment and decline, incident AD and MCI, vascular dementia, other dementias, and AD pathologic conditions in older persons with and without dementia; frail women are at higher risk of incident AD than frail men.[8,46,47] The reciprocal relationship, that cognitive impairment predicts future physical frailty, has also been reported in samples of community-dwelling older adults.[48] While frailty and cognitive impairment have been viewed as 2 independent concepts in which both predict adverse outcomes,[49] when they coexist, cumulative negative effects are often detected.[50] In support of a cognitive frailty phenotype, Bu and colleagues'[51] meta-analysis found that among older adults living in communities, cognitive frailty was a significant predictor of all-cause mortality and dementia, and that cognitive frailty was a better predictor of all-cause mortality and dementia than frailty alone. However, several studies found no relationship between physical frailty and cognition.[48] Thus, some investigators suggest that frailty syndrome and neurocognitive disorders should be treated as distinct conditions that may interact bidirectionally.[42]

Xie and coauthors[52] found that advanced age, depression, and insomnia were significantly associated with higher rates of cognitive frailty. Indeed, several investigators postulated that physical frailty, cognitive impairment, and depression are interrelated constructs.[52] Vaughan and colleagues[35] and Brown and colleagues[13] concluded that there is a bidirectional relationship between depression and physical frailty, and together they increase the risk of dementia, suicidality, and mortality.

A systematic review of social frailty by McKelvie and colleagues[12] showed that it led to various health problems late in life. Compared with those who do not exhibit social frailty, older adults with this condition have been found to have significantly lower physical and cognitive functioning and a significantly higher risk of future incident disability.[40] For example, Teo and colleagues[40] found that social frailty independently predicted adverse health outcomes such as functional and severe disability, nursing home referral, and mortality; combining social frailty with physical frailty increased the prediction of adverse outcomes. Social frailty predicted physical and cognitive decline in Japanese community-dwelling older adults, and social frailty had more impact on depression than physical or cognitive frailty.[30]

Several studies have supported the conceptual framework that the frailty domains are related but largely independent of each other and that each domain incrementally increased risk estimates of various adverse health outcomes. Vermeiren and colleagues[53] showed that combining various frailty dimensions increased mortality hazard ratios (HRs); HRs associated with 1, 2, and 3 frailty dimensions were 1.9, 3.9, and 10.4, respectively.

Despite evidence of the close relationship between the various frailty domains, the mechanisms involved in this association have not yet been determined.[42] All the domains are complex and have multifactorial influences. Fabricio and colleagues[42] proposed that the pathophysiologic mechanisms for these domains overlap considerably and may develop positive feedback loops. Mechanisms involved in the onset of the physical frailty syndrome are also found to promote neurodegeneration (eg, chronic inflammation and oxidative stress), and many of these risk factors are also found in

Table 2
Risk factors/markers for development and progression of various cognitive domains and potential treatment approaches

Biological Factors	Description	Possible Treatment Approach
Inflammation	High levels of C-Reactive Protein, Interleukin-6, TumorNecrosis Factor -alpha	Exercise, healthy diet, smoking cessation, treatment of medical illnesses, pharmacological agents with anti-inflammatory effects
Mitochondrial bioenergetics	Diminished functioning	Aerobic exercise interventions have resulted in improved muscle oxidative capacity and upregulated mitochondrial genes, improved skeletal muscle mitochondrial content in sedentary older adults, and are effective for improving physical functioning in frail elders
Dopamine dysfunction	Diminution	Pharmacologic augmentation of dopaminergic neurotransmission may be beneficial to ameliorating cognitive and physical slowing and depressive symptoms in adults within the depressed frail phenotype.
Hypothalamic Pituitary Adrenal axis dysfunction	Especially hypercortisol and hypocortisol dysfunction	Assessment and medical treatment
Epigenetic changes	Frailty is associated with epigenetically accelerated aging measured by the difference between predicted DNA methylation age and chronologic age	Exercise, psychosocial, and nutritional interventions are potential therapeutic targets. Additional study is needed.
Undernutrition/ Micronutrient deficits	Protein-energy undernutrition is associated with poorer cognitive performance. Weight loss, reduced caloric intake, and the reduced intake or deficits of specific micronutrients (eg, carotenoids, Vitamin	Nutrient supplementation

(continued on next page)

Table 2
(continued)

Biological Factors	Description	Possible Treatment Approach
	B6, Vitamin D, Vitamin E) are associated with detectable changes in body composition and physical function characterizing the transition from independence to disability, with weight loss also proposed as a dementia risk factor	
Low testosterone	Testosterone may promote hippocampal synaptic plasticity and regulate amyloid deposition, whereas age-related depletion may be associated with frailty by reducing muscle mass and strength	Exogenous testosterone increases physical performance and strength in older testosterone-deficient men. Testosterone may decrease depressive symptoms in men with late-life depression
Increased volumes of white matter hyperintensities; loss of structure of the thalamus and hippocampus on MRI	Found in cognitively frail and prefrail persons	Cardiovascular risk prevention, reduction, and treatment strategies; cognitive exercises
Clinical Factors		
Diabetes and hyperinsulinemia	Elevated Hemoglobin A1C, obesity	Medication, dietary changes, and exercise
Cardiovascular risk factors	Atrial fibrillation congestive heart failure cerebral vascular accident, hypoxia, peripheral vascular disease, hypertension, hypercholesterolemia, smoking, high-fat diets	Cardiovascular risk prevention, reduction, and treatment strategies including appropriate medication, lifestyle changes, and dietary modificatons including the Mediterranean diet, smoking cessation, and exercise
Sarcopenia	Decline in skeletal mass and function	Physical exercise and strength training in combination with protein supplementation
Miscellaneous physical markers and symptoms	Anemia, low serum albumin, low glomerular filtration rate, sensory deficits, pain	Determine cause and treat

(continued on next page)

Table 2 (continued)		
Biological Factors	**Description**	**Possible Treatment Approach**
Depression	Associated with physical and cognitive frailty	Psychotherapy and/or pharmacotherapy; ameliorate environmental stressors
Environmental Factors		
Social and demographic risk factors	Social isolation, loneliness, low income, housing insecurity, low education, advanced age, female gender, unmarried, rural residence, low-income neighborhood, low quality of life	Promotion of emotional resilience, active and socially integrated lifestyles; enhance safety net for at-risk older adults
Lifestyle Factors	Low physical activity, smoking, high alcohol consumption	Individual and group exercise, balance, and strength training; counseling and pharmacologic interventions regarding smoking and alcohol intake

References: Kelaiditi et al;[9] Panza et al;[8] Brown et al;[13] Fabricio et al ;[42] Briej et al;[2] Vatatabe et al;[43] Feng et al;[44] Elwood et al;[33] Facal et al.[45]

late-life depression. Other clinical conditions can increase the risk of both frailty and dementia, such as heart failure, peripheral vascular disease, diabetes, and hypertension. Therefore, it is likely that physical frailty, neurocognitive disorders, and depression share common risk factors and biological mechanisms.

Finally, frailty is a dynamic state with heterogeneous outcomes, although most persons remain in their baseline state and a substantial percentage die (about one-third), on 4 to 5-year mean follow-up, up to 37% experienced transitions in their status, either improvement or decline.[3] Notably, several investigators found improvement rates among frail elders of between 15.5% and 27%[53–56]; 12% of pre-frail improved.[54]

TREATMENT AND PREVENTION

Dent and colleagues[1] reviewed the treatment literature and found that the "certainty of evidence" for any management strategy was low. The main strategies have included physical activities (aerobic training, resistance-based, balance coordination) in individual or group sessions, health behavior advice, protein and micronutrient supplementation, social support strategies, hormonal therapy, cognitive training, comprehensive geriatric assessments, and multicomponent packages. First-line management has focused primarily on physical activities and adequate protein intake. These approaches are listed in **Table 2**.

Primary prevention of frailty has focused on changing unhealthy lifestyles and behaviors, identifying and modifying various risk factors for frailty, and conducting regular screenings for physical frailty, cognitive decline, mood changes, and social and functional decline.[3] A patient-centered (personalized) clinical approach is essential, and it is necessary to identify the relevant risk factors across domains for each patient. These are summarized in **Table 2**. An especially challenging and understudied topic is how to reorganize healthcare systems to focus on frailty assessment and management. There is increasing evidence that many of the risk factors emerge in midlife, so early interventions are desirable.[3]

UNRESOLVED ISSUES

1. Virtually every review article bemoans the lack of consensus regarding the definition of frailty within all domains. Physical frailty is dominated by 2 distinct competing paradigms—the phenotype model and the deficit accumulation model. Sometimes, hybrid approaches have been used or alternative frameworks based on resiliency have been proposed. Researchers in cognitive frailty debate whether to include subjective cognitive frailty as a "prefrail" measure but the definitions of SCI are varied, and it is unclear if it is a valid clinical concept. Similarly, definitions of psychological frailty usually include mood but may include cognition, anxiety, and motivation; social frailty tends to focus on social supports and activities but may encompass safety net issues such as income, housing insecurity, and the like.

2. Frailty was originally conceived as a physical condition. However, in recent years a broader biopsychosocial approach has been proffered. Frailty has evolved from a

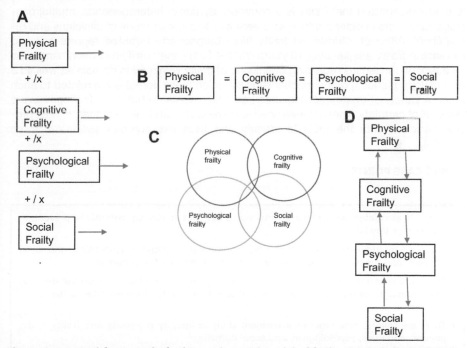

Fig. 1. Conceptual frameworks for biopsychosocial model of frailty. (*A*) Each frailty domain is largely independent of the other domains but may have additive (+) or interactive (x) effects with the other domains on outcome measures. (*B*) Each domain is part of a singular phenotype that has a common underlying mechanism. (*C*) Each domain may have some overlapping features and some underlying mechanisms with the other domains. (*D*) Each domain is largely separate but has unidirectional or bidimensional effects on other domains. (*Modified from* Brown et al, 2016.[13])

biological/physical entity to encompass cognitive brain functions and psychological conditions that involve emotions and socially mediated elements such as language and thoughts. Moreover, social frailty focuses on the social domain and doesn't typically require the co-occurrence of physical frailty. Conversely, the biopsychosocial model proposes that the external social domain affects the internal domain, that is, it must be "embodied." This broader biopsychosocial conceptualization of frailty is not universally accepted or widely used and understanding the complexities of how the 4 domains interact is daunting.

3. How the different domains relate to each other is another contested area. One possibility is that each domain is a separate clinical entity and that each has independent additive or interactive (nonlinear) effects on outcome measures such as disability and mortality (**Fig. 1**A). A second possibility is that several or all of them have common underlying mechanisms and could therefore be considered a single phenotype (**Fig. 1**B). A third possibility is that they are separate entities with some common underlying pathogenesis (**Fig. 1**C). A fourth possibility is that they are separate entities that can affect each other, either unidirectionally, or most likely, bidirectionally, perhaps through some underlying common pathways (**Fig. 1**D). Developing appropriate prevention measures and treatment will depend on resolving these issues.

SUMMARY

It is now recognized that frailty is a common, dynamic, heterogeneous, multidimensional syndrome in older adults that is germane to a broad range of clinicians and researchers. Although studies on frailty have burgeoned—PubMed reports a 6-fold increase in frailty articles over 10 years (2012–2021)—their utility has been hampered by a lack of consensus regarding definitions of frailty within each domain as well as a lack of understanding of the mechanisms by which these domains are related to each other. A variety of treatment measures has been evaluated but most findings have a low level of certainty. These issues need to be resolved, and future research must provide clinicians with the tools to identify and treat this complex syndrome more precisely.

CLINICS CARE POINTS

- Frailty is associated with many serious outcomes, but it can be potentially prevented, reversed, or slowed.
- Frailty is a multidimensional concept affecting physical, cognitive, psychological, and social domains, and the more domains that are affected, the worse the prognosis.
- The frailty domains are interrelated and addressing one domain may improve the status of other domains; conversely, the worsening of one domain may adversely affect other domains.
- There are simple, time-efficient assessment tools to identify pre-frailty and frailty in the physical, cognitive, psychological, and social domains.

DISCLOSURE

The authors have nothing to disclose.

REFERENCES

1. Dent E, Martin FC, Bergman H, et al. Management of frailty: opportunities, challenges, and future directions. Lancet 2019;394(10206):1376–86.
2. de Breij S, van Hout HPJ, de Bruin SR, et al. Predictors of frailty and vitality in older adults aged 75 years and over: results from the longitudinal aging study amsterdam. Gerontology 2021;67(1):69–77.
3. Hoogendijk EO, Afilalo J, Ensrud KE, et al. Frailty: implications for clinical practice and public health. Lancet 2019;394(10206):1365–75.
4. Boers M, Cruz Jentoft AJ. A new concept of health can improve the definition of frailty. Calcified Tissue Int 2015;97(5):429–31.
5. Cesari M, Gambassi G, Abellan van Kan G, et al. The frailty phenotype and the frailty index: different instruments for different purposes. Age and Ageing 2014; 43(1):10–2.
6. Rockwood K, Mitnitski A. Frailty in relation to the accumulation of deficits. J Gerontol Ser A Biol Sci Med Sci 2007;62(7):722–7.
7. Fried LP, Tangen CM, Walston J, et al. Frailty in Older Adults: Evidence for a Phenotype. J Gerontol Ser A Biol Sci Med Sci 2001;56(3):M146–57.
8. Panza F, Lozupone M, Solfrizzi V, et al. Different cognitive frailty models and health-and cognitive-related outcomes in older age: from epidemiology to prevention. J Alzheimer's Dis 2018;62(3):993–1012.
9. Kelaiditi E, Cesari M, Canevelli M, et al. Cognitive frailty: Rational and definition from an (I.A.N.A./I.A.G.G.) International Consensus Group. J Nutr Health Aging 2013;17(9):726–34.
10. Ruan Q, Xiao F, Gong K, et al. Prevalence of cognitive frailty phenotypes and associated factors in a community-dwelling elderly population. J Nutr Health Aging 2020;24(2):172–80.
11. Bunt S, Steverink N, Olthof J, et al. Social frailty in older adults: a scoping review. Eur J Ageing 2017;14(3):323–34.
12. Mckelvie M, Donnelly M, O'Reilly D, et al. P35 Psychological frailty and social frailty in older adults: a scoping review. BMJ 2021. https://doi.org/10.1136/jech-2021-ssmabstracts.123. A58.1-A58.
13. Brown PJ, Rutherford BR, Yaffe K, et al. The depressed frail phenotype: the clinical manifestation of increased biological aging. Am J Geriatr Psychiatry 2016; 24(11):1084–94.
14. Morley JE, Malmstrom TK, Miller DK. A simple frailty questionnaire (FRAIL) predicts outcomes in middle aged African Americans. J Nutr Health Aging 2012; 16(7):601–8.
15. Mitnitski AB, Mogilner AJ, Rockwood K. Accumulation of deficits as a proxy measure of aging. Sci World J 2001;1:323–36.
16. Rolfson DB, Majumdar SR, Tsuyuki RT, et al. Validity and reliability of the Edmonton Frail Scale. Age and Ageing 2006;35(5):526–9.
17. Gobbens RJJ, van Assen MALM, Luijkx KG, et al. The Tilburg frailty indicator: psychometric properties. J Am Med Directors Assoc 2010;11(5):344–55.
18. Borson S, Scanlan J, Brush M, et al. The Mini-Cog: a cognitive 'vital signs' measure for dementia screening in multi-lingual elderly. Int J Geriatr Psychiatry 2000; 15(11):1021–7.
19. Folstein MF, Folstein SE, McHugh PR. Mini-mental state." A practical method for grading the cognitive state of patients for the clinician. J Psychiatr Res 1975;12: 189–98.

20. Teng EL, Chui HC. The Modified Mini-Mental State (3MS) examination. J Clin Psychiatry 1987;48(8):314–8.
21. Nasreddine ZS, Phillips NA, Bédirian V, et al. The Montreal Cognitive Assessment, MoCA: a brief screening tool for mild cognitive impairment. J Am Geriatr Soc 2005;53(4):695–9.
22. Coblentz JM. Presenile dementia. Arch Neurol 1973;29(5):299.
23. Rosen WG, Mohs RC, Davis KL. A new rating scale for Alzheimer's disease. Am J Psychiatry 1984;141(11):1356–64.
24. Moms JC, Heyman A, Mohs RC, et al. The Consortium to Establish a Registry for Alzheimer's Disease (CERAD). Part I. Clinical and neuropsychological assessment of Alzheimer's disease. Neurology 1989;39(9):1159.
25. Rami L, Mollica MA, García-Sanchez C, et al. The Subjective Cognitive Decline Questionnaire (SCD-Q): a validation study. J Alzheimer's Dis 2014;41(2):453–66.
26. Pashmdarfard M, Azad A. Assessment tools to evaluate activities of daily living (ADL) and instrumental activities of daily living (IADL) in older adults: A systematic review. Med J Islamic Republic Iran 2020;34(1).
27. Yesavage JA, Brink TL, Rose TL, et al. Development and validation of a geriatric depression screening scale: A preliminary report. J Psychiatr Res 1982;17(1):37–49.
28. Radloff LS. The CES-D Scale. Appl Psychol Meas 1977;1(3):385–401.
29. Malmstrom TK, Morley JE. Frailty and cognition: Linking two common syndromes in older persons. J Nutr Health Aging 2013;17(9):723–5.
30. Tsutsumimoto K, Doi T, Makizako H, et al. Social frailty has a stronger impact on the onset of depressive symptoms than physical frailty or cognitive impairment: a 4-year follow-up longitudinal cohort study. J Am Med Directors Assoc 2018;19(6):504–10.
31. Siriwardhana DD, Hardoon S, Rait G, et al. Prevalence of frailty and prefrailty among community-dwelling older adults in low-income and middle-income countries: A systematic review and meta-analysis. BMJ Open 2018;8(3). https://doi.org/10.1136/bmjopen-2017-018195.
32. Delrieu J, Andrieu S, Pahor M, et al. Neuropsychological profile of "cognitive frailty" subjects in MAPT study. J Prev Alzheimer's Dis 2016;1–9. https://doi.org/10.14283/jpad.2016.94.
33. Ellwood A, Quinn C, Mountain G. Psychological and social factors associated with coexisting frailty and cognitive impairment: a systematic review. Res Aging 2021. https://doi.org/10.1177/01640275211045603.
34. Yamada M, Arai H. Social Frailty Predicts Incident Disability and Mortality Among Community-Dwelling Japanese Older Adults. J Am Med Directors Assoc 2018;19(12):1099–103.
35. Vaughan L, Corbin AL, Goveas JS. Depression and frailty in later life: A systematic review. Clin Interventions Aging 2015;10:1947–58.
36. Clegg A, Young J, Iliffe S, et al. Frailty in elderly people. Lancet 2013;381:752–62.
37. Sukkriang N, Punsawad C. Comparison of geriatric assessment tools for frailty among community elderly. Heliyon 2020;6(9). https://doi.org/10.1016/j.heliyon.2020.e04797.
38. Tariq SH, Tumosa N, Chibnall JT, et al. Comparison of the saint louis university mental status examination and the mini-mental state examination for detecting dementia and mild neurocognitive disorder—a pilot study. Am J Geriatr Psychiatry 2006;14(11):900–10.

39. Rabin LA, Wang C, Mogle JA, et al. An approach to classifying subjective cognitive decline in community-dwelling elders. Alzheimer's Demen Diagn Assess Dis Monit 2020;12(1).
40. Teo N, Yeo PS, Gao Q, et al. A bio-psycho-social approach for frailty amongst Singaporean Chinese community-dwelling older adults-evidence from the Singapore Longitudinal Aging Study. BMC Geriatr 2019;19(1).
41. Jung H, Kim M, Lee Y, et al. Prevalence of physical frailty and its multidimensional risk factors in Korean community-dwelling older adults: Findings from Korean frailty and aging cohort study. Int J Environ Res Public Health 2020;17(21):1–20.
42. Fabrício D de M, Chagas MHN, Diniz BS. Frailty and cognitive decline. Translational Res 2020;221:58–64.
43. Vatanabe IP, Pedroso RV, Teles RHG, et al. A systematic review and meta-analysis on cognitive frailty in community-dwelling older adults: risk and associated factors. Aging Ment Health 2021. https://doi.org/10.1080/13607863.2021.1884844.
44. Feng Z, Lugtenberg M, Franse C, et al. Risk factors and protective factors associated with incident or increase of frailty among community-dwelling older adults: A systematic review of longitudinal studies. PLoS One 2017;12(6). https://doi.org/10.1371/journal.pone.0178383.
45. Facal D, Burgo C, Spuch C, et al. Cognitive frailty: an update. Front Psychol 2021;12. https://doi.org/10.3389/fpsyg.2021.813398.
46. Kulmala J, Nykänen I, Mänty M, et al. Association between frailty and dementia: a population-based study. Gerontology 2014;60(1):16–21.
47. Kim S, Park JL, Hwang HS, et al. Correlation between frailty and cognitive function in non-demented community dwelling older koreans. Korean J Fam Med 2014;35(6):309.
48. Robertson DA, Savva GM, Kenny RA. Frailty and cognitive impairment-A review of the evidence and causal mechanisms. Ageing Res Rev 2013;12(4):840–51.
49. Jacobs JM, Cohen A, Fin-Mor E, et al. Frailty, cognitive impairment and mortality among the oldest old. J Nutr Health Aging 2011;15(8):678–82.
50. St. John PD, Tyas SL, Griffith LE, et al. The cumulative effect of frailty and cognition on mortality – results of a prospective cohort study. Int Psychogeriatrics 2017;29(4):535–43.
51. Bu ZH, Huang A le, Xue MT, et al. Cognitive frailty as a predictor of adverse outcomes among older adults: A systematic review and meta-analysis. Brain Behav 2021;11(1). https://doi.org/10.1002/brb3.1926.
52. Xie B, Ma C, Chen Y, et al. Prevalence and risk factors of the co-occurrence of physical frailty and cognitive impairment in Chinese community-dwelling older adults. Health Soc Care Community 2021;29(1):294–303.
53. Gill TM, Gahbauer EA, Allore HG, et al. Transitions between frailty states among community-living older persons. Arch Intern Med 2006;166(4):418–23.
54. Trevisan C, Veronese N, Maggi S, et al. Factors influencing transitions between frailty states in elderly adults: the Progetto Veneto Anziani longitudinal study. J Am Geriatr Soc 2017;65(1):179–84.
55. Pollack LR, Litwack-Harrison S, Cawthon PM, et al. Patterns and predictors of frailty transitions in older men: the osteoporotic fractures in men study. J Am Geriatr Soc 2017;65(11):2473–9.
56. Qui Y, Li G, Wang X, et al. Prevalence of cognitive frailty among community-dwelling older adults: A systematic review and meta-analysis. Int J Nurs Stud 2022;125:104112.

Printed and bound by CPI Group (UK) Ltd, Croydon, CR0 4YY

03/10/2024

01040477-0001